Essentials of Mechanical Ventilation

Essentials of Mechanical Ventilation
Third Edition

DEAN R. HESS, PhD, RRT
Associate Professor of Anaesthesia
Harvard Medical School
Assistant Director of Respiratory Care Services
Massachusetts General Hospital
Boston, Massachusetts

ROBERT M. KACMAREK, PhD, RRT
Professor of Anaesthesia
Harvard Medical School
Director of Respiratory Care Services
Massachusetts General Hospital
Boston, Massachusetts

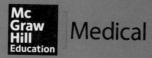 Medical

New York Chicago San Francisco Athens London Madrid
Mexico City Milan New Delhi Singapore Sydney Toronto

Essentials of Mechanical Ventilation

34567890 DOC/DOC 098765

ISBN 978-0-07-177151-1
MHID 0-07-177151-4

This book was set in Minion by Cenveo© Publisher Services.
The editors were Andrew Moyer and Christina M. Thomas
Project supervision was carried out by Sandhya Gola, Cenveo Publisher Services.
The production supervisor was Richard Ruzycka.
The cover designer was Paul McCarthy.
RRD Crawfordsville was printer and binder.
This book is printed on acid-free paper.

Library of Congress Cataloging-in-Publication Data

Hess, Dean, auhor.
  Essentials of mechanical ventilation / Dean R. Hess, Robert M. Kacmarek. —Third edition.
      p. ; cm.
  Includes bibliographical references and index.
  ISBN 978-0-07-177151-1 (pbk. : alk. paper)—ISBN 0-07-177151-4
  I. Kacmarek, Robert M., auhor.   II. Title.
  [DNLM: 1. Respiration, Artificial. 2. Ventilators, Mechanical. WF 145]
  RC87.9
  615.8′36—dc23
                                                                                          2013042070

International Edition ISBN 978-1-259-25151-1; MHID 1-259-25151-9.
Copyright © 2014. Exclusive rights by McGraw-Hill Education, for manufacture and export. This book cannot be re-exported from the country to which it is consigned by McGraw-Hill Education. The International Edition is not available in North America.

Dedication

For Susan, Terri, Rob, Max, Abby, Lauren, and Matt—who make every day enjoyable.
D.R.H.

For my children Robert, Julia, Katie, and Callie, who make it all worthwhile.
R.M.K.

Contents

Preface

Mechanical ventilation is an integral part of the care of many critically ill patients. It is also provided at sites outside the ICU and outside the hospital, including long-term acute care hospitals and the home. A thorough understanding of the essentials of mechanical ventilation is requisite for respiratory therapists and critical care physicians. A general knowledge of the principles of mechanical ventilation is also required of critical care nurses and primary care physicians whose patients occasionally require ventilatory support.

This book is intended to be a practical guide to adult mechanical ventilation. We have written this book from our perspective of over 75 years of experience as clinicians, educators, researchers, and authors. We have made every attempt to keep the topics current and with a distinctly clinical focus. As in the previous editions, we have kept the chapters short, focused, and practical.

There have been many advances in the practice of mechanical ventilation over the past 10 years. Hence, much of the book is rewritten. Like previous editions, the book is divided into four parts. Part 1, *Principles of Mechanical Ventilation*, describes basic principles of mechanical ventilation and then continues with issues such as indications for mechanical ventilation, appropriate physiologic goals, and weaning from mechanical ventilation. Part 2, *Ventilator Management*, gives practical advice for ventilating patients with a variety of diseases. Part 3, *Monitoring During Mechanical Ventilation*, discusses blood gases, hemodynamics, mechanics, and waveforms. In the final part, *Topics Related to Mechanical Ventilation*, we discuss issues such as airway management, aerosol delivery, extracorporeal life support, and miscellaneous ventilatory techniques.

This is a book about mechanical ventilation and not mechanical ventilators. We do not describe the operation of any specific ventilator (although we do discuss some modes specific to some ventilator types). We have tried to keep the material covered in this book generic and it is, by and large, applicable to any adult mechanical ventilator. We do not cover issues related to pediatric and neonatal mechanical ventilation. Because these topics are adequately covered in pediatric and neonatal respiratory care books, we decided to limit the focus of this book to adult mechanical ventilation. Although we provide a short bibliography at the end of each chapter, we have specifically tried to make this a practical book and not an extensive reference book.

This book is written for all clinicians caring for mechanically ventilated patients. We believe that it is unique and hope you will enjoy reading it as much as we have enjoyed writing it.

Dean R. Hess, PhD, RRT
Robert M. Kacmarek, PhD, RRT

Abbreviations

A/C	Assist/control		CPP	Cerebral perfusion pressure
AG	Anion gap		CPR	Cardiopulmonary resuscitation
APRV	Airway pressure release ventilation		CSV	Continuous spontaneous ventilation
ARDS	Acute respiratory distress syndrome		CT	Computed tomography
ARDSnet	ARDS network		$C\bar{v}o_2$	Mixed venous oxygen content
AVAPS	Average volume assured pressure support		CVP	Central venous pressure
BAL	Bronchoalveolar lavage		C_W	Chest wall compliance
BE	Base excess		Do_2	Oxygen delivery
BEE	Basal energy expenditure		EAdi	Electrical activity of the diaphragm
BSA	Body surface area		ECLS	Extracorporeal life support
CCI	Chronic critical illness		ECMO	Extracorporeal membrane oxygenation
Cao_2	Oxygen content of arterial blood		EELV	End-expiratory lung volume
$Cc'o_2$	Pulmonary capillary oxygen content		EPAP	Expiratory positive airway pressure
CDC	Centers for Disease Control and Prevention		f_b	Frequency of breathing; respiratory rate
CI	Cardiac index		f_c	Heart rate
C_L	Lung compliance		Fio_2	Fraction of inspired oxygen
Cl^-	Chloride ion		FRC	Functional residual capacity
CMV	Continuous mandatory ventilation		Hb	Hemoglobin
CO	Carbon monoxide		HbCO	Carboxyhemoglobin
Co_2	Oxygen content of the blood		HCO_3^-	Bicarbonate concentration
COPD	Chronic obstructive pulmonary disease		HFJV	High frequency jet ventilation
			HFOV	High frequency oscillatory ventilation
CPAP	Continuous positive airway pressure		HFPPV	High frequency positive pressure ventilation

HFV	High frequency ventilation		ΔP_L	Transpulmonary pressure
HME	Heat and moisture exchanger		ΔPOP	Plethysmographic waveform amplitude
Hz	Hertz		ΔPpl	Change in pleural pressure
I:E	Inspiratory time to expiratory time ratio		$P(a\text{-}et)CO_2$	Difference between arterial and end-tidal Pco_2
IBW	Ideal body weight (sometimes called predicted body weight)		Pao_2/PAO_2	Ratio of arterial PO_2 to alveolar Po_2
ICP	Intracranial pressure		Pao_2/Fio_2	Ratio of arterial Po_2 to Fio_2
ICU	Intensive care unit		$P(A\text{-}a)O_2$	Difference between alveolar Po_2 and arterial Po_2
IMV	Intermittent mandatory ventilation		$Paco_2$	Partial pressure of carbon dioxide in arterial blood
iNO	Inhaled nitric oxide		$\overline{P}alv$	Mean alveolar pressure
IPAP	Inspiratory positive airway pressure		$Palv$	Alveolar pressure
ISB	Isothermal saturation boundary		Pao_2	Partial pressure of oxygen in arterial blood
IVAC	Infection related ventilator associated condition		PAO_2	Alveolar Po_2
j	Joules		PAP	Pulmonary artery pressure
LV	Left ventricle		PAV	Proportional-assist ventilation
LVSWI	Left ventricular stroke work index		$\overline{P}aw$	Mean airway pressure
MAP	Mean arterial pressure		Pb	Barometric pressure
MDI	Metered-dose inhaler		Pbo_2	Brain Po_2
MIC	Maximum insufflation capacity		PC-CMV	Continuous mandatory ventilation with pressure control
MIE	Mechanical insufflation–exsufflator		PC-IMV	Pressure-controlled intermittent mandatory ventilation
MMV	Mandatory minute ventilation		PCIRV	Pressure-controlled inverse ration ventilation
MODS	Multiple organ dysfunction syndrome		Pco_2	Partial pressure of carbon dioxide
MPAP	Mean pulmonary artery pressure		PCV	Pressure-controlled ventilation
NO	Nitric oxide		PCWP	Pulmonary capillary wedge pressure
Na^+	Sodium			
NAVA	Neurally adjusted ventilatory assist		Pdi	Transdiaphragmatic pressure
NIV	Noninvasive ventilation		$P\overline{E}co_2$	Mixed exhaled Pco_2
NPE	Neurogenic pulmonary edema		PH_2O	Water vapor pressure
OI	Oxygenation index		PEEP	Positive end-expiratory pressure
ΔPaw	Change in airway pressure			

PEG	Percutaneous endoscopic gastrostomy
Peso	Esophageal pressure
Petco$_2$	End-tidal Pco$_2$
Pexhco$_2$	Measured mixed exhaled Pco$_2$ including gas compressed in the ventilator circuit
pH	Negative log of the hydrogen ion concentration
PI	Plethysmographic perfusion index
PI$_{max}$	Maximum inspiratory pressure
PI$_{min}$	Minimal value of the plethysmographic perfusion index
PIP	Peak inspiratory pressure
Pmus	Pressure generated by the respiratory muscles
PMV	Prolonged mechanical ventilation
Po$_2$	Partial pressure of oxygen
Pplat	Plateau pressure
PPV	Arterial pulse pressure variation
PRVC	Pressure-regulated volume control
PSV	Pressure support ventilation
Ptcco$_2$	Transcutaneous Pco$_2$
Ptco$_2$	Transcutaneous Po$_2$
P$\bar{v}$co$_2$	Mixed venous Pco$_2$
Pvent	Pressure-generated by the ventilator
PVI	Plethysmographic variability index
P$\bar{v}$o$_2$	Mixed venous Po$_2$
PVR	Pulmonary vascular resistance
$\dot{Q}$c	Cardiac output
$\dot{Q}_s/\dot{Q}_T$	Pulmonary shunt
R	Respiratory quotient

R$_E$	Expiratory resistance
REE	Resting energy expenditure
REM	Rapid eye movement
R$_I$	Inspiratory resistance
RSBI	Rapid shallow breathing index
RVSWI	Right ventricular stroke work index
Sao$_2$	Hemoglobin oxygen saturation of arterial blood
SBT	Spontaneous breathing trial
Scvo$_2$	Central venous oxygen saturation
SID	Strong ion difference
SIMV	Synchronized intermittent mandatory ventilation
Sjvo$_2$	Jugular venous oxygen saturation
Spco	Carbon monoxide measured by pulse oximetry
SpHb	Hemoglobin measured by pulse oximetry
SpMet	Methemoglobin measured by pulse oximetry
Spo$_2$	Hemoglobin oxygen saturation measured by pulse oximetry
SVI	Stroke volume index
S$\bar{v}$o$_2$	Mixed venous oxygen saturation
SVR	Systemic vascular resistance
SVRI	Systemic vascular resistance index
T$_E$	Expiratory time
T$_I$	Inspiratory time
T$_T$	Total cycle time
UUN	Urine urea nitrogen
$\dot{V}$	Flow
$\dot{V}$a	Alveolar ventilation
$\dot{V}/\dot{Q}$	Ratio of ventilation to blood flow

VAC	Ventilator-associated condition	VC-IMV	volume-controlled intermittent mandatory ventilation
VAE	Ventilator-associated event	V_D/V_T	Dead space to tidal volume ratio
VAP	Ventilator-associated pneumonia	VILI	Ventilator-induced lung injury
VC	Vital capacity	$\dot{V}_{O_2}$	Oxygen consumption
$\dot{V}_{CO_2}$	Carbon dioxide production	VS	Volume support
$\dot{V}_D$	Dead space ventilation	V_T	Tidal volume
$\dot{V}_E$	Minute ventilation	W	Work
$\dot{V}_I$	Inspiratory flow	τ	Time constant
VCV	Volume-controlled ventilation		
VC-CMV	Continuous mandatory ventilation with volume control		

Part 1
Principles of Mechanical Ventilation

Chapter 1
Physiologic Effects of Mechanical Ventilation

Objectives

1. List the factors affecting mean airway pressure during positive pressure ventilation.
2. Describe the effects of positive pressure ventilation on shunt and dead space.
3. Discuss the roles of alveolar overdistention and opening/closing on ventilator-induced lung injury.
4. Discuss the physiologic effects of positive pressure ventilation on the pulmonary, cardiac, renal, hepatic, gastric, and neuromuscular function.
5. Discuss the effects of positive pressure ventilation on nutrition, the airway, and sleep.
6. Describe methods that can be used to minimize the harmful effects of positive pressure ventilation.

Introduction

Ventilators used in adult acute care use positive pressure applied to the airway opening to inflate the lungs. Although positive pressure is responsible for the beneficial effects of mechanical ventilation, it is also responsible for many potentially deleterious side effects. Application of mechanical ventilation requires an understanding of both its beneficial and adverse effects. In the care of an individual patient, this demands application of strategies that maximize the potential benefit of mechanical ventilation while minimizing the potential for harm. Due to the homeostatic interactions between the lungs and other body systems, mechanical ventilation can affect nearly every organ system of the body. This chapter provides an overview of the beneficial and adverse physiologic effects of mechanical ventilation.

Mean Airway Pressure

During normal spontaneous breathing, intrathoracic pressure is negative throughout the ventilatory cycle. Intrapleural pressure varies from about -5 cm H_2O during exhalation to -8 cm H_2O during inhalation. Alveolar pressure fluctuates from $+1$ cm H_2O during exhalation to -1 cm H_2O during inhalation. The decrease in intrapleural pressure during inhalation facilitates lung inflation and venous return. Transpulmonary pressure is the difference between proximal airway pressure and intrapleural pressure. The greatest static transpulmonary pressure that can be generated normally during spontaneous inspiration is less than 35 cm H_2O.

Intrathoracic pressure fluctuations during positive pressure ventilation are opposite to those that occur during spontaneous breathing. During positive pressure ventilation, the mean intrathoracic pressure is usually positive. Intrathoracic pressure increases during inhalation and decreases during exhalation. Thus, venous return is greatest during exhalation and it may be decreased if expiratory time is too short or mean alveolar pressure is too high.

Many of the beneficial and adverse effects associated with mechanical ventilation are related to mean airway pressure. Mean airway pressure is the average pressure applied to the airway during the ventilatory cycle. It is related to both the amount and duration of pressure applied during the inspiratory phase (peak inspiratory pressure, inspiratory pressure waveform, and inspiratory time) and the expiratory phase (positive end-expiratory pressure [PEEP] and respiratory rate).

Pulmonary Effects

Shunt

Shunt is perfusion (blood flow) without ventilation (Figure 1-1). Pulmonary shunt occurs when blood flows from the right heart to the left heart without participating in gas exchange. The result of shunt is hypoxemia. Shunt can be either capillary shunt or anatomic shunt. Capillary shunt results when blood flows past unventilated alveoli. Examples of capillary shunt are atelectasis, pneumonia, pulmonary edema, and acute respiratory distress syndrome (ARDS). Anatomic shunt occurs when blood flows from the right heart to the left heart and completely bypasses the lungs. Normal anatomical shunt occurs due to the Thebesian veins and the bronchial circulation. Abnormal anatomic shunt occurs with congenital cardiac defects. Total shunt is the sum of the capillary and anatomic shunt.

Positive pressure ventilation usually decreases shunt and improves arterial oxygenation. An inspiratory pressure that exceeds the alveolar opening pressure expands a collapsed alveolus, and an expiratory pressure greater than alveolar closing pressure prevents its collapse. By maintaining alveolar recruitment with an adequate expiratory pressure setting, arterial oxygenation is improved. However, if positive pressure ventilation produces overdistention of some lung units, this may result in redistribution of pulmonary blood flow to unventilated regions (Figure 1-2). In this case, positive pressure ventilation paradoxically results in hypoxemia.

Although positive pressure ventilation may improve capillary shunt, it may worsen anatomic shunt. An increase in alveolar pressure may increase pulmonary vascular resistance, which could result in increased flow through the anatomic shunt, decreased flow through the lungs, and worsening hypoxemia. Thus, mean airway pressure should be kept as low as possible if an anatomic right-to-left shunt is present.

A relative shunt effect can occur with poor distribution of ventilation, such as might result from airway disease. With poor distribution of ventilation, some alveoli are underventilated relative to perfusion (shunt-like effect and low ventilation-perfusion ratio), whereas other alveoli are

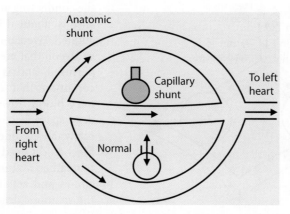

Figure 1-1 Schematic illustration of anatomic shunt and capillary shunt.

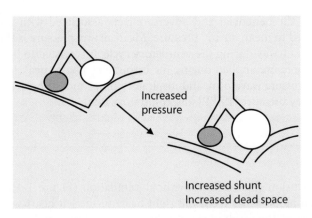

Figure 1-2 Alveolar overdistention, resulting in redistribution of pulmonary blood flow to unventilated units and an increased shunt.

overventilated (dead space effect and high ventilation-perfusion ratio). Positive pressure ventilation may improve the distribution of ventilation, particularly by improving the ventilation of previously underventilated areas of the lungs.

Ventilation

Ventilation is the movement of gas into and out of the lungs. Tidal volume (V_T) is the amount of gas inhaled or exhaled with a single breath and minute ventilation ($\dot{V}_E$) is the volume of gas breathed in 1 minute. Minute ventilation is the product of tidal volume (V_T) and respiratory frequency (f_b):

$$\dot{V}_E = V_T \times f_b$$

Ventilation can be either dead space ventilation ($\dot{V}_D$) or alveolar ventilation ($\dot{V}_A$). Minute ventilation is the sum of dead space ventilation and alveolar ventilation:

$$\dot{V}_E = \dot{V}_D + \dot{V}_A$$

Alveolar ventilation participates in gas exchange (Figure 1-3), whereas dead space ventilation does not. In other words, dead space is ventilation without perfusion. Anatomic dead space is the volume of the conducting airways of the lungs, and is about 150 mL in normal adults. Alveolar dead space refers to alveoli that are ventilated but not perfused, and is increased by any condition that decreases pulmonary blood flow. Total physiologic dead space fraction (V_D/V_T) is normally about one-third of the $\dot{V}_E$. Mechanical dead space refers to the rebreathed volume of the ventilator circuit and acts as an extension of the anatomic dead space. Due to the

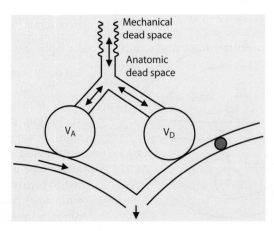

Figure 1-3 Schematic illustration of mechanical dead space, anatomic dead space, and alveolar dead space.

fixed anatomic dead space, a low tidal volume increases the dead space fraction and decreases alveolar ventilation. An increased dead space fraction will require a greater minute ventilation to maintain alveolar ventilation (and $Paco_2$).

Because mechanical ventilators provide a tidal volume and respiratory rate, any desired level of ventilation can be provided. The level of ventilation required depends upon the desired $Paco_2$, alveolar ventilation, and tissue CO_2 production ($\dot{V}co_2$). This is illustrated by the following relationships (note that the factor 0.863 is not used if the measurements are made at the same conditions and using the same units):

$$Paco_2 \propto \dot{V}co_2/\dot{V}_A$$

and

$$Paco_2 = (\dot{V}co_2 \times 0.863)/(\dot{V}_E \times [1 - V_D/V_T])$$

A higher $\dot{V}_E$ will be required to maintain $Paco_2$ if $\dot{V}co_2$ is increased, such as occurs with fever and sepsis. If dead space is increased, a higher $\dot{V}_E$ is required to maintain the same level of $\dot{V}_A$ and $Paco_2$. If this level of ventilation is undesirable due to its injurious effects on the lungs and hemodynamics, $Paco_2$ can be allowed to increase (permissive hypercapnia). Mechanical ventilation can produce overdistention of normal alveoli, resulting in alveolar dead space. Mechanical ventilation can also distend airways, increasing anatomic dead space.

Atelectasis

Atelectasis is a common complication of mechanical ventilation. This can be the result of preferential ventilation of nondependent lung zones with passive ventilation, the weight of the lungs causing compression of dependent regions or airway obstruction. Breathing 100% oxygen may produce absorption atelectasis, and should be avoided if possible. Use of PEEP to maintain lung volume is effective in preventing atelectasis.

Barotrauma

Barotrauma is alveolar rupture due to overdistention. Barotrauma can lead to pulmonary interstitial emphysema, pneumomediastinum, pneumopericardium, subcutaneous emphysema, and pneumothorax (Figure 1-4). Pneumothorax is of greatest clinical concern, because it can progress rapidly to life-threatening tension pneumothorax. Pneumomediastinum and subcutaneous emphysema rarely have major clinical consequences.

Ventilator-Induced Lung Injury

Alveolar overdistention causes acute lung injury. Alveolar distention is determined by the difference between intra-alveolar pressure and the intrapleural pressure. The peak alveolar pressure (end-inspiratory plateau pressure) should ideally be as low as possible and less than 30 cm H_2O. Alveolar distention is also affected by intrapleural pressure. Thus, a stiff chest wall may be protective against alveolar overdistention. Overdistention is minimized by limiting tidal volume (eg, 4-8 mL/kg ideal body weight) and alveolar distending pressure (< 25 cm H_2O). Ventilator-induced lung injury can also

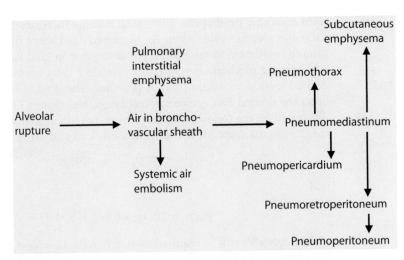

Figure 1-4 Barotrauma-related injuries that can occur as the result of alveolar rupture.

result from cyclical alveolar collapse during exhalation and re-opening during subsequent inhalation. This injury is ameliorated by the application of PEEP to avoid alveolar derecruitment. Ventilating the lungs in a manner that promotes alveolar overdistention and derecruitment increases inflammation in the lungs (biotrauma). Inflammatory mediators may translocate into the pulmonary circulation, resulting in systemic inflammation. An important characteristic of the lungs of mechanically ventilated patients is heterogeneity; that is, some lung units are prone to overdistention and others are prone to collapse.

Pneumonia

Ventilator-associated pneumonia (VAP) can occur during mechanical ventilation; this is more common during invasive ventilation than with noninvasive ventilation. VAP most often results from aspiration of oropharyngeal secretions around the cuff of the endotracheal tube. A number of prevention strategies can be bundled to reduce the risk of VAP.

Hyperventilation and Hypoventilation

Hyperventilation lowers $Paco_2$ and increases arterial pH. This should be avoided because of the injurious effects of alveolar overdistention and an alkalotic pH. Respiratory alkalosis causes hypokalemia, decreased ionized calcium, and increased affinity of hemoglobin for oxygen (left shift of the oxyhemoglobin dissociation curve). Relative hyperventilation can occur when mechanical ventilation is provided for patients with chronic compensated respiratory acidosis; if a normal $Paco_2$ is established in such patients, the result is an elevated pH. Hypercapnia during mechanical ventilation may be less injurious than the traumatic effects of high levels of ventilation to normalize the $Paco_2$. A modest elevation of $Paco_2$ (50-70 mm Hg) may not be injurious and a pH as low as 7.20 is well tolerated by most patients.

Oxygen Toxicity

A high inspired oxygen concentration is considered toxic. What is less clear is the level of oxygen that is toxic. Oxygen toxicity is probably related to F_{IO_2} as well as the amount of time that the elevated F_{IO_2} is breathed. Although the clinical evidence is weak, it is commonly recommended that an F_{IO_2} greater than 0.6 be avoided, particularly if breathed for a period more than 48 hours. High F_{IO_2} levels can result in a higher than normal P_{aO_2}. A high P_{aO_2} may produce an elevation in P_{aCO_2} due to the Haldane effect (ie, unloading CO_2 from hemoglobin), due to improving blood flow to low-ventilation lung units (ie, relaxing hypoxic pulmonary vasoconstriction), and due to suppression of ventilation (less likely). However, this is usually not an issue during mechanical ventilation because ventilation can be controlled. A high P_{aO_2} can produce retinopathy of prematurity in neonates, but this is not known to occur in adults.

Cardiac Effects

Positive pressure ventilation can decrease cardiac output, resulting in hypotension and potential tissue hypoxia. This effect is greatest with high mean airway pressure, high lung compliance, and low circulating blood volume. Increased intrathoracic pressure decreases venous return and right heart filling, which may reduce cardiac output. With spontaneous breathing, venous return to the right atrium is greatest during inhalation, when the intrathoracic pressure is lowest. During positive pressure ventilation, venous return is greatest during exhalation.

Positive pressure ventilation may increase pulmonary vascular resistance. The increase in alveolar pressure, particularly with PEEP, has a constricting effect on the pulmonary vasculature. The increase in pulmonary vascular resistance decreases left ventricular filling and cardiac output. Increased right ventricular afterload can result in right ventricular hypertrophy, with ventricular septal shift and compromise of left ventricular function. Increased pulmonary vascular resistance with PEEP produces a West Zone 1 effect, which increases dead space, and thus results in less alveolar ventilation and a higher P_{aCO_2}.

The adverse cardiac effects of positive pressure ventilation are ameliorated by lower mean airway pressure. When high mean airway pressure is necessary, circulatory volume loading and administration of vasopressors may be necessary to maintain cardiac output and arterial blood pressure.

Renal Effects

Urine output can decrease secondary to mechanical ventilation. This is partially related to decreased renal perfusion due to decreased cardiac output, and may also be related to elevations in plasma antidiuretic hormone and reductions in atrial natriuretic peptide that occur with mechanical ventilation. Fluid overload frequently occurs during mechanical ventilation, due to decreased urine output, excessive intravenous fluid administration, and elimination of insensible water loss from the respiratory tract due to humidification of the inspired gas.

Gastric Effects

Patients being mechanically ventilated may develop gastric distention (meteorism). Stress ulcer formation and gastrointestinal bleeding can also occur in mechanically ventilated patients, and stress ulcer prophylaxis should be provided.

Nutritional Effects

Appropriate nutritional support is problematic in mechanically ventilated patients. Underfeeding can result in respiratory muscle catabolism and increases the risk of pneumonia and pulmonary edema. Overfeeding increases metabolic rate and thus increases the required minute ventilation. Overfeeding with carbohydrates increases $\dot{V}_{CO_2}$, further increasing the ventilation requirement.

Neurologic Effects

In patients with head injury, positive pressure ventilation might increase intracranial pressure. This is related to a decrease in venous return, which increases intracranial blood volume and pressure. If high mean airway pressure is used, cerebral perfusion can also be compromised due to arterial hypotension.

Delirium is common in mechanically ventilated patients. The mnemonic ABCDE has been proposed to remind clinicians of important steps of care in mechanically ventilated patients (Awakening and Breathing, Choice of sedative and analgesic, Delirium monitoring, and Early mobilization). Such an evidence-based protocol may improve patient outcome, including mortality. Benzodiazepine-based sedation may increase the risk of delirium, when compared with agents such as dexmedetomidine.

Neuromuscular Effects

Mechanically ventilated patients are at increased risk of critical illness and weakness (polyneuropathy and polymyopathy). If the respiratory muscles are not used during mechanical ventilation (ie, paralysis), ventilator-induced diaphragm dysfunction can occur. On the other extreme, excessive respiratory muscle activity can result in muscle fatigue. Thus, an appropriate balance between respiratory muscle activity and support from the ventilator is important. Mobilization of mechanically ventilated patients is used increasingly to address generalized weakness in this patient population.

Hepatosplanchnic Effects

PEEP can reduce portal blood flow. However, the clinical importance of the effects of positive pressure ventilation on hepatosplanchnic perfusion is unclear.

Airway Effects

Critically ill patients are usually mechanically ventilated through an endotracheal or tracheostomy tube. This puts these patients at risk for all of the complications of artificial airways such as laryngeal edema, tracheal mucosal trauma, contamination of the lower respiratory tract, sinusitis, loss of the humidifying function of the upper airway, and communication problems.

Sleep Effects

Mechanically ventilated patients may not have normal sleep patterns. Sleep deprivation can produce delirium, patient-ventilator asynchrony, and sedation-induced ventilator dependency.

Patient-Ventilator Asynchrony

Lack of synchrony between the breathing efforts of the patient and the ventilator may be due to poor trigger sensitivity, auto-PEEP, incorrect inspiratory flow or time setting, inappropriate tidal volume, or inappropriate mode. Asynchrony can also be caused by nonventilator issues such as pain, anxiety, and acidosis.

Mechanical Malfunctions

A variety of mechanical complications can occur during mechanical ventilation. These include accidental disconnection, leaks in the ventilator circuit, loss of electrical power, and loss of gas pressure. The mechanical ventilator system should be monitored frequently to prevent mechanical malfunctions.

> **Points to Remember**
>
> - Many of the beneficial and adverse effects of mechanical ventilation are related to mean airway pressure.
> - Positive pressure ventilation usually improves arterial P_{O_2} and P_{CO_2}, but may increase shunt and dead space under some conditions.

- Atelectasis, barotrauma, acute lung injury, pneumonia, hypoventilation or hyperventilation, and oxygen toxicity are pulmonary complications of positive pressure ventilation.
- Positive pressure ventilation can produce adverse cardiac, renal, nutritional, neurologic, hepatic, and airway effects.
- An ABCDE approach (Awakening and Breathing, Choice of sedative and analgesic, Delirium monitoring, and Early mobilization) may improve outcomes of mechanically ventilated patients.
- Asynchrony commonly occurs and should be corrected by use of appropriate ventilator settings and by addressing nonventilator issues leading to asynchrony.

Additional Reading

Blot S, Lisboa T, Angles R, Rello J. Prevention of VAP: is zero rate possible? *Clin Chest Med.* 2011;32:591-599.

Brower RG, Rubenfeld GD. Lung-protective ventilation strategies in acute lung injury. *Crit Care Med.* 2003;31:S312-S316.

Cabello B, Parthasarathy S, Mancebo J. Mechanical ventilation: let us minimize sleep disturbances. *Curr Opin Crit Care.* 2007;13:20-26.

Dueck R. Alveolar recruitment versus hyperinflation: a balancing act. *Curr Opin Anaesthesiol.* 2006;19:650-654.

Frontera JA. Delirium and sedation in the ICU. *Neurocrit Care.* 2011;14:463-474.

Gattinoni L, Carlesso E, Caironi P. Stress and strain within the lung. *Curr Opin Crit Care.* 2012;18:42-47.

Gattinoni L, Carlesso E, Caironi P, et al. Ventilator-induced lung injury: the anatomical and physiological framework. *Crit Care Med.* 2010;38:S539-S548.

Griffiths RD, Hall JB. Intensive care unit-acquired weakness. *Crit Care Med.* 2010;38:779-787.

Haitsma JJ. Diaphragmatic dysfunction in mechanical ventilation. *Curr Opin Anaesthesiol.* 2011;24:214-218.

Haitsma JJ. Physiology of mechanical ventilation. *Crit Care Clin.* 2007;23:117-134.

Hess DR. Approaches to conventional mechanical ventilation of the patient with acute respiratory distress syndrome. *Respir Care.* 2011;56:1555-1572.

Jubran A. Critical illness and mechanical ventilation: effects on the diaphragm. *Respir Care.* 2006;51:1054-1064.

Luecke T, Pelosi P. Clinical review: positive end-expiratory pressure and cardiac output. *Crit Care.* 2005;9:607-621.

MacIntyre NR. Current issues in mechanical ventilation for respiratory failure. *Chest.* 2005; 128:561S-567S.

Morandi A, Brummel NE, Ely EW. Sedation, delirium and mechanical ventilation: the 'ABCDE' approach. *Curr Opin Crit Care.* 2011;17:43-49.

Mutlu GM, Mutlu EA, Factor P. Prevention and treatment of gastrointestinal complications in patients on mechanical ventilation. *Am J Respir Med.* 2003;2:395-411.

Patel SB, Kress JP. Sedation and analgesia in the mechanically ventilated patient. *Am J Respir Crit Care Med.* 2012;185:486-497.

Pierson DJ. Respiratory considerations in the patient with renal failure. *Respir Care.* 2006;51:413-422.

Pinsky MR. Cardiovascular issues in respiratory care. *Chest.* 2005;128:592S-597S.

Ramnath VR, Hess DR, Thompson BT. Conventional mechanical ventilation in acute lung injury and acute respiratory distress syndrome. *Clin Chest Med.* 2006;27:601-613.

Ricard JD, Dreyfuss D, Saumon G. Ventilator-induced lung injury. *Eur Respir J Suppl.* 2003;42:2s-9s.

Schweickert WD, Kress JP. Implementing early mobilization interventions in mechanically ventilated patients in the ICU. *Chest.* 2011;140:1612-1617.

Steingrub JS, Tidswell M, Higgins TL. Hemodynamic consequences of heart-lung interactions. *J Intensive Care Med.* 2003;18:92-99.

Yilmaz M, Gajic O. Optimal ventilator settings in acute lung injury and acute respiratory distress syndrome. *Eur J Anaesthesiol.* 2008;25:89-96.

Young N, Rhodes JK, Mascia L, Andrews PJ. Ventilatory strategies for patients with acute brain injury. *Curr Opin Crit Care.* 2010;16:45-52.

Chapter 2
Physiologic Goals of Mechanical Ventilation

Introduction

Many clinical management decisions are designed to return abnormal physiologic function to normal or to return abnormal laboratory data to normal. However, during mechanical ventilation, it may not be prudent to target normal blood gas values irrespective of the tidal volume (V_T) delivered, pressure applied, or F_{IO_2} used. The inappropriate use of the ventilator may cause lung injury, activate inflammatory mediators, and potentially cause or extend multisystem organ failure. Of particular concern are patients with acute respiratory distress syndrome (ARDS), asthma, or chronic obstructive pulmonary disease (COPD), whose lungs have abnormal mechanics. Regardless of the pathophysiology requiring ventilatory support, the primary goals of mechanical ventilation should be to (1) cause no additional injury, avoiding ventilator-induced lung injury by minimizing lung stress and strain, (2) maintain gas exchange and acid-base balance at a level appropriate for the specific patient, accepting hypercapnia and hypoxemia where indicated, and (3) ensure patient-ventilator synchrony, selecting the mode and ventilator settings that best match the patient's respiratory drive while ensuring lung protection.

Tidal Volume and Alveolar Distending Pressure

Tidal Volume

In the past, approaches to mechanical ventilation suggested V_T of 10 to 15 mL/kg of ideal body weight (IBW). We now know that these V_T are excessive for any patient who requires mechanical ventilation. A V_T of greater than 10 mL/kg IBW should be avoided in all acutely ill patients regardless of their lung mechanics. Since it is impossible to clinically detect localized overdistention, an acceptable V_T in a given patient must be judged relative to alveolar distending pressure.

Alveolar Distending Pressure

Alveolar distending pressure is assessed by measuring end-inspiratory plateau pressure (Pplat), which reflects mean peak alveolar pressure. To measure Pplat, a 0.5- to 2-second end-inspiratory breath-hold is applied. Pplat should be limited to 30 cm H_2O if chest wall compliance is normal. This is generally achieved by using a V_T of 4 to 8 mL/kg IBW for patients with ARDS and a V_T no greater than 10 mL/kg IBW for any patient requiring acute mechanical ventilation. Exceeding this Pplat target should be avoided in the absence of a stiff chest wall.

Positive End-Expiratory Pressure

The recommended level of positive end-expiratory pressure (PEEP) is 8 to 15 cm H_2O for mild ARDS and 10 to 20 cm H_2O for moderate to severe ARDS, which is needed to maintain lung recruitment. If PEEP is set at 10 to 20 cm H_2O and Pplat is limited to 30 cm H_2O, then only 10 to 20 cm H_2O ventilating pressure (driving pressure) is available. This may result in a V_T of only 4 to 6 mL/kg IBW. In this case, minute ventilation is adjusted by increasing the respiratory rate, provided that air trapping does not occur.

For patients with flow limitation (eg, COPD) and auto-PEEP, applied PEEP may be useful to improve the ability of the patient to trigger the ventilator. For most other patients, a PEEP of 5 cm H_2O is reasonable to maintain functional residual capacity and prevent atelectasis. This level of PEEP will usually have no adverse affects. However, PEEP levels as low as 0 may be necessary for patients who are hemodynamically unstable, or who have a large bronchopleural fistula.

Permissive Hypercapnia

Permissive hypercapnia is the deliberate limitation of ventilator support to avoid alveolar overdistension, allowing $Paco_2$ levels greater than normal (50-100 mm Hg). Allowing the $Paco_2$ to rise to these levels should be considered when the only alternative is a potentially dangerous increase in alveolar distending pressure or significant levels of auto-PEEP. The potential adverse effects of an elevated $Paco_2$ are listed in Table 2-1. Most of the more important clinical problems occur at $Paco_2$ levels above 150 mm Hg. However, even small increases in $Paco_2$ increase cerebral blood flow and permissive hypercapnia is generally contraindicated when intracranial pressure is increased (eg, acute head injury). Elevated $Paco_2$ also stimulates ventilation and may contribute to asynchrony, but patients are usually sedated when permissive hypercapnia is used.

Table 2-1 Physiologic Effects of Permissive Hypercapnia

- Shift of the oxyhemoglobin dissociation curve to the right
- Decreased alveolar Po_2
- Stimulation and depression of the cardiovascular system
- Central nervous system depression
- Increased ventilatory drive
- Pulmonary vasoconstriction (pulmonary hypertension)
- Systemic vasodilatation (systemic hypotension)
- Increased intracranial pressure
- Anesthesia ($Paco_2 > 200$ mm Hg)
- Decreased renal blood flow ($Paco_2 > 150$ mm Hg)
- Leakage of intracellular potassium ($Paco_2 > 150$ mm Hg)

Permissive hypercapnia may adversely affect oxygenation in some patients. Elevated $Paco_2$ and acidosis shift the oxyhemoglobin dissociation curve to right. This decreases the affinity of hemoglobin for oxygen, decreasing oxygen loading in the lungs but facilitating unloading of oxygen at the tissues. As illustrated by the alveolar gas equation, an increase in alveolar Pco_2 results in a decrease in alveolar Po_2. For each $Paco_2$ rise of 1 mm Hg, the Pao_2 decreases by about 1 mm Hg. When permissive hypercapnia is allowed, optimal efforts to maximize oxygenation should be used.

As illustrated in Figure 2-1, carbon dioxide stimulates or depresses some parts of the cardiovascular system, but opposite effects can occur via stimulation of the autonomic nervous system. It is thus difficult to predict the precise response of the cardiovascular system to permissive hypercapnia. An increase in Pco_2 might cause pulmonary hypertension and it might affect cardiac output. Rarely, pharmaceutical agents might need to be adjusted in the presence of permissive hypercapnia, but this is usually the result of acidosis and not the elevated Pco_2 per se.

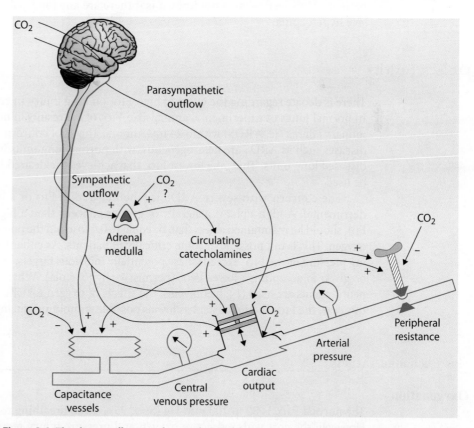

Figure 2-1 This diagram illustrates the complexity of the mechanisms by which carbon dioxide influences the circulatory system. See text for details. (Reproduced with permission from Nunn JF. Carbon dioxide. In: Nunn JF, ed. *Applied Respiratory Physiology*. 2nd ed. London, UK: Butterworth and Co.; 1977:334-374.)

The primary factor limiting permissive hypercapnia is the acidosis that results. Patients without significant comorbid conditions usually tolerate a pH as low as 7.20, and previously healthy patients may tolerate an even lower pH. The specific acceptable pH needs to be determined on an individual patient basis. If $Paco_2$ increases gradually, renal compensation can occur. Abrupt changes in ventilation that result in rapid and marked elevation of $Paco_2$ are more poorly tolerated.

Whether buffers should be administered to manage the acidosis induced by permissive hypercapnia is debatable. The use of sodium bicarbonate in the setting of permissive hypercapnia has not been extensively studied. One might expect a short-term increase in carbon dioxide load when sodium bicarbonate is administered, which is exhaled over time if the level of ventilation is held constant. An alternative buffer is THAM, which does not generate CO_2 and produces intracellular as well as extracellular buffering of pH. THAM can actually result in a decrease in Pco_2.

Cautious use of permissive hypercapnia is recommended only when the V_T and Pplat targets have been met and respiratory rate cannot be increased further. There does not seem to be any significant short-term adverse effect in the majority of patients. However, what is not known is if there are any long-term effects of permissive hypercapnia.

Oxygen Toxicity

There is debate regarding the effect of high FIO_2 on lung injury in critically ill patients. In normal lungs of experimental animals, an FIO_2 of 1.0 results in noncardiogenic pulmonary edema (ie, ARDS) within 24 to 48 hours. This is of concern because acute lung diseases such as ARDS are heterogeneous, with normal lung units interspersed among diseased lung units. Thus, the lowest FIO_2 that achieves the desired Pao_2 should always be used.

The concern with severe ARDS is whether a high FIO_2 or a high Pplat is more detrimental. A high Pplat is generally of greater concern than a high FIO_2. Ideally, the FIO_2 should be maintained at less than or equal to 0.6 to avoid the potential toxic effects of oxygen. This is not possible in some critically ill patients. As either the alveolar distending pressure or the FIO_2 exceeds these potentially injurious targets, consideration should be given to accepting a lower Pao_2 (permissive hypoxemia). When some chemotherapeutic agents are used (eg, bleomycin), the effects of oxygen toxicity are exaggerated. In this case, the FIO_2 should be kept as low as possible without producing tissue hypoxia.

Gas Exchange Targets

Oxygenation

The normal Pao_2 is 80 to 100 mm Hg (Spo_2 95%-98%) breathing room air at sea level. However, the cost with respect to oxygen and pressure injury requires adjustment of this target in many critically ill patients. Table 2-2 lists target Pao_2 associated with severity of pulmonary disease. In the ARDSNet study, the target Pao_2 was 55 to 80 mm Hg

Table 2-2 **Gas Exchange Targets**

Condition	Target value
Pao$_2$	
Normal lungs	> 80 mm Hg
ARDS	55-80 mm Hg
COPD	50-65 mm Hg
Paco$_2$	
Normal lungs	35-45 mm Hg
Lung injury	< 80 mm Hg
pH	
Normal lungs	7.35-7.45
Lung injury	≥ 7.20

(Spo$_2$ 88%-95%). At higher altitude, the target can be further decreased. In patients with COPD, a reasonable Pao$_2$ target is 50 to 65 mm Hg (Spo$_2$ 88%-92%).

Ventilation

Normal Paco$_2$ is 35 to 45 mm Hg, and this should be the target in mechanically ventilated patients unless the risks of high Pplat and V$_T$ outweigh the benefit of a normal Paco$_2$. The Paco$_2$ can be allowed to increase to as high as 80 to 100 mm Hg if necessary, provided increased intracranial pressure is not of concern and marked metabolic acidosis is not present. Paco$_2$ levels more than 100 mm Hg are almost never necessary.

Acid-Base Balance

In most mechanically ventilated patients, the target pH is 7.35 to 7.45. However, when Pplat and V$_T$ are limited and Paco$_2$ is allowed to increase, the potential for respiratory acidosis exists. If the rise in Paco$_2$ is gradual and renal and cardiovascular function are adequate, a pH of 7.20 to 7.30 is usually well tolerated, although a rapid rise in Paco$_2$ may cause a marked decrease in pH. Many patients tolerate well a pH as low as 7.25. Allowing the pH to fall below 7.20 may be tolerated in some patients.

Respiratory alkalosis should be avoided. Many clinicians have traditionally regarded respiratory alkalosis as benign. However, respiratory alkalosis is associated with a variety of potential problems, including electrolyte disturbances (eg, hypokalemia, decreased ionized calcium), seizures, decreased oxygen unloading from hemoglobin (ie, left-shifted oxyhemoglobin dissociation curve), and decreased cerebral blood flow.

Patient-Ventilator Synchrony

Asynchrony is defined as a lack of coordination between a patient's respiratory center output and the response of the ventilator. Asynchrony is a potential problem regardless of mode of ventilation selected. This is a concern because it increases oxygen consumption, carbon dioxide production, hemodynamic instability, sedation requirement, and may contribute to ventilator-induced lung injury by producing high alveolar distending pressures and excessive V_T.

Asynchrony manifests as missed triggering, auto-triggering, double-triggering, inability of the ventilator to meet the inspiratory flow demand of the patient, or failure of the ventilator to cycle to exhalation at the patient's neural inspiratory time. Assessment of the ventilator settings should occur before sedation is used to improve synchrony.

Points to Remember

- The concept of physiologic normal must be reconsidered during mechanical ventilation.
- To reduce the risk of ventilator-induced lung injury, Pplat should be kept less than or equal to 30 cm H_2O.
- V_T in patients with acute or chronic lung disease should be 4 to 8 mL/kg IBW.
- V_T should not exceed 10 mL/kg IBW.
- In early ARDS, PEEP is set to maintain lung recruitment (10-20 cm H_2O).
- Permissive hypercapnia is the deliberate adjustment of mechanical ventilation to allow the $Paco_2$ to rise above 40 mm Hg.
- Most patients tolerate a pH as low as 7.20 if no significant comorbid condition is present.
- The Fio_2 should be kept as low as possible with a target of less than or equal to 0.6.
- It is more important to limit Pplat and V_T than to limit Fio_2.
- The Pao_2 target should be decreased as the severity of acute lung disease increases.
- Patient-ventilator asynchrony can occur in any mode of ventilation.
- Before administering sedatives to correct asynchrony, assess the ventilator settings.

Additional Reading

Abdelsalam M, Cheifetz IM. Goal-directed therapy for severely hypoxic patients with acute respiratory distress syndrome: permissive hypoxemia. *Respir Care.* 2010;55:1483-1490.

Brochard L. New goals for positive end-expiratory pressure in acute respiratory distress syndrome: a paradigm shift or the end of an area of uncertainty? *Am J Respir Crit Care Med.* 2010;181:528-530.

Chiumello D, Carlesso E, Cadringher P, et al. Lung stress and strain during mechanical ventilation of the acute respiratory distress syndrome. *Am J Respir Crit Care Med.* 2008;178:346-355.

Chonghaile M, Higgins B, Laffey J. Permissive hypercapnia: role in protective lung ventilatory strategies. *Curr Opin Crit Care.* 2005;11:56-62.

De Prost N, Dreyfuss D. How to prevent ventilator-induced lung injury? *Minerva Anestesiol.* 2012;78:1054-1066.

de Wit M, Miller KB, Green DA, et al. Ineffective triggering predicts increased duration of mechanical ventilation. *Crit Care Med.* 2009;37:2740-2745.

Hager DN, Krishnan JA, Hayden DL, Brower RG. Tidal volume reduction in patients with acute lung injury when plateau pressures are not high. *Am J Respir Crit Care Med.* 2005;172: 1241-1245.

Kallet RH, Matthay MM. Hyperoxic acute lung injury. *Respir Care.* 2013;58:123-140.

MacIntyre NR. Supporting oxygenation in acute respiratory failure. *Respir Care.* 2013;58: 142-148.

Phoenix SI, Paravastu S, Columb M, et al. Does a higher positive end expiratory pressure decrease mortality in acute respiratory distress syndrome? A systematic review and meta-analysis. *Anesthesiology.* 2009;110:1098-1105.

Serpa Neto A, Cardoso SO, Manetta JA, et al. Association between use of lung-protective ventilation with lower tidal volumes and clinical outcomes among patients without acute respiratory distress syndrome. *JAMA.* 2012;308:1651-1659.

The Acute Respiratory Distress Syndrome Network. Ventilation with lower tidal volumes as compared with traditional tidal volumes for acute lung injury and the acute respiratory distress syndrome. *N Engl J Med.* 2000;342:1301-1308.

Thille AW, Rodriguez P, Cabello B, et al. Patient-ventilator asynchrony during assisted mechanical ventilation. *Intensive Care Med.* 2006;32:1515-1522.

Villar J, Kacmarek RM, Perez-Mendez L, Aguirre-Jaime A. A high positive end-expiratory pressure, low tidal volume ventilatory strategy improves outcome in persistent acute respiratory distress syndrome: a randomized, controlled trial. *Crit Care Med.* 2006;34:1311-1318.

subcutaneous emphysema. It is reasonable to assume that the higher the ventilating pressure, the greater the likelihood of barotrauma. Early reports on ARDS and asthma where unlimited peak airway pressure was applied resulted in a higher incidence of barotrauma than more recent case series where high pressure and overdistention of the lungs was avoided. No clear, specific relationship between applied pressure and barotrauma is available. However, many clinicians agree that barotrauma occurs in the lungs ventilated with high alveolar pressures and large tidal volumes (V_T). The specific volume and pressure required to develop barotrauma is likely patient-specific.

Oxygen Toxicity

High concentrations of inhaled oxygen result in the formation of oxygen-free radicals (eg, superoxide, hydrogen peroxide, hydroxyl ion). These free radicals can cause ultrastructural changes in the lung similar to acute lung injury. In animal models, inhalation of 100% oxygen causes death within 24 to 48 hours. Human volunteers breathing 100% oxygen develop inflammatory airway changes and bronchitis within 24 hours. There are also laboratory data to suggest that former exposure to bacterial endotoxin, inflammatory mediators, and sublethal levels of oxygen ($\leq 85\%$) protect the lung from further injury when inspiring a high F_{IO_2}.

Concern for oxygen toxicity should never prevent the use of a high F_{IO_2} in a patient who is hypoxemic. An F_{IO_2} of 1.0 should be administered whenever there is uncertainty about the Pa_{O_2} and pulse oximetry is not available. However, F_{IO_2} should be lowered to the level resulting in a Pa_{O_2} of 55 to 80 mm Hg (SpO_2 88%-95%). The target F_{IO_2} is less than or equal to 0.60. Few clinicians feel the concern of oxygen toxicity is greater than the concern of tissue hypoxia. An exception is the patient treated with bleomycin. The combination of bleomycin and oxygen results in marked injury to the lungs. In this setting, the lowest F_{IO_2} should be used, tolerating a Pa_{O_2} as low as 50 mm Hg (Spo_2 85%-88%).

Stress and Strain

Primary determinants of lung injury are stress and strain. Stress is defined as the internal counterforce per unit area that balances an external load on a structure or the pressure gradient across a structure. Strain is the resulting deformation of the system as a result of the external load or the change in size or shape of the structure. From a pulmonary perspective, stress is the alveolar distending pressure (alveolar pressure minus pleural pressure) and strain is the ratio of volume change (V_T plus volume increase caused by positive end-expiratory pressure [PEEP]) to functional residual capacity during the application of the stress.

Lung strain of more than 2 is considered injurious to the lungs. Stress and strain are related by the specific lung elastance of 13.5 cm H_2O/mL. Thus, lung stress 13.5 cm H_2O/mL times lung strain. From a bedside perspective the surrogates for stress and strain are plateau pressure (Pplat) and V_T. Thus the highest alveolar distending pressure that theoretically prevents disruption of the alveolar capillary membrane is 27 cm H_2O; thus the Pplat limit of 30 cm H_2O is in close agreement with this value when the chest wall compliance is normal. In passively ventilated critically ill patients, the alveolar distending pressure never exceeds the (Pplat) and in most settings the (Pplat) is at least a few cm H_2O greater than the alveolar distending pressure.

Volutrauma

Volutrauma refers to lung parenchymal damage caused by mechanical ventilation that is similar to ARDS (see Figure 3-1). Volutrauma is VILI manifested by an increase in the permeability of the alveolar capillary membrane, the development of pulmonary edema, the accumulation of neutrophils and proteins, the disruption of surfactant production, the development of hyaline membranes, and a decrease in compliance of the respiratory system (Table 3-2). The term *volutrauma* is used because the induced injury is the result of alveolar overdistention. Clinically, volume is used as a surrogate for pressure as it is impossible to measure local overdistention at the bedside. The pressure that has been used as a surrogate for local overdistention is Pplat. A Pplat more than 30 cm H_2O increases the likelihood of VILI; Pplat should be kept as low as possible.

Chest Wall Compliance

Because alveolar distention is determined by the difference between alveolar and pleural pressure, the chest wall has a role in determining the extent of overdistention. When the chest wall is stiff (low compliance), a high Pplat may be associated with less risk of overdistention. That is, a stiff chest wall (eg, abdominal distention, massive fluid resuscitation, chest wall deformity, chest wall burns, morbid obesity) protects the lungs from VILI.

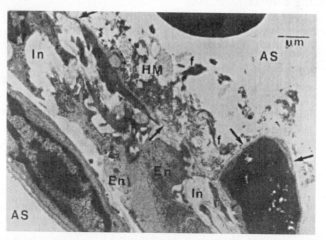

Figure 3-1 Electron microscopic view of the cross section of the alveolar-capillary complex of a rat ventilated with large volumes at a peak pressure of 45 cm H_2O with 0 PEEP. Markedly altered alveolar septum with three capillaries. At the right side, the epithelial lining is destroyed, denuding the basement membrane (arrows). Hyaline membrane (HM) composed of cell debris and fibrin (f) are present. Two endothelial cells (En) of another capillary are visible inside the interstitium (In). At the lower left side, a monocyte fills the lumen of a third capillary with a normal blood-air barrier. (Reproduced with permission from Dreyfuss D, Basset G, Soler P, Saumon G. Intermittent positive-pressure hyperventilation with high inflation pressures produces pulmonary microvascular injury in rats. *Am Rev Respir Dis.* 1985; Oct; 132(4):880-884.)

Table 3-2 **The Spectrum of Lung Injury Induced by Mechanical Ventilation**

- Atelectasis
- Alveolar hemorrhage
- Alveolar neutrophil infiltration
- Alveolar macrophage accumulation
- Decreased compliance
- Detachment of endothelial cells
- Denuding of basement membranes
- Emphysematous changes
- Pulmonary edema
- Hyaline membrane formation
- Interstitial edema
- Increased interstitial albumin levels
- Interstitial lymphocyte infiltration
- Intracapillary bleeding
- Pneumothorax
- Severe hypoxemia
- Subcutaneous emphysema
- Systemic gas embolism
- Tension cyst formation
- Type II pneumocyte proliferation

Active Breathing Efforts

The alveolar distending pressure can change markedly on a breath-by-breath basis in a spontaneous breathing patient. This most commonly occurs in pressure-targeted ventilation with high inspiratory efforts by the patient. When the airway pressure is constant and the patient forcefully inhales, the alveolar distending pressure may exceed what is expected by the airway pressure setting. For example, if the pressure control is 25 cm H_2O and the patient's effort decreases the pleural pressure to -10 cm H_2O, alveolar distending pressure is 35 cm H_2O, 10 cm H_2O greater than expected with an airway pressure setting of 25 cm H_2O. During pressure-targeted ventilation, the contribution of patient's effort to alveolar distending pressure must be appreciated.

Preexisting Injury

Preexisting injury increases the likelihood of VILI. This is called the two-hit process of lung injury. Previous injury predisposes the lungs to a greater likelihood of ventilator-induced injury. The use of lung-protective ventilatory strategies is thus necessary for all patients. The risk of developing ARDS is reduced if lung-protective ventilation strategies are implemented from the onset of mechanical ventilation (eg, volume and pressure limitation).

Atelectrauma

Another mechanism for the development of VILI is the repetitive recruitment and derecruitment (opening and closing) of unstable lung units (atelectrauma) during each

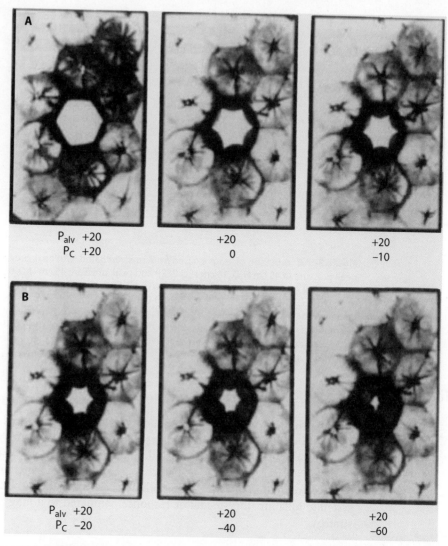

Figure 3-2 Illustration of the stress across a fully collapsed and fully expanded alveolus. P_{alv}, pressure inside surrounding alveolar units; P_c, pressure inside central alveolus. (Reproduced with permission from Mead J, Takishima T, Leith D. Stress distribution in lungs: a model of pulmonary elasticity. *J Appl Physiol.* 1970; May; 28(5):596-608.)

ventilatory cycle. The junction between an open and a closed alveolus serves as a stress riser (Figure 3-2). It has been estimated that more than 100 cm H_2O of stress is created when 30 cm H_2O alveolar distending pressure is applied adjacent to a collapsed alveolus. As illustrated in Figure 3-3, when PEEP is applied, the effect of a given distending pressure is attenuated and the extent of VILI reduced. The method used to determine the amount of PEEP in ARDS that prevents de-recruitment in a given alveolar unit is controversial. However, the best PEEP level prevents de-recruitment at end exhalation.

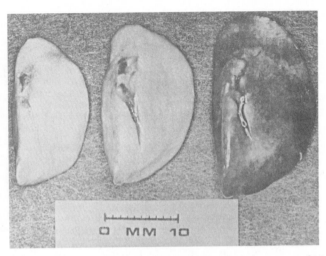

Figure 3-3 Comparison of lungs excised from rats ventilated with peak pressure of 14 cm H_2O, 0 PEEP; peak pressure of 45 cm H_2O, 10 cm H_2O PEEP and peak pressure 45 cm H_2O, 0 PEEP (left to right). The perivascular groove is distended with edema in the lungs from rats ventilated with peak pressures of 45 cm H_2O. The lung ventilated at 45 cm H_2O, 0 PEEP is grossly hemorrhaged. This injury is attenuated with the addition of PEEP of 10 cm H_2O (cneter). (Reproduced with permission from Webb HH, Tierney DF. Experimental pulmonary edema due to intermittent positive pressure ventilation with high inflation pressures. Protection by positive end-expiratory pressure. *Am Rev Respir Dis.* 1974; Nov; 110(5):556-565.)

Biotrauma

Overdistending V_T and repetitive opening and closing of unstable alveoli result in the activation of inflammatory mediators within the lung. Numerous proinflammatory (cytokines, chemokines) and anti-inflammatory mediators are activated by injurious ventilatory patterns. These mediators increase edema formation, neutrophil migration, and relaxation of vascular smooth muscle. Injurious ventilatory patterns increase systemic inflammatory-mediator response compared to a lung protective ventilation strategy.

Translocation of Cells

Bacteria instilled into the lungs of otherwise healthy animals produce bacteremia when inappropriate ventilatory patterns are employed. Translocation of bacteria is minimized if lung-protective ventilatory strategies are used.

Other Mechanisms

Preliminary and controversial animal data suggest a role for vascular volume, ventilator rate, and body temperature on VILI. Higher vascular infusion volumes, rapid respiratory rates, and high body temperature potentially cause greater injury. These potentially injurious factors are probably most important in the presence of nonprotective ventilatory strategies.

Ventilator-Induced Lung Injury and Multiple Organ Dysfunction Syndrome

Injurious ventilatory patterns not only cause VILI but may also cause or extend multiple organ dysfunction syndrome (MODS). Disruption of the alveolar-capillary membrane allows leakage of pulmonary inflammatory mediators into the bloodstream, allowing downstream organ failures (Figure 3-4).

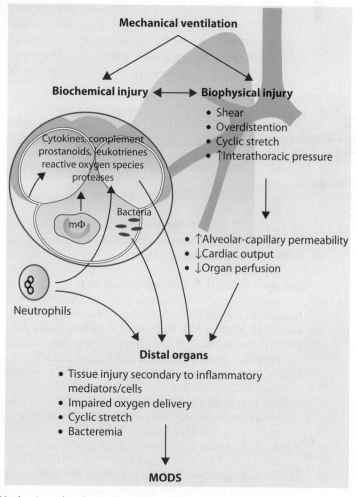

Figure 3-4 Mechanism whereby mechanical ventilation may contribute to MODS. (Reproduced with permission from Slutsky A, Tremblay L. Multiple system organ failure: Is mechanical ventilation a contributing factor? *Am J Respir Crit Care Med.* 1998; Jun; 157(6 Pt 1):1721-1725.)

Points to Remember

- The higher the Pplat, the larger the V_T, and the more severe the disease, the greater the likelihood for barotrauma.
- Oxygen toxicity should never prevent the appropriate administration of oxygen to avoid tissue hypoxemia.
- Lung stress is the transalveolar pressure (alveolar pressure minus pleural pressure).
- Lung strain is the volume change (V_T plus volume established by PEEP) to functional residual capacity (FRC) ratio during the application of the stress.
- Lung injury is caused by large V_T, Pplat, and low PEEP.
- PEEP prevents de-recruitment and attenuates volutrauma.
- Pplat determines the level of overdistention.
- Inflammatory mediators are activated by inappropriate ventilatory strategies.
- MODS can be caused by inappropriate ventilatory patterns.
- VILI can be avoided by a lung protective ventilation strategy: small V_T (4-8 mL/kg), low alveolar distending pressure (< 27 cm H_2O; Pplat < 30 cm H_2O), and sufficient PEEP to prevent de-recruitment (8-20 cm H_2O for ARDS).

Additional Reading

Adeniji K, Steel AC. The pathophysiology of perioperative lung injury. *Anesthesiol Clin.* 2012;30:573-579.

Calzia E, Asfar P, Hauser B, Matejovic M, et al. Hyperoxia may be beneficial. *Crit Care Med.* 2010;38:S559-S568.

de Prost N, Ricard JD, Saumon G, Dreyfuss D. Ventilator-induced lung injury: historical perspectives and clinical implications. *Ann Intensive Care.* 2011;1:28.

Della Rocca G, Coccia C. Acute lung injury in thoracic surgery. *Curr Opin Anaesthesiol.* 2013;26:40-46.

Gattinoni L, Protti A, Caironi P, Carlesso E. Ventilator-induced lung injury: the anatomical and physiological framework. *Crit Care Med.* 2010;38:S539-S548.

Heffner JE. The story of oxygen. *Respir Care.* 2013;58:18-31.

Kallet RH, Matthay MA. Hypoxemic acute lung injury. *Respir Care.* 2013;58:123-141.

Pelosi P, Rocco PR. Ventilator-induced lung injury in healthy and diseased lungs: better to prevent than cure! *Anesthesiology.* 2011;115:923-925.

Pierson DJ. Oxygen in respiratory care: a personal perspective from 40 years in the field. *Respir Care.* 2013;58:196-204.

Ranieri VM, Suter PM, Tortorella C, et al. Effect of mechanical ventilation on inflammatory mediators in patients with acute respiratory distress syndrome: a randomized controlled trial. *JAMA.* 1999;282:54-61.

Slutsky A, Tremblay L. Multiple system organ failure: Is mechanical ventilation a contributing factor? *Am J Respir Crit Care Med.* 1998;157:1721-1725.

The Acute Respiratory Distress Syndrome Network. Ventilation with lower tidal volumes as compared with traditional tidal volumes for acute lung injury and the acute respiratory distress syndrome. *N Engl J Med.* 2000;342:1301-1308.

Chapter 4
Ventilator-Associated Pneumonia

Introduction

Although the term *ventilator-associated pneumonia* (VAP) implies that the ventilator is the cause of the nosocomial pneumonia, a more appropriate term is *artificial airway-associated pneumonia*. Although contamination of the ventilator circuit may cause VAP, the most common cause is aspiration of contaminated oral secretions (Figure 4-1). VAP has become an increasing concern because it is not only associated

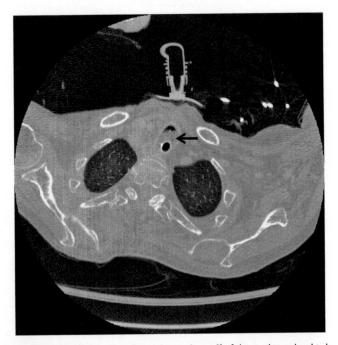

Figure 4-1 Computed tomography taken from above the cuff of the endotracheal tube. Note the accumulation of secretions above the cuff (arrow), which can potentially be aspirated into the trachea.

with increased cost, but also with increased time on the ventilator, morbidity, and possibly mortality. It has been estimated that VAP results in an additional cost of about $50,000 per case. Thus third-party payers are evaluating whether the hospital should assume the cost of this iatrogenic infection. Therefore, VAP has become a major concern for hospitals, physicians, respiratory therapists, and nurses caring for ventilated patients. There has been much investigation of risk factors for VAP and effective strategies to decrease VAP rate. In this chapter the definition of VAP, causes of VAP, and strategies to reduce VAP are discussed.

Etiology of VAP

Ventilator Circuit Versus the Artificial Airway

VAP is the result of organisms introduced into the respiratory tract during mechanical ventilation. This can arise from the ventilator circuit or by aspiration of contaminated secretions from above the cuff of the artificial airway. If a clean circuit is used and the patient is never disconnected, the organisms that accumulate in the circuit arise from the patient. However, if the circuit is disconnected and care is not taken to avoid contamination, the circuit could potentially cause VAP. This, however, is less likely to occur than the aspiration of contaminated oropharyngeal secretions.

The primary source of VAP is the aspiration of contaminated oropharyngeal secretions around the airway cuff (Figure 4-2). This occurs because of longitudinal folds that develop in inflated cuffs. To minimize this leakage, it is important to avoid accumulation of secretions above the cuff and to ensure that gastric contents do not move into the pharynx.

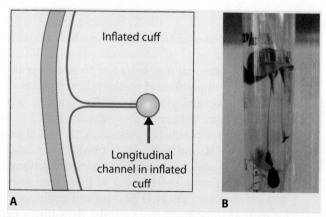

Figure 4-2 (A) Diagram illustrating folding of an artificial airway cuff creating a channel allowing fluid to move past the cuff. (B) Simulated microaspiration using dye to illustrate movement of secretions through the longitudinal folds of the endotracheal tube cuff. (Reproduced with permission from Deem S, Treggiari MM. New endotracheal tubes designed to prevent ventilator-associated pneumonia: do they make a difference? *Respir Care.* 2010; Aug; 55(8):1046-1055.)

Early Versus Late VAP

VAP has frequently been categorized as early or late. Early VAP is considered the result of the aspiration of oral secretions and, as a result, is caused by organisms usually found in the month or gastrointestinal tract (gram-positive cocci, *Haemophilus influenzae*, or gram-negative enteric bacteria). Late VAP is caused by the same bacteria that frequently cause nosocomial infections in other organ systems (methicillin-resistant *Staphylococcus aureus*, *Pseudomonas aeruginosa*, *Acinetobacter* species, and other gram-negative organisms). Based on the type of organism involved, early VAP is usually the result of aspiration of oral secretions, while late VAP is more likely a result of cross-contamination by poor infection control procedures. Early VAP usually occurs in the first 5 to 7 days of mechanical ventilation and late VAP occurs after this period.

Identification of VAP

Many of the approaches to VAP surveillance used in the past have been subjective. In 2013, the Centers for Disease Control and Prevention (CDC) established new objective guidelines designing to make the reporting more precise and consistent across institutions.

Historical Approach

Historically, the identification of VAP was not objective. The criteria used were evaluation of chest X-rays, changes in body temperature, white cell count, and the quantity and quality of respiratory secretions. As a result, reported VAP rates varied considerably. Some institutions indicated a zero VAP rate, causing many to question the subjective nature of these criteria. Moreover, the results of VAP surveillance were often not consistent with the diagnosis of VAP used in clinical care of patients.

CDC 2013 Guidelines

In 2013, the National Healthcare Safety Network of the CDC introduced a new surveillance approach for ventilator-associated events (VAEs). A VAE is defined as deterioration in patient's status that may be caused by an iatrogenic event, including not only VAP but also other complications of mechanical ventilation. This tiered approach first identifies ventilator-associated conditions (VACs). If a VAC is present, evaluation for an infection-related ventilator-associated complication (IVAC) is done. If an IVAC is present, evaluation is made for possible or probable VAP. This objective surveillance approach calls for reporting of VAC and IVAC, but not VAP. The intent of these guidelines is to make reporting of VAE an objective approach to compare performance between institutions.

A VAC is an increase in FIO_2 of more than or equal to 0.2 or an increase of more than or equal to 3 cm H_2O positive end-expiratory pressure (PEEP) that is sustained for more than or equal to 2 calendar days after a period of stability (Figure 4-3). The period of stability is defined as more than or equal to 2 calendar days where the FIO_2 and PEEP are stable or decreasing. The period of stability may be at the onset of intubation or any time during the course of invasive ventilation. VAC rate is reportable to external agencies.

Patient has a baseline period of stability or improvement on the ventilator, defined by ≥2 calendar days of stable or decreasing daily minimum FIO_2 or PEEP values. The baseline period is defined as the 2 calendar days immediately preceding the first day of increased daily minimum PEEP or FIO_2.

AND

After a period of stability or improvement on the ventilator, the patient has at least one of the following indicators of worsening oxygenation:

(1) Increase in daily minimum FIO_2 of ≥0.20 over the daily minimum FIO_2 in the baseline period, sustained for ≥2 calendar days.

(2) Increase in daily minimum PEEP values of ≥3 cm H_2O over the daily minimum PEEP in the baseline period, sustained for ≥2 calendar days.

Figure 4-3 Ventilator-associated condition. (From CDC Guidelines Device Associated Events: Ventilator Associated Events (VAE) January 2013. http://www.cdc.gov/nhsn/PDFs/pscManual/10-VAE_FINAL.pdf.)

There is evaluation for IVAC if VAC criteria are met (Figure 4-4). IVAC occurs on or after day 3 of mechanical ventilation and within 2 calendar days before or after the onset of worsening oxygenation, if both of the following criteria are met: (1) temperature more than 38°C or less than 36°C, or white cell count more than or equal to 12,000 cells/mm³ or less than or equal to 4000 cells/mm³ and (2) a new antimicrobial agent is started and continued for more than or equal to 4 calendar days. IVAC is reportable to external agencies.

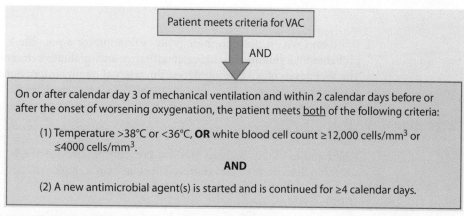

Patient meets criteria for VAC

AND

On or after calendar day 3 of mechanical ventilation and within 2 calendar days before or after the onset of worsening oxygenation, the patient meets <u>both</u> of the following criteria:

(1) Temperature >38°C or <36°C, **OR** white blood cell count ≥12,000 cells/mm³ or ≤4000 cells/mm³.

AND

(2) A new antimicrobial agent(s) is started and is continued for ≥4 calendar days.

Figure 4-4 Infection-related ventilator-associated condition. (From CDC Guidelines Device Associated Events: Ventilator Associated Events (VAE) January 2013. http://www.cdc.gov/nhsn/PDFs/pscManual/10-VAE_FINAL.pdf.)

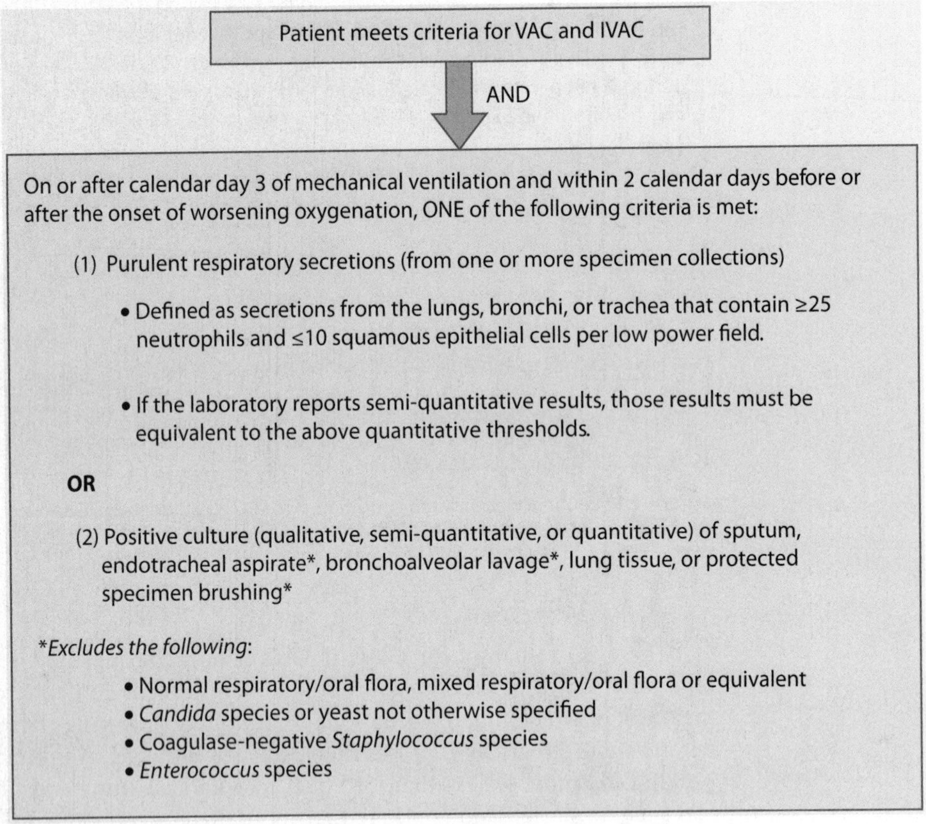

Figure 4-5 Possible ventilator-associated pneumonia. (From CDC Guidelines Device Associated Events: Ventilator Associated Events (VAE) January 2013. http://www.cdc.gov/nhsn/PDFs/pscManual/10-VAE_FINAL.pdf.)

If an IVAC is present, there is an evaluation for a possible VAP (Figure 4-5) and probable VAP (Figure 4-6) using quantitative and qualitative microbiologic techniques. The VAP levels of VAE are designed for internal quality improvement initiatives.

Prevention of VAP

VAP bundles (Table 4-1) are used for prevention. The use of a bundle recognizes that a combination of strategies is more effective than a single strategy for VAP prevention.

Hand Hygiene and Related Precautions

The basic tenant of infection control is to ensure that organisms are not transferred from one patient to another. This dictates proper hand hygiene before and after all patient contacts. Gloves should be worn during the patient interaction if there is potential for

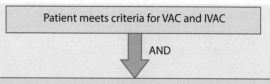

Patient meets criteria for VAC and IVAC

AND

On or after calendar day 3 of mechanical ventilation and within 2 calendar days before or after the onset of worsening oxygenation, ONE of the following criteria is met:

(1) Purulent respiratory secretions (from one or more specimen collections—and defined as for possible VAP)

AND one of the following:

- Positive culture of endotracheal aspirate*, $\geq 10^5$ CFU/mL or equivalent semi-quantitative result
- Positive culture of bronchoalveolar lavage*, $\geq 10^4$ CFU/mL or equivalent semi-quantitative result
- Positive culture of lung tissue, $\geq 10^4$ CFU/g or equivalent semi-quantitative result
- Positive culture of protected specimen brush*, $\geq 10^3$ CFU/mL or equivalent semi-quantitative result

Same organism exclusions as noted for possible VAP.

OR

(2) One of the following (without requirement for purulent respiratory secretions):

- Positive pleural fluid culture (where specimen was obtained during thoracentesis or initial placement of chest tube and NOT from an indwelling chest tube)
- Positive lung histopathology
- Positive diagnostic test for *Legionella* spp.
- Positive diagnostic test on respiratory secretions for influenza virus, respiratory syncytial virus, adenovirus, parainfluenza virus, human metapneumovirus, coronavirus

Figure 4-6 Probable ventilator-associated pneumonia. (From CDC Guidelines Device Associated Events: Ventilator Associated Events (VAE) January 2013. http://www.cdc.gov/nhsn/PDFs/pscManual/10-VAE_FINAL.pdf.)

contact with body secretions. Depending on the infectious condition of the patient, additional precautions such as gown, gloves, and/or a mask may be necessary. Reusable equipment must be cleaned and disinfected appropriately before it is used on another patient.

Care of the Artificial Airway

Orotracheal intubation is preferred over nasotracheal intubation. The cuff on the artificial airway should be inflated to 20 to 30 cm H_2O during exhalation to minimize aspiration of secretions and to minimize tracheal injury. However, even at this pressure, microaspiration can occur through the longitudinal folds in the cuff. To minimize pooling of

---

Table 4-1 **Elements Commonly Included in a VAP Prevention Bundle**

- Appropriate hand hygiene.
- Precautions based on specific infection.
- Use noninvasive ventilation.
- Head elevated > 30 degrees.
- Routine oral care.
- Use cuff pressure of 20-30 cm H_2O.
- Use inline suction catheters.
- Do no routinely change ventilator circuits.
- Remove ventilator circuit condensate away from the patient.
- Use orotracheal instead of nasotracheal intubation.
- Use subglottic suction systems and cuffs that minimize aspiration.
- Rinse nebulizers with sterile water (or saline) between treatments and allow to air dry.
- Deliver aerosolized medications using methods that do not break the circuit.
- Reduce colonization of gastrointestinal tract; peptic ulcer prophylaxis.
- Avoid gastric overdistention.
- Ensure adequate nutrition.
- Perform daily spontaneous awaking trials and spontaneous breathing trials.
- Use positive end-expiratory pressure of at least 5 cm H_2O.
- Minimize transports out of the unit for diagnostic studies.

---

secretions above the cuff, deep pharyngeal suctioning should be performed on a regular basis and before movement of the patient. Use of endotracheal tubes with subglottic suction ports may reduce the risk of VAP, but care is necessary to prevent occlusion of the suction port. Concern has been raised about the potential for tracheal injury due to the suction and the potential for laryngeal injury due to the rigidity of the tube. Endotracheal tubes coated with silver and the use of devices that scrape the inside of the tube to remove secretions are also available. Newer tapered cuff designs and cuff material (ultrathin polyurethane) may reduce microaspiration. The cost-effectiveness, however, of these newer tube designs and devices is yet to be determined.

Care of the Ventilator Circuit

Ventilator circuits do not need to be changed on a routine basis. Not breaking the circuit is important so that the interior of the circuit is not contaminated. An important part of this practice is use of inline suction catheters. Inline catheters become part of the circuit and do not need to be changed routinely. Any condensate that accumulates in the circuit should be removed away from the patient and from the circuit aseptically. The type of humidification, whether active or passive, does not affect VAP rates. If aerosolized medications are delivered, a device that remains in the ventilator circuit should be used (spacer for metered-dose inhaler, mesh nebulizer, or T-connector with a valve for jet nebulizers). Reusable nebulizers should be rinsed with sterile water (or saline) between treatments and allowed to air dry.

Oral Hygiene

Important to VAP prevention is oral hygiene. The goal is to reduce the bacterial load in the mouth and pharynx. This includes suctioning of the oropharynx, teeth brushing, and the use of chlorhexidine wash.

Noninvasive Ventilation

Use noninvasive ventilation (NIV) when appropriate to decrease the risk of VAP. NIV reduces the risk of VAP because intubation is avoided.

Minimize the Duration of Mechanical Ventilation

The shorter the time that a patient remains intubated, the lower the risk of VAP. Thus, daily spontaneous awaking trials and spontaneous breathing trials should be used to identify extubation readiness. Re-intubation is also associated with VAP risk, so efforts should be used to minimize extubation failure such as the use of NIV in patients at risk.

Positive End-Expiratory Pressure

The use of positive end-expiratory pressure (PEEP) has been shown to reduce VAP rate. The mechanism is that the positive tracheal pressure inhibits microaspiration past the cuff on the artificial airway.

Avoid Unnecessary Transport

Transport of ventilated patients out of the ICU has been shown to increase the risk of VAP. Thus, patient transports for diagnostic tests should be minimized, and care should be taken to avoid contamination of the airway during transport.

Patient Position

Mechanically ventilated patients should be positioned with the head elevated to more than 30 degrees unless there is a contraindication to this position. This is to avoid reflux of gastric contents into the oropharynx and its subsequent aspiration. Some investigators, however, believe that prone position or lateral Trendelenburg position may be more effective in removing secretions and preventing aspiration.

Management of the Gastrointestinal Tract

Reduction of the bacterial load of the gastrointestinal tract affects the risk of VAP. Peptic ulcer prophylaxis is recommended. Appropriate nutritional support should be maintained, but gastric overdistention should be avoided to reduce the risk of regurgitation. Selective decontamination of the gastrointestinal tract has been used in Europe, but this approach has not been widely adopted elsewhere.

Points to Remember

- Ventilator-associated pneumonia (VAP) should more appropriately be called artificial airway-associated pneumonia.
- The lower respiratory tract is infected primarily by aspiration past an inflated cuff.
- Aspiration occurs through channels created by the folds in the cuff when it is inflated.
- The new CDC guidelines focus on ventilator-associated events.

- A ventilator-associated condition is defined as a sustained F_{IO_2} or PEEP increase following a period of stability.
- Hand hygiene should be performed before and after patient contact.
- The head should be elevated to more than 30 degrees.
- Routine oral hygiene should be preformed.
- Airway cuffs should be inflated to 20 to 30 cm H_2O.
- Inline suction catheters should be used on all intubated patients.
- Ventilator circuits and inline suction catheters should not be changed routinely.
- The cost-effectiveness of subglottic suction systems is unclear.
- Nebulizers should be rinsed with sterile water (or saline) between treatments and allowed to air dry.
- Peptic ulcer prophylaxis should be used with all ventilated patients.
- Gastric overdistention should be avoided.
- Use noninvasive ventilation whenever possible.
- Perform daily spontaneous awakening trials and spontaneous breathing trials.

Additional Reading

Bird D, Zambuto A, O'Donnell C, et al. Adherence to ventilator-associated pneumonia bundle and incidence of ventilator-associated pneumonia in the surgical intensive care unit. *Arch Surg*. 2010;145:465-470.

Bouadma L, Mourvillier B, Deiler V, et al. A multifaceted program to prevent ventilator-associated pneumonia: impact on compliance with preventive measures. *Crit Care Med*. 2010;38:789-796.

Bouadma L, Wolff M, Lucet JC. Ventilator-associated pneumonia and its prevention. *Curr Opin Infect Dis*. 2012;25:395-404.

Caserta RA, Marra AR, Durão MS, et al. A program for sustained improvement in preventing ventilator associated pneumonia in an intensive care setting. *BMC Infect Dis*. 2012;12:234-239.

CDC Guidelines Device Associated Events: Ventilator Associated Events (VAE) January 2013. http://www.cdc.gov/nhsn/PDFs/pscManual/10-VAE_FINAL.pdf. Viewed on February 20th, 2013.

Coffin SE, Klompas M, Classen D, Arias KM, et al. Strategies to prevent ventilator-associated pneumonia in acute care hospitals. *Infect Control Hosp Epidemiol*. 2008;29:S31-S40.

Deem S, Treggiari MM. New endotracheal tubes designed to prevent ventilator-associated pneumonia: do they make a difference? *Respir Care*. 2010;55:1046-1055.

Fernandez JF, Levine SM, Restrepo MI. Technologic advances in endotracheal tubes for prevention of ventilator-associated pneumonia. *Chest*. 2012;142:231-238.

Gentile MA, Siobal MS. Are specialized endotracheal tubes and heat-and-moisture exchangers cost-effective in preventing ventilator associated pneumonia? *Respir Care*. 2010;55:184-197.

Han J, Liu Y. Effect of ventilator circuit changes on ventilator-associated pneumonia: a systematic review and meta-analysis. *Respir Care*. 2010;55:467-474.

Harbrecht BG. Head of bed elevation and ventilator-associated pneumonia. *Respir Care*. 2012;57:659-560.

Hess DR. Noninvasive positive-pressure ventilation and ventilator-associated pneumonia. *Respir Care*. 2005;50:924-931.

Hess DR, Kallstrom TJ, Mottram CD, et al. Care of the ventilator circuit and its relation to ventilator-associated pneumonia. *Respir Care.* 2003;48:869-879.

Hillier B, Wilson C, Chamberlain D, King L. Preventing ventilator-associated pneumonia through oral care, product selection, and application method: a literature review. *AACN Adv Crit Care.* 2013;24:38-58.

Kaynar AM, Mathew JJ, Hudlin MM, et al. Attitudes of respiratory therapists and nurses about measures to prevent ventilator-associated pneumonia: a multicenter, cross-sectional survey study. *Respir Care.* 2007;52:1687-1694.

Klompas M, Magill S, Robicsek A, et al. Objective surveillance definitions for ventilator-associated pneumonia. *Crit Care Med.* 2012;40:3154-3161.

Mietto C, Pinciroli R, Patel N, Berra L. Ventilator associated pneumonia: evolving definitions and preventive strategies. *Respir Care.* 2013;58:990-1007.

Morris AC, Hay AW, Swann DG, et al. Reducing ventilator-associated pneumonia in intensive care: impact of implementing a care bundle. *Crit Care Med.* 2011;39:2218-2224.

O'Grady NP, Murray PR, Ames N. Preventing ventilator-associated pneumonia: does the evidence support the practice? *JAMA.* 2012;307:2534-2539.

Pérez-Granda M, Muñoz P, Heras C, et al. Prevention of ventilator-associated pneumonia: can knowledge and clinical practice be simply assessed in a large institution? *Respir Care.* 2013;58:1213-1219.

Pneumatikos IA, Dragoumanis CK, Bouros DE. Ventilator-associated pneumonia or endotracheal tube-associated pneumonia? An approach to the pathogenesis and preventive strategies emphasizing the importance of endotracheal tube. *Anesthesiology.* 2009;110:673-680.

Rosenthal VD, Rodrigues C, Álvarez-Moreno C, et al. Effectiveness of a multidimensional approach for prevention of ventilator-associated pneumonia in adult intensive care units from 14 developing countries of four continents: findings of the International Nosocomial Infection Control Consortium. *Crit Care Med.* 2012;40:3121-3128.

Sinuff T, Muscedere J, Cook DJ, et al. Implementation of clinical practice guidelines for ventilator-associated pneumonia: a multicenter prospective study. *Crit Care Med.* 2013;41:15-23.

Torres A, Bassi GL, Ferrer M. Diagnosis of ventilator-associated pneumonia: do we need surrogate parameters? *Crit Care Med.* 2012;40:3311-3312.

Trouillet JL. Ventilator-associated pneumonia: a comprehensive review. *Hosp Pract (Minneap).* 2012;40:165-175.

Chapter 5
Ventilator Mode Classification

Objectives

1. Distinguish between the pneumatic and electronic powering systems of the ventilator.
2. Describe the variables, breath sequence, and targeting scheme used to control mechanical ventilator operation.
3. Compare pressure control, volume control, flow control, and time control.
4. Distinguish between trigger, limit, and cycle.
5. Define spontaneous and mandatory breath types.
6. Compare continuous mandatory ventilation, intermittent mandatory ventilation, and continuous spontaneous ventilation.
7. Compare set point, dual servo, adaptive, optimal, and intelligent targeting schemes.
8. Use the equation of motion to describe patient-ventilator interaction.

Introduction

Current generation mechanical ventilators are sophisticated life support devices. The ventilator must be reliable, flexible, and relatively easy to use by the skilled clinician. This chapter describes the ventilator system, and then covers ventilator classification and breath types during mechanical ventilation.

The Ventilator Powering Systems

Because ventilators deliver gases to the patient, they must have a pneumatic component. First-generation ventilators were typically pneumatically powered, using gas pressure to power the ventilator as well as ventilate the patient. Current generation ventilators are electronically controlled with the aid of a microprocessor. A generic block diagram of a ventilator is shown in Figure 5-1.

Pneumatic System

The pneumatic system is responsible for delivery of a gas mixture to the patient. Room air and 100% oxygen are delivered to the ventilator at 50 lb/in². The ventilator reduces this pressure and mixes these gases to provide a prescribed F_{IO_2} and flow into the ventilator circuit. The ventilator circuit not only delivers gas to the patient, but also filters, warms, and humidifies the inspired gas. During exhalation, gas flows through the expiratory limb of the circuit, a filter, the exhalation valve, and then into the atmosphere. The exhalation valve closes during inspiration to allow inflation of the lungs and is responsible for controlling positive end-expiratory pressure (PEEP). In the past, the exhalation valve was closed completely during the inspiratory phase. Newer-generation ventilators use an active exhalation valve during pressure-controlled ventilation, meaning that it opens if the pressure exceeds the pressure set during the inspiratory phase.

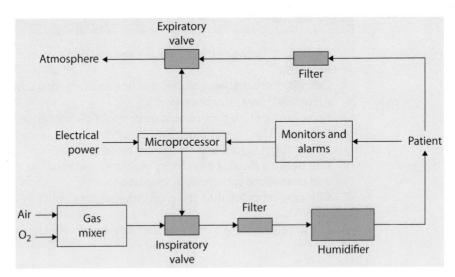

Figure 5-1 A simplified generic block diagram of the ventilator system.

The pneumatic system can be either single circuit or double circuit. With single-circuit ventilators, the gas that powers the ventilator is the same gas that is delivered to the patient. With double-circuit ventilators, the gas delivered to the patient is separate from the gas that powers the pneumonic system.

Ventilators can be positive-pressure or negative-pressure generators. Positive-pressure ventilators apply a positive pressure to the airway. Negative-pressure ventilators apply a negative pressure to the chest wall. Critical care ventilators are positive-pressure generators. Negative-pressure ventilators are used infrequently, but may be used in some patients receiving prolonged mechanical ventilation.

Electronic System

Current-generation mechanical ventilators are microprocessor-controlled. The microprocessor controls the inspiratory and expiratory valves. It also controls the flow of information from the monitoring system of the ventilator (eg, pressure, flow, volume) and the display of that information. Ventilator alarms are also controlled by the microprocessor.

Classification of Mechanical Ventilators

Ventilator classification describes how the ventilator works. The classification schemes described here are general enough to be applied to any commercially available ventilator. The components of a ventilator classification system are the control variables, breath sequence, and targeting scheme (Table 5-1).

Control Variables

Control variables describe how the ventilator manages pressure, volume, and flow during the inspiratory phase. The control variable remains constant as the ventilatory load

Table 5-1 **Ventilator Classification System**

- **Control variable**
  - Pressure
  - Volume
- **Breath sequence**
  - Continuous mandatory ventilation (CMV): actual rate may be greater than the set rate with the patient-triggered breaths; backup rate is the minimum value in case of apnea.
  - Intermittent mandatory ventilation (IMV): spontaneous breaths allowed between mandatory breaths; backup rate is the minimum value if apnea occurs.
  - Continuous spontaneous ventilation (CSV): all breaths are patient-triggered.
- **Targeting scheme**
  - Set point
  - Dual
  - Servo
  - Adaptive
  - Optimal
  - Intelligent

changes. Specific control variables are pressure, volume, flow, and time (Figure 5-2). Modern ventilators control either flow or pressure during the inspiratory phase. Moreover, the ventilator can only control flow or pressure at any time. Dual control occurs in situations where inspiration starts out as volume control and then switches to pressure control before the end of the breath (or vice versa).

A ventilator is a pressure controller if the pressure waveform is not affected by changes in resistance and compliance. If the volume waveform remains unchanged with changes in resistance and compliance, the ventilator can be either a volume controller or a flow controller. The ventilator is a volume controller if volume is measured and used to control the volume waveform. If volume is not used as a feedback signal, but the volume

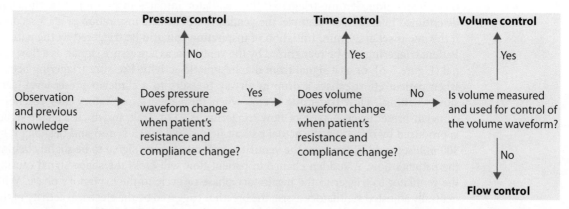

Figure 5-2 Criteria used to determine the control variable during inspiration. (Reproduced with permission from Chatburn RL. Classification of mechanical ventilators. *Respir Care.* 1992; Sep; 37(9):1009-1025.)

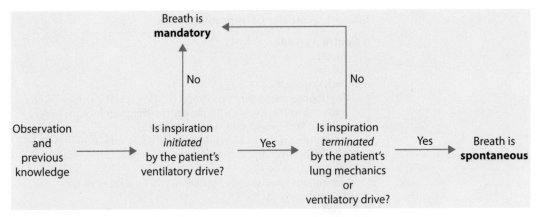

Figure 5-3 Criteria used to determine breath types during mechanical ventilation. (Reproduced with permission from Chatburn RL. Classification of mechanical ventilators. *Respir Care.* 1992; Sep; 37(9):1009-1025.)

waveform remains constant, then the ventilator is a flow controller. A ventilator is a time controller if inspiratory and expiratory times are the only variables that are controlled.

Breath Sequence

Two clinically different breath types can be provided during mechanical ventilation: mandatory or spontaneous breaths (Figure 5-3). A spontaneous breath is both initiated and terminated by the patient. If the ventilator determines either the beginning and/ or the end of the breath, it is mandatory. The three types of breath sequences during mechanical ventilation are continuous mandatory ventilation, intermittent mandatory ventilation, and continuous spontaneous ventilation (Figure 5-4). All ventilator modes can be identified by one of breathing patterns given in Table 5-2.

Operational Algorithms

Phase variables are used to initiate some phase of the ventilatory cycle. Specifically, these are the trigger, limit, and cycle variables (Figure 5-5). The trigger variable initiates inspiration. If time-triggered, the ventilator initiates inspiration at a clinician-determined interval. For example, the ventilator will initiate inspiration every 3 seconds if the rate is set at 20/min. Initiation of inspiration can also be triggered by the patient. Patient triggering can be recognized by the ventilator as a pressure signal, as a flow signal (Figure 5-6), or as a signal from diaphragmatic activity. Pressure triggering occurs when patient effort causes a drop in airway pressure to a clinician-preset level (sensitivity setting). Flow triggering occurs when the patient's inspiratory flow reaches a clinician-preset level. A type of flow triggering is Auto-Trak, in which a shape signal is produced by offsetting the actual patient flow signal by 15 L/min and delaying it by 300 milliseconds. This causes the ventilator-generated shape signal to be slightly behind the patient's flow. A sudden change in patient flow will cross the shape signal causing the ventilator to trigger to the inspiratory phase or cycle to the expiratory phase. With neutrally adjusted ventilatory assist, the breath is triggered by the electrical activity of the diaphragm.

The limit variable is the pressure, volume, or flow that cannot be exceeded during the inspiratory phase. Inspiration is not necessarily terminated when the limit variable

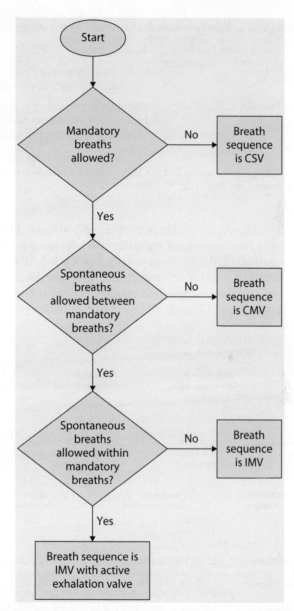

Figure 5-4 Breath sequence during mechanical ventilation. CMV, continuous spontaneous ventilation; CSV, continuous spontaneous ventilation; IMV, intermittent mandatory ventilation. (Adapted from Chatburn RL. Classification of ventilator modes: update and proposal for implementation. *Respir Care* 2007; Mar; 52(3):301-323.)

is reached. Pressure-controlled ventilation is pressure limited because the pressure limit is reached before inspiration ends. For some ventilators, the inspiratory flow, inspiratory time, and tidal volume are set separately. In this case, the ventilator is volume limited because tidal volume is delivered before inspiration ends.

Table 5-2 **Ventilation Modes Identified by Breathing Patterns**

Breath-control variable	Breath sequence	Acronym
Volume	Continuous mandatory ventilation	VC-CMV
	Intermittent mandatory ventilation	VC-IMV
Pressure	Continuous mandatory ventilation	PC-CMV
	Intermittent mandatory ventilation	PC-IMV
	Continuous spontaneous ventilation	PC-CSV (ie, pressure support ventilation

Adapted from CHATBURN RL. Classification of ventilator modes: update and proposal for implementation. Respir Care. 2007; Mar; 52(3):301-323.

The cycle variable is the pressure, volume, flow, or time that terminates inspiration. First-generation ventilators were typically pressure-cycled. With pressure support ventilation, the breath is usually flow-cycled. With volume-controlled ventilation, the breath is volume or time-cycled. With pressure-controlled ventilation, the breath is time-cycled. The baseline variable is what is controlled during the expiratory phase, and is the PEEP or continuous positive airway pressure setting.

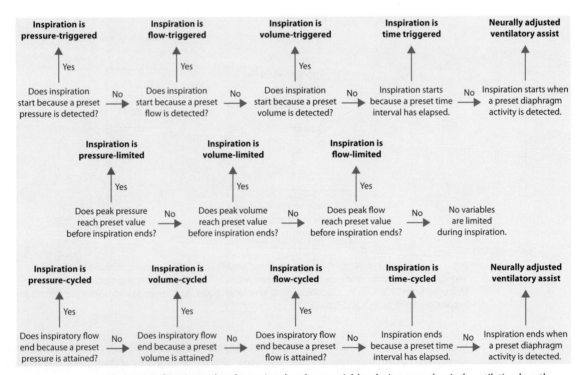

Figure 5-5 Criteria used to determine the phase variables during a mechanical ventilation breath. (From Chatburn RL. Classification of mechanical ventilators. *Respir Care.* 1992; Sep; 37(9):1009-1025.)

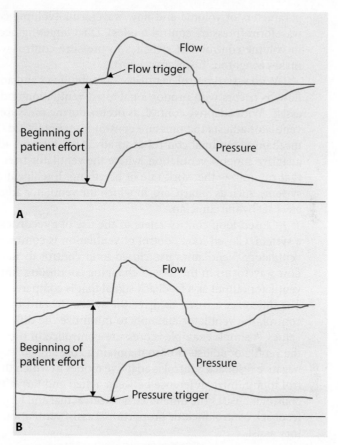

Figure 5-6 Flow (A) and pressure (B) triggering. With flow triggering, the ventilator responds to a change in flow. With pressure triggering, the ventilator responds to a decrease in airway pressure.

Conditional variables are used by the operational logic system of the ventilator to make decisions on how to manage control and phase variables. Conditional variables are if/then statements. For example, *if* minute ventilation is below the set threshold, *then* deliver a mandatory breath (eg, mandatory minute ventilation). Computational logic is a description of the relationship between ventilator settings, feedback signals, and breathing pattern to add detail about how the mode operates that is not given in the other components of the mode specification (eg, adaptive support ventilation).

Targeting Scheme

The targeting scheme determines the feedback-control algorithm used by the ventilator. For set point targeting, the clinician adjusts specific static set points such as the pressure limit, tidal volume, and inspiratory flow. Set point targeting occurs with conventional modes such as volume-controlled ventilation, pressure-controlled ventilation, and pressure support ventilation. For set point targeting, the clinician sets all parameters of volume and flow waveforms (volume control modes) or the pressure waveform (pressure control modes). Dual targeting occurs when the breath starts out in volume control, but switches to pressure control within the breath if the patient makes a vigorous inspiratory effort.

With servo control, ventilator output follows and amplifies the patient's inspiratory flow, as occurs with proportional assist ventilation and neutrally adjusted ventilatory assist. With adaptive control, as occurs during pressure-regulated volume control, the ventilator adjusts the pressure control to maintain tidal volume with changes in lung mechanics. Optimal control is an advanced form of adaptive control, as occurs with adaptive support ventilation, where the ventilator tries to achieve a breathing pattern that minimizes the work rate of breathing. Intelligent control uses rule-based expert systems, such as SmartCare, in which the ventilator adjusts its output based on parameters set by the clinician.

Closed-loop control refers to the use of a feedback signal to adjust the output of a system. Closed-loop control of ventilation is commonly used in current-generation ventilators. Ventilators use closed-loop control to maintain consistent pressure and flow waveforms in the face of changing conditions. This is accomplished by using the ventilator output as a feedback signal that is compared to the input set by the clinician. The difference is used to drive the system toward the desired output. With negative control, the ventilator attempts to minimize the difference between target and actual values. A simple example is pressure-controlled or pressure support ventilation, where the ventilator adjusts flow to maintain a constant airway pressure. Another example of negative feedback control is adaptive modes in which there is a change in pressure control to minimize difference between actual and target tidal volume. Positive-feedback control increases the difference between actual and target values. Examples of positive-feedback control include proportional assist ventilation and neutrally adjusted ventilatory assist.

Equation of Motion

Inflation of the lungs is explained by the equation of motion, which states that the pressure required to deliver a breath is determined by the elastic (volume and compliance) and resistive (flow and resistance) properties of the respiratory system. The pressure can be either that applied to the airway (P_{vent}) by the ventilator or the pressure generated by the respiratory muscles (P_{mus}), or a combination of both. Mathematically, this becomes:

$$P_{vent} + P_{mus} = V/C + \dot{V}R$$

During volume-controlled ventilation, flow and volume delivery from the ventilator are fixed. If the patient generates an inspiratory effort (increased P_{mus}) during volume-controlled ventilation, the airway pressure drops—a common sign of patient-ventilator asynchrony. During pressure-controlled ventilation, P_{airway} is fixed. If the patient generates an inspiratory effort during pressure-controlled ventilation, flow and volume delivery increase, which may improve patient-ventilator synchrony but might also contribute to overdistension lung injury.

Points to Remember

- The ventilator system consists of a pneumatic component and an electronic component.
- The variable that the ventilator manipulates during the inspiratory phase is the control variable.
- Phase variables initiate a phase of the ventilatory cycle (inspiration or expiration).
- The inspiratory phase can be triggered by time, changes in pressure or flow at the proximal airway, or electrical activity of the diaphragm.
- The cycle variable is the pressure, volume, flow, or time that terminates inspiration.
- Two clinically different breath types that can be delivered during mechanical ventilation are mandatory breaths and spontaneous breaths.
- Targeting schemes used during mechanical ventilation are set point, dual servo, adaptive, optimal, and intelligent.
- Ventilators use closed-loop control to maintain consistent pressure and flow waveforms in the face of changing conditions.
- The equation of motion can be used to describe the effects of patient-ventilator interactions.

Additional Reading

Branson RD. Techniques for automated feedback control of mechanical ventilation. *Semin Respir Crit Care Med.* 2000;21:203-209.

Branson RD, Chatburn RL. Controversies in the critical care setting. Should adaptive pressure control modes be utilized for virtually all patients receiving mechanical ventilation? *Respir Care.* 2007;52(4):478-488.

Branson RD, Davis K Jr. Does closedloop control of assist control ventilation reduce ventilator-induced lung injury? *Clin Chest Med.* 2008;29:343-350.

Branson RD, Johannigman JA, Campbell RS, Davis K Jr. Closed-loop mechanical ventilation. *Respir Care.* 2002;47:427-513.

Chatburn RL. Classification of ventilator modes: update and proposal for implementation. *Respir Care.* 2007;52:301-323.

Chatburn RL. Understanding mechanical ventilators. *Expert Rev Respir Med.* 2010;4:809-819.

Chatburn RL, Mireles-Cabodevila E. Closed-loop control of mechanical ventilation: description and classification of targeting schemes. *Respir Care.* 2011;56:85-102.

Chatburn RL, Primiano FP Jr. A new system for understanding modes of mechanical ventilation. *Respir Care.* 2001;46:604-621.

Mireles-Cabodevila E, Diaz-Guzman E, Heresi GA, Chatburn RL. Alternative modes of mechanical ventilation: a review for the hospitalist. *Cleve Clin J Med.* 2009;76:417-430.

Mireles-Cabodevila E, Hatipoglu U, Chatburn RL. A rational framework for selecting modes of ventilation. *Respir Care.* 2013;58:348-366.

Volsko TA, Hoffman J, Conger A, Chatburn RL. The effect of targeting scheme on tidal volume delivery during volume control mechanical ventilation. *Respir Care.* 2012;57:1297-1304.

Chapter 6
Traditional Modes of Mechanical Ventilation

Objectives

1. Compare pressure-controlled and volume-controlled ventilation.
2. Distinguish between continuous mandatory ventilation, continuous spontaneous ventilation, and synchronized intermittent mandatory ventilation.
3. Compare continuous positive airway pressure and pressure support ventilation.
4. Compare full and partial ventilatory support.

Introduction

The relationship between breath types and phase variables is referred to as a mode of ventilation. During mechanical ventilation, the mode is one of the principal ventilator settings. Although many modes are available, the choice of mode is usually based on clinician's preference or institutional bias, since evidence is lacking that one mode is clearly superior to others. This chapter describes traditional ventilator modes (Table 6-1), which include continuous mandatory ventilation (CMV), continuous spontaneous ventilation (CSV), and synchronized intermittent mandatory ventilation (SMV).

Volume-Controlled Versus Pressure-Controlled Ventilation

The two general approaches to ventilatory support are volume-controlled ventilation and pressure-controlled ventilation. At any time, the ventilator controls either volume (flow) or pressure applied to the airway. Some volume-targeted modes such as pressure-regulated volume control and adaptive support ventilation actually adjust the level of pressure control to achieve the set tidal volume. Although the term *volume control* is usually used, in reality the ventilator controls the inspiratory flow. The important

Table 6-1 Ventilator Modes

Mode	Control variable; Mandatory breath	Control variable; Spontaneous breath	Name
CMV	Volume	None	VC-CMV
	Pressure	None	PC-CMV
CSV	None	Pressure	CPAP or PSV
SIMV	Volume	Pressure	VC-SIMV
	Pressure	Pressure	PC-SIMV

Abbreviations: CMV, continuous mandatory ventilation; CPAP, continuous positive airway pressure; CSV, continuous spontaneous ventilation; PC-CMV, pressure-controlled continuous mandatory ventilation; PC-SIMV, pressure-controlled synchronized intermittent mandatory ventilation; PSV, pressure support ventilation; SIMV, synchronized intermittent mandatory ventilation; VC-CMV, volume-controlled continuous mandatory ventilation; VC-SIMV, volume-controlled synchronized mandatory ventilation.

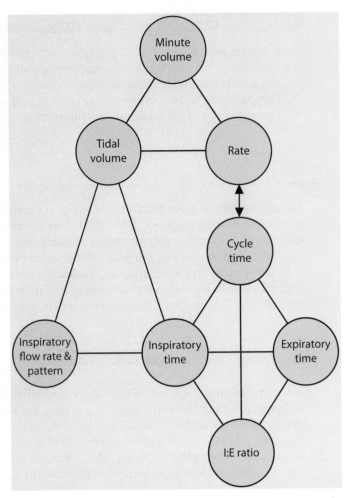

Figure 6-1 Important variables and their interaction during volume-controlled ventilation. (Adapted from Chatburn RL. A new system for understanding mechanical ventilators. *Respir Care* 1991;36:1123-1155.)

variables for volume-controlled ventilation are shown in Figure 6-1. During pressure-controlled ventilation, the inspiratory flow decreases as the alveolar pressure approaches the pressure applied to the airway. The important variables affecting pressure-controlled ventilation are illustrated in Figure 6-2.

Continuous Mandatory Ventilation

A minimal rate is set with CMV (Figure 6-3). The patient can trigger the ventilator at a more rapid rate, but every breath delivered is a mandatory breath type. Note that the mandatory breaths can be either volume-controlled or pressure-controlled. CMV is commonly called assist/control (A/C) ventilation—the terms CMV and A/C

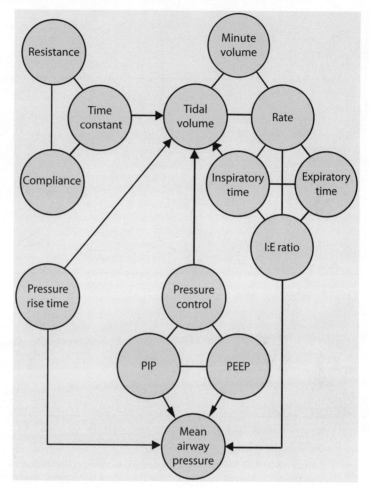

Figure 6-2 Important variables and their interaction during pressure-controlled ventilation. (Adapted from Chatburn RL. A new system for understanding mechanical ventilators. *Respir Care* 1991;36:1123-1155.)

are used interchangeably. Note that, from the perspective of the ventilator, there is no controlled-mechanical ventilation mode. If the patient's breathing is completely controlled by the ventilator, this is the result of pharmacologic support or pathophysiology, not the ventilator mode. Also note that the ventilator always assists the patient's breathing regardless of the ventilator mode.

Continuous Spontaneous Ventilation

With CSV, every breath is a spontaneous type; ie, every breath is triggered and cycled by the patient. The two most common forms of CSV are continuous positive airway pressure (CPAP) and pressure support ventilation (PSV).

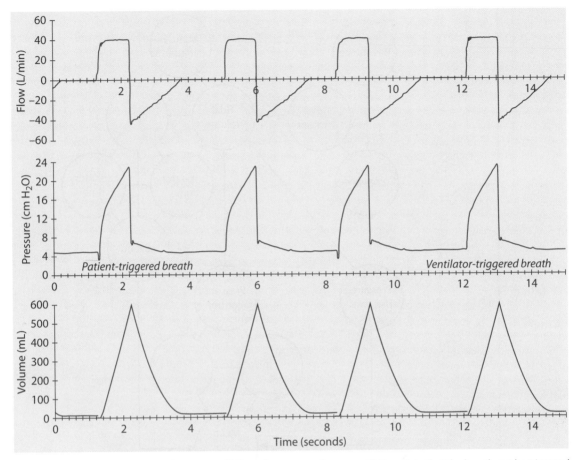

Figure 6-3 Volume-controlled continuous mandatory ventilation. Note that the breath can be triggered by the patient or the ventilator. After the breath is triggered, every breath type is mandatory.

Continuous Positive Airway Pressure

This is a spontaneous breathing mode; no mandatory breaths are delivered (Figure 6-4). A clinician-determined level of positive pressure is maintained throughout the ventilatory cycle. However, it is possible to set CPAP to 0, where the pressure applied to the airway is ambient. The CPAP mode is most commonly used to evaluate whether the patient can be liberated from the ventilator. It is interesting to note that the performance of many current generation ventilators is such that a small level of PSV (1-2 cm H_2O) is applied during CPAP. Ventilator performance during CPAP is better with flow-triggering than with pressure-triggering. For that reason, flow-triggering is recommended when CPAP is used.

Pressure Support Ventilation

The patient's inspiratory effort is assisted by the ventilator at a preset level of inspiratory pressure with PSV. Inspiration is triggered and cycled by patient's effort. During PSV, the

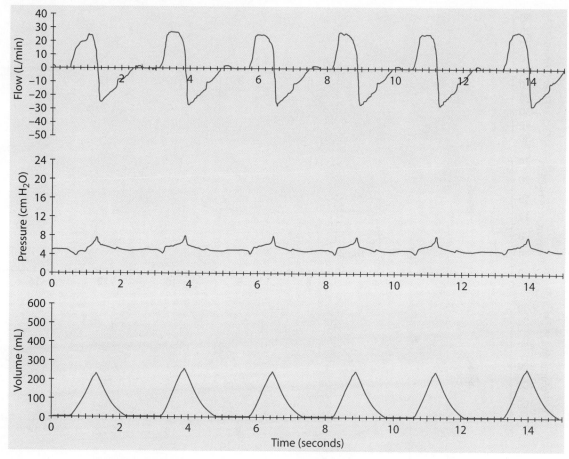

Figure 6-4 Continuous positive airway pressure. Note that every breath is spontaneous.

patient determines the respiratory rate, inspiratory time, and tidal volume (Figure 6-5). Current generation ventilators provide backup ventilation (volume-controlled or pressure-controlled CMV) should apnea occur during PSV, but this is an alarm condition. PSV is normally flow-cycled. Secondary cycling mechanisms with PSV are pressure and time. In other words, PSV will cycle to the expiratory phase when the flow decreases to a ventilator-determined level, when the pressure rises to a ventilator-determined level, or when the inspiratory time reaches a ventilator-determined limit. The flow at which the ventilator cycles to the expiratory phase can be either a fixed flow, a flow based on the peak inspiratory flow, or a flow based on peak inspiratory flow and elapsed inspiratory time. Newer generation ventilators allow the clinician to adjust the termination flow at which the ventilator cycles to a level appropriate for the patient. Newer generation ventilators also allow adjustment of rise time at the beginning of the pressure support breath and the maximum time of the inspiratory phase. Rise time is the amount of time required to reach the pressure support level at the beginning of inspiration.

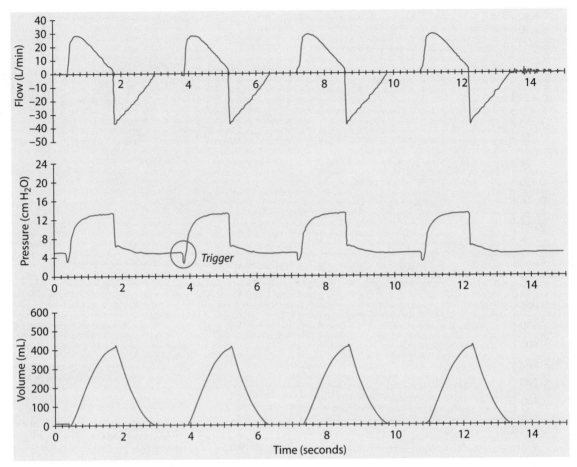

Figure 6-5 Pressure support ventilation. Note that every breath is triggered by the patient and is flow-cycled.

Synchronized Intermittent Mandatory Ventilation

Synchronized intermittent mandatory ventilation (SIMV) is a ventilator mode where mandatory breaths are delivered intermittently with volume-controlled or pressure-controlled ventilation. Between the mandatory breaths, the patient is allowed to breathe spontaneously. The ventilator delivers the mandatory breaths in *synchrony* with the patient's inspiratory effort (Figure 6-6). If no inspiratory effort is detected, the ventilator delivers a mandatory breath at the scheduled time. This is usually achieved by use of an assist window (Figure 6-7). This window opens at intervals determined by the SIMV rate, and remains open for a manufacturer-specific period of time. If a patient-generated effort is detected while this window is open, a mandatory breath is delivered. If no patient effort is detected in the time that the window is open, the ventilator delivers a mandatory breath. With SIMV, the spontaneous breaths are usually

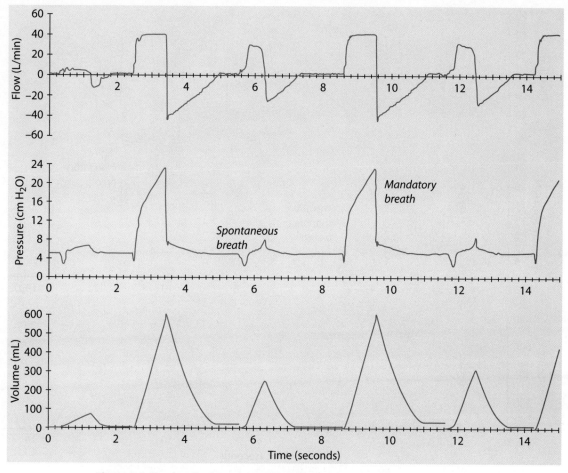

Figure 6-6 Synchronized intermittent mandatory ventilation illustrating mandatory and spontaneous breaths. The mandatory breaths are volume-controlled.

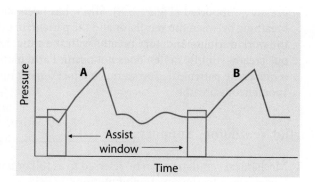

Figure 6-7 Pressure waveform for synchronized intermittent mandatory ventilation illustrating the assist window for synchronization of mandatory breaths.

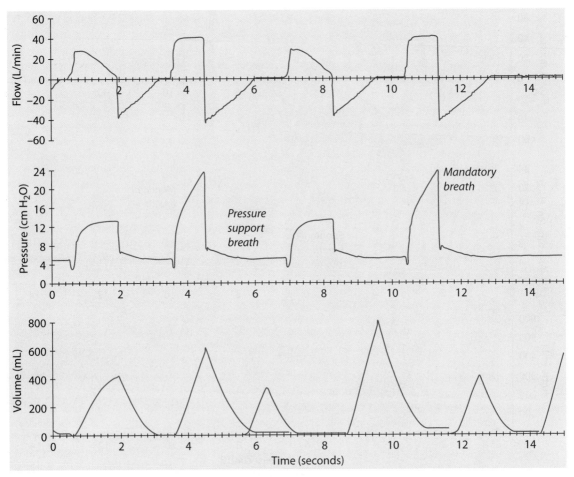

Figure 6-8 Synchronized intermittent mandatory ventilation with pressure support for the spontaneous breaths. The mandatory breaths are volume-controlled.

pressure-supported (Figure 6-8). SIMV has been suggested to partition the work-of-breathing between the ventilator and the patient; in other words, for the ventilator to do the work during mandatory breaths with the patient doing the work during spontaneous breaths. But this often does not occur. Particularly at a low mandatory rate, SIMV requires the patient to exert as much effort during the mandatory breath as during the spontaneous breaths.

Full Versus Partial Ventilatory Support

Mechanical ventilation can be referred to as full or partial ventilatory support. This can be described by the equation of motion:

$$P_{vent} + P_{mus} = V/C + \dot{V}R$$

With full support, there is no respiratory muscle activity and thus Pmus is 0. With partial support, there is a contribution by the respiratory muscles, and thus, Pmus makes a contribution to the equation of motion.

With full support, the ventilator does all of the work needed for ventilation of the patient; the patient does *not* trigger the ventilator or breathe spontaneously. This can be achieved as the result of the patient's primary disease process (eg, neuromuscular disease), pharmacologic therapy (eg, paralysis), or a minute ventilation high enough to suppress the patient's respiratory drive (eg, hyperventilation). Full support is often preferred for patients who are severely ill to decrease the oxygen cost of breathing and achieve control of the patient's ventilatory pattern. Full support is provided by CMV.

With partial support, some of the work-of-breathing is provided by the ventilator and the remainder is provided by the patient. Partial ventilatory support is commonly used during weaning from mechanical ventilation. Partial support is also preferred by clinicians who believe that this maintains respiratory muscle tone, allows the patient to maintain some control of the ventilatory pattern, and improves patient comfort and synchrony. Total respiratory muscle suppression can quickly lead to atrophy and weakness. Partial ventilatory support can be achieved with CMV, SIMV, or PSV.

Points to Remember

- With continuous mandatory ventilation, all breaths are mandatory volume-controlled or pressure-controlled breaths.
- All breaths are spontaneous with continuous positive airway pressure.
- The patient's inspiratory effort is assisted by a preset level of inspiratory pressure during pressure support ventilation.
- With synchronized intermittent mandatory ventilation, both spontaneous and mandatory breaths are delivered and the mandatory breaths are synchronized to patient effort.
- With full ventilatory support, the ventilator does all of the work of breathing for the patient.
- With partial ventilatory support, some of the work is provided by the ventilator and the remainder is provided by the patient.

Additional Reading

Chatburn RL. Classification of ventilator modes: update and proposal for implementation. *Respir Care.* 2007;52:301-323.

Mireles-Cabodevila E, Hatipoglu U, Chatburn RL. A rational framework for selecting modes of ventilation. *Respir Care.* 2013;58:348-366.

Chapter 7
Pressure and Volume Ventilation

Objectives

1. Discuss the gas delivery patterns during volume-controlled ventilation (VCV) and pressure-controlled ventilation (PCV).
2. Describe the effect of varying rise time and inspiratory cycle criteria during pressure support ventilation and PCV.
3. Describe how an end-inspiratory plateau can be achieved with PCV.
4. Describe approaches to monitor gas delivery during PCV and VCV.
5. Contrast the advantages and disadvantages of PCV and VCV.

Introduction

Controversy has always followed the introduction of new modes of ventilation. In the late 1970s it was assist/control (continuous mandatory ventilation [CMV]) versus intermittent mandatory ventilation (IMV). In the mid- to late-1980s, it was IMV versus pressure support ventilation. A debate today is whether gas delivery should be volume-controlled or pressure-controlled.

Volume-Controlled Ventilation

All of these first-generation ICU ventilators only provided VCV, and until the 1970s, it was without the option for patient-triggered breaths. Pressure-limited ventilators (eg, Bird and Puritan-Bennett machines) have been available since the 1950s, but they were not designed for continuous ventilatory support.

With VCV, the variable that is constant during each breath is tidal volume. With this approach, there is a variable inspiratory pressure. With changes in respiratory mechanics (eg, resistance, compliance) and patient's effort, airway pressure varies because volume delivery is constant. With VCV, the clinician sets tidal volume (V_T), flow pattern, peak inspiratory flow, rate, and trigger sensitivity. In some ventilators, inspiratory time, minute volume, and I:E ratio are set instead of V_T and flow. In other ventilators, both inspiratory time and flow are set; if the inspiratory time is longer than the time required to deliver the V_T, an end-inspiratory pause will result. In practice, modern ventilators provide VCV by controlling the inspiratory flow. VCV can be applied as CMV or as synchronized IMV (CMV-IMV).

Pressure-Controlled Ventilation

With pressure-controlled ventilation (PCV), a fixed pressure is applied during the inspiratory phase. In addition, inspiratory time, or I:E ratio, and trigger sensitivity are set. As respiratory mechanics (eg, resistance, compliance) and patient's effort change, V_T must vary because pressure is constant. As noted in Table 7-1, the primary

Table 7-1 PCV Versus VCV

	PCV	*VCV*
V_T	Variable	Constant
PIP	Constant	Variable
Pplat	Constant	Variable
Flow pattern	Variable	Set
Peak flow	Variable	Set
Inspiratory time	Set	Set
Minimum rate	Set	Set

Abbreviations: PCV, pressure-controlled ventilation; VCV, volume-controlled ventilation.

difference between these VCV and PCV is a fixed V_T or a fixed peak inspiratory pressure (PIP), respectively. In newer generation ventilators, the clinician may also set the rise time, which is the time required for the set pressure to be reached. This occurs by varying the slope of the flow increase from baseline to peak flow.

Pressure Support Ventilation

Pressure support ventilation (PSV) is pressure-limited, but it is different from PCV. Traditionally, the only set variable with PSV is the pressure support level. Respiratory rate, inspiratory time, inspiratory flow, and V_T are patient-controlled.

In newer generation ventilators, the clinician also sets the rise time with PSV. With some ventilators, the pressure setting can be achieved within in as little as 50 milliseconds, whereas with others, the pressure setting cannot be achieved until near the end of the inspiratory phase (Figure 7-1). The ventilator cycles to exhalation when inspiratory flow decreases to a predetermined level. Inspiratory cycle criteria on most current generation ICU ventilators is clinician-adjustable as a percentage of peak flow.

The most appropriate rise time and inspiratory termination criteria should be set to enhance patient comfort. Rise time should be set to satisfy patient peak inspiratory demand. An initial overshoot in pressure above the set pressure support level indicates that the rise time is too short (flow is too rapid), whereas a concave rise in initial airway pressure usually indicates the rise time is too long (flow is too slow). The inspiratory termination criteria should be adjusted so that the patient does not double-trigger or activate expiratory muscles to terminate the breath; in other words, so that the ventilator response matches the patient's neural inspiratory time. An end-inspiratory pressure spike that exceeds the set level indicates that the patient has actively exhaled before the ventilator reached its inspiratory termination criteria.

Rise time, inspiratory termination criteria, and the pressure support level are interrelated. Peak flow increases with a faster rise time or higher set pressure. As a result, there will be a greater flow for inspiratory termination if the ventilator determines cycle criteria based on a percent of peak flow. Thus, if any of these three variables are changed (pressure, rise time, and termination flow), the other two should be re-evaluated.

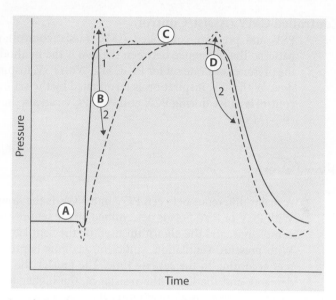

Figure 7-1 Design characteristics of a pressure supported breath. The inspiratory pressure is triggered at point A by a patient effort resulting in an airway pressure decrease. Demand valve sensitivity and responsiveness are characterized by the depth and duration of this negative pressure. The rise to pressure (line B) is provided by a fixed high initial flow delivery into the airway. Note that if flows exceed patient demand, initial pressure exceeds set level (B1), whereas if flows are less than patient demand, a very slow (concave) rise to pressure can occur (B2). The plateau of pressure support (line C) is maintained by servo control of flow. A smooth plateau reflects appropriate responsiveness to patient demand, fluctuations would reflect less responsiveness of the servo mechanisms. Termination of pressure support occurs at point D and should coincide with the end of the spontaneous inspiratory effort. If termination is delayed, the patient actively exhales (bump in pressure above plateau) (D1); if termination is premature, the patient will have continued inspiratory efforts (D2). (Reproduced with permission from McIntyre N, et al. The Nagoya conference on system design and patient-ventilator interactions during pressure support ventilation. *Chest.* 1990; Jun; 97(6):1463-1466.)

Airway pressure graphics are helpful to properly set rise time and inspiratory termination criteria.

A lengthy inspiratory time, beyond the patient's neural inspiratory time, may occur with PSV whenever a leak is present or the termination criteria is set too low. Cuff leaks, bronchopleural fistulae, or circuit leaks can all prolong inspiration because they may prevent the inspiratory termination criteria from being met. That is, flow will be unable to decrease to the level required to initiate expiration. Whenever lengthy inspiratory times are observed with pressure support, a system leak or inappropriately set termination criteria should be suspected.

Another issue related to PSV is periodic breathing, which can result due to lack of a set rate. Wakefulness drive to breathe and the pressure assist with PSV can lead to respiratory alkalosis. This can result in apnea—particularly during sleep. When apnea occurs, the ventilator alarms and this stimulates the patient to breathe. Arousals may be more common with PSV than ventilator modes with a backup rate. This can be addressed by using a lower level of pressure support, by using a mode with a rate, or by using a mode such as proportional-assist ventilation.

Pressure-Controlled CMV (Assist/Control)

PSV and pressure-controlled CMV (assist/control) provide a similar gas delivery pattern. The difference between the two is the method of terminating inspiration and the presence of a rate set for PC-CMV. With PSV, inspiration is normally terminated by flow. With PCV, inspiration is terminated by the set inspiratory time. The rise in time control is active during PCV and PSV. PCV can also be used during synchronized IMV (PC-IMV).

Flow and Flow Pattern

A major difference between PCV and VCV is the flow pattern. With VCV, flow is set. With PCV or PSV, flow is determined by the set pressure, patient's demand, resistance, compliance, and the algorithm used by the ventilator to establish the pressure target. With pressure ventilation, sufficient gas flow is provided so that the set pressure is met according to the set rise time. The greater the pressure, the greater the patient's demand, and the lower the resistance, the higher is the peak inspiratory flow. With some ventilators, peak inspiratory flows may exceed 180 L/min during pressure ventilation. In experimental models, a high flow at the onset of inspiration is associated with increased lung injury, but the clinical relevance of this is unclear.

A distinctive flow pattern occurs with PCV. Because the set pressure is met by establishing a high initial flow rate and the pressure applied is constant, flow decreases exponentially as inspiratory time proceeds. The rate of decrease depends on the pressure set, the patient's inspiratory demand, and respiratory mechanics. When the set pressure is low, inspiratory demand is low, compliance is low, or resistance is high, the flow decrease occurs rapidly. When the set pressure is low, inspiratory demand is low, compliance is high, or resistance is low, the rate of flow decrease is slow.

With VCV, a precise gas flow pattern is set on the ventilator. Various flow patterns (eg, rectangular, ramp) can be set during VCV. Airway pressure during VCV decreases as the inspiratory demand increases, resistance decreases, and compliance increases. PIP increases as compliance decreases or resistance increases. As shown in Figure 7-2, when a descending ramp flow pattern is chosen, PCV and VCV cannot be easily distinguished if set to deliver gas in a similar manner provided inspiratory demand, compliance, and resistance remain constant.

End-Inspiratory Pause

With PCV and no patient triggering, inspiratory time or I:E is set and the gas flow pattern responds to the set pressure and respiratory mechanics. For a specific pressure and lung mechanics, there is an inspiratory time beyond which there is zero flow. Decreasing inspiratory time below the point of zero flow eliminates the plateau and decreases the delivered V_T. With VCV the clinician must set an end-inspiratory pause to achieve this effect. With VCV, the plateau remains constant unless changed by the clinician. With PCV the length of the end-inspiratory plateau changes with changes in

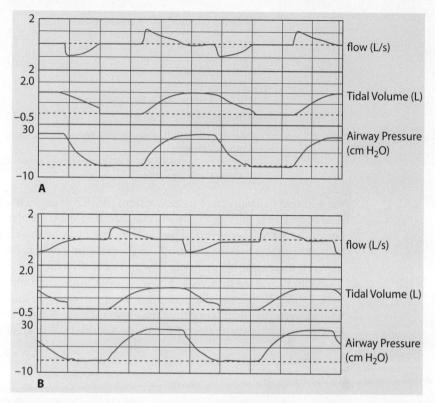

Figure 7-2 (A) Pressure-controlled ventilation. (B) Volume-controlled ventilation. Pressure and volume-controlled modes generated on a lung model. Volume control was set to match pressure control flow delivery pattern; same peak flow, same inspiratory time, and same end-inspiratory pause time. The two delivery patterns are virtually indistinguishable.

lung mechanics. As compliance decreases, the end-inspiratory plateau time increases. As resistance increases, the plateau time decreases. A descending flow pattern with either VCV or PCV has the effect of delivering the majority of the V_T early in the inspiratory phase (Figure 7-2). This may result in better distribution of the inspired gas, a higher Pao_2 and a lower $Paco_2$, although the effect is usually small.

Inspiratory Time and Air Trapping

Increasing inspiratory time and changing the inspiratory flow pattern are the only manipulations of the gas delivery pattern that result in an increase in mean airway pressure ($\bar{P}aw$) without increasing peak alveolar pressure (Table 7-2). Increasing inspiratory time has been used to improve gas exchange in the management of severe acute respiratory failure. However, the effect is usually only a small increase in Pao_2.

With VCV, inspiratory time can be increased by decreasing the flow setting, increasing the tidal volume setting, or adding an end-inspiratory pause. Of these, only

---

Table 7-2 Methods of Increasing P̄aw

- Increase PEEP
- Increase V_T
- Increase rate
- Increase PIP
- Select descending ramp flow pattern[a]
- Increase inspiratory time[a]

Abbreviations: PEEP, positive end-expiratory pressure; PIP, peak inspiratory pressure.

[a]Only methods that do not affect peak alveolar pressure, or level of ventilation (provided auto-PEEP does not occur).

the addition of a pause maintains constant the PIP to increases the P̄aw. Decreasing the flow increases inspiratory time without affecting the peak alveolar pressure. However, because it decreases the rate of gas delivery, the increase in P̄aw as a result of increasing inspiratory time may be offset by the decrease in P̄aw associated with the slower gas delivery. Increasing V_T increases P̄aw and peak alveolar pressure.

With PCV, P̄aw is increased by increasing inspiratory time or increasing the pressure setting. Increasing the pressure setting increases V_T and peak alveolar pressure, while increasing inspiratory time may also increase V_T as P̄aw is increased. As noted in Figure 7-3, as inspiratory time increases tidal volume increases to a point, then

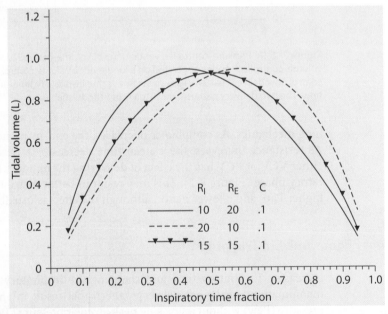

Figure 7-3 Relationship of inspiratory time fraction to tidal volume (pressure target = 20 cm H_2O). When inspiratory (R_I) and expiratory (R_E) resistance are equal, optimal duration (D) = 0.5. When $R_I > R_E$, more inspiratory time is required, and optimal D > 0.5. Conversely, when $R_E > R_I$, optimal D < 0.5. (Reproduced with permission from Marini JJ, Crooke PS, Truwit JD. Determinants and limits of pressure-preset ventilation. A mathematical model of pressure control. *J Appl Physiol.* 1989; Sep; 67(3):1081-1092.)

Table 7-3 Effects of the Development of Auto-PEEP

Pressure ventilation	*Volume ventilation*

• No change:
  – Peak alveolar pressure
  – PIP
	• No change:
	  – Tidal volume

• Decrease:
  – Tidal volume
	• Increased:
	  – Peak alveolar pressure
	  – Peak airway pressure

Abbreviations: PEEP, positive end-expiratory pressure; PIP, peak inspiratory pressure.

decreases. The specific inspiratory time where this change occurs is dependent on resistance and compliance. If compliance is low, maximum V_T will occur at a shorter inspiratory time. If resistance is high, a longer inspiratory time is needed to maximize tidal volume delivery. Once flow decreases to 0, V_T remains constant with PCV until inspiratory time is increased enough to cause air trapping and auto-positive end-expiratory pressure (auto-PEEP) (Table 7-3), at which point V_T decreases.

There is an inspiratory time at which expiratory time is too short to prevent air trapping. When air trapping develops, VCV and PCV respond differently. With VCV, since V_T is constant, the development of air trapping and auto-PEEP results in an increase in PIP and Pplat. With PCV, air trapping and auto-PEEP result in a decrease in the delivered V_T with peak alveolar pressure remaining constant.

Transition to Controlled Ventilation

When patients are transitioned to pharmacologically controlled ventilation, the response differs for VCV and PCV. PSV cannot be used due to the lack of a set backup rate. With the loss of active breathing efforts, tidal volume may decrease in the setting of PCV. With VCV and with PCV, synchrony will improve. With VCV, airway pressures decrease due to loss chest wall muscle tone.

Work-of-Breathing

Pressure modes may result in less patient work than volume modes. With pressure ventilation, delivered flow varies with patient's demand. Increased demand results in greater delivered flow. However, this has the potential to result in excessive tidal volume and increased risk of ventilator-induced lung injury. During pressure ventilation, alveolar stretch (stress) is determined by the pressure setting on the ventilator and the decrease in pleural pressure decrease generated by the patient's respiratory muscles. With VCV, flow should be set high enough to meet patient's demand. For VCV and PCV, inspiratory time should set to avoid double-triggering or active exhalation at the end of the inspiratory phase.

Table 7-4 **Monitoring during pressure and volume ventilation**

Volume ventilation – Monitor pressure	Pressure ventilation – Monitor volume

• Ventilator-triggered breaths:
  – PIP alarm 5 cm H_2O above average PIP
• Patient-triggered breaths:
  – PIP alarm 10 cm H_2O above average PIP
	• Ventilator-triggered breaths:
	  – Low V_T or $\dot{V}_E$ alarms 50% below average volume
	• Patient-triggered breaths:
	  – Low V_T alarm 50% below average V_T

Abbreviation: PIP, peak inspiratory pressure.

Monitoring

With VCV, monitoring should focus on airway pressure. PIP, Pplat, and $\overline{\text{Paw}}$ change with alterations in resistance and compliance. Of primary concern is the rapid identification of elevated pressures in the presence of a pneumothorax or airway obstruction. Patients who are not actively breathing, alarms should be set about 5 to 10 cm H_2O above the average PIP. In actively breathing patients, alarms should be set about 10 cm H_2O above the average PIP (Table 7-4).

With PCV, monitoring should focus on V_T and $\dot{V}_E$ changes. For patients without spontaneous breathing efforts, low V_T or $\dot{V}_E$ alarms should be set 50% lower than the average V_T or $\dot{V}_E$. For patients who are actively breathing, low V_T alarms are more appropriate than low $\dot{V}_E$ alarms. Patients may compensate for the decreased V_T by increasing their respiratory rate to keep $\dot{V}_E$ constant. In this setting, low V_T alarms should be set 50% lower than the average V_T.

Of concern with PCV is the recognition of a pneumothorax or major airways obstruction. Since PIP is constant, V_T decreases as the pneumothorax increases, but its decrease is limited by the eventual equilibration of pressure in the thorax and in the airway. That is, the pneumothorax may not extend to the degree seen with VCV and the level of hemodynamic compromise with PCV may be less than with VCV. With PCV, the first indication of a problem is deterioration in gas exchange. With VCV the effects of a tension pneumothorax are immediate, dramatic, and rapidly recognized. However, with PCV the response is less dramatic, more difficult to recognize and may go unrecognized until a routine chest X-ray or arterial blood gases are obtained.

PCV Versus VCV

There are advantages and disadvantages of both PCV and VCV. The decision to employ one or the other approach is generally based on personal bias and, which of the advantages or disadvantages are considered most important for an individual patient. Physiologic effects, lung injury, synchrony, and patient outcomes are similar for PCV and VCV. This is particularly true when PCV is compared with VCV with a descending ramp flow.

PCV: Advantages and Disadvantages

The major advantage of PCV is that PIP and peak alveolar pressures are kept at a constant level. Flow also varies with patient's demand, potentially decreasing the likelihood of asynchrony. However, increased patient demand increases the potential for delivery of injurious tidal volumes. A major disadvantage is that V_T varies as respiratory mechanics changes, increasing the likelihood of blood gas changes and making it more difficult to rapidly identify major alterations in mechanics.

VCV: Advantages and Disadvantages

The major advantage of VCV is the delivery of a constant V_T. This ensures a consistent level of alveolar ventilation and results in easily identifiable changes in PIP and Pplat as respiratory mechanics change. But flow pattern is fixed, potentially contributing to asynchrony. However, unlike PCV, V_T cannot exceed safe limits with active inspiratory efforts, but this might contribute to asynchrony.

Points to Remember

- With volume-controlled ventilation (VCV), V_T is constant but pressure varies with changes in respiratory mechanics and patient's demand.
- With pressure-controlled ventilation (PCV), airway pressure is constant but V_T varies with changes in respiratory mechanics and patient's demand.
- Pressure support ventilation (PSV) is a pressure mode in which inspiratory time is not set.
- Rise time is adjustable on most ventilators during PCV and PSV.
- Inspiratory termination criteria can be adjusted during PSV on most modern ventilators.
- Gas delivery patterns during PSV and PCV are similar.
- Due to the lack of a set rate, periodic breathing can occur with PSV.
- With pressure ventilation, a decreasing flow pattern is observed, while with VCV the flow pattern is set on the ventilator.
- With pressure ventilation, an end-inspiratory plateau may occur, dependent on the pressure, inspiratory time, resistance, and compliance.
- With a descending ramp flow pattern the majority of the V_T is delivered early in inspiration.
- PCV and VCV are available in continuous mandatory ventilation (A/C) and synchronized intermittent mandatory ventilation modes.
- For a set flow pattern, the only method of increasing P̄aw that does not affect peak alveolar pressure is increasing inspiratory time.
- Increasing inspiratory time can result in air-trapping.
- With active inspiratory effort, pressure ventilation may unload the work-of-breathing to a greater extent than VCV.
- Monitoring of airway pressure is necessary with VCV, while monitoring of V_T is necessary with pressure ventilation.

- If a leak is present (eg, bronchopleural fistula), inspiration may be prolonged during PSV.
- When transitioning to pharmacologically controlled ventilation, V_T may decrease with PCV and peak airway pressure may decrease with VCV.

Additional Reading

Bosma K, Ferreyra G, Ambrogio C, et al. Patient-ventilator interaction and sleep in mechanically ventilated patients: pressure support versus proportional assist ventilation. *Crit Care Med.* 2007;35:1048-1054.

Chatmongkolchart S, Williams P, Hess DR, Kacmarek RM. Evaluation of inspiratory rise time and inspiration termination criteria in new-generation mechanical ventilators: a lung model study. *Respir Care.* 2001;46:666-677.

Chiumello D, Pelosi P, Taccone P, et al. Effect of different inspiratory rise time and cycling off criteria during pressure support ventilation in patients recovering from acute lung injury. *Crit Care Med.* 2003;31:2604-2610.

Chiumello D, Polli F, Tallarini F, et al. Effect of different cycling-off criteria and positive end-expiratory pressure during pressure support ventilation in patients with chronic obstructive pulmonary disease. *Crit Care Med.* 2007;35:2547-2552.

Garnero AJ, Abbona H, Gordo-Vidal F, et al. Pressure versus volume controlled modes in invasive mechanical ventilation. *Med Intensiva.* 2013;37:292-298.

Hess DR. Ventilator waveforms and the physiology of pressure support ventilation. *Respir Care.* 2005;50:166-186.

Kallet RH, Campbell AR, Dicker RA, et al. Work of breathing during lung-protective ventilation in patients with acute lung injury and acute respiratory distress syndrome: a comparison between volume and pressure-regulated breathing modes. *Respir Care.* 2005;50: 1623-1631.

Kallet RH, Hemphill JC 3rd, Dicker RA, et al. The spontaneous breathing pattern and work of breathing of patients with acute respiratory distress syndrome and acute lung injury. *Respir Care.* 2007;52:989-995.

MacIntyre N. Counterpoint: is pressure assist-control preferred over volume assist-control mode for lung protective ventilation in patients with ARDS? No. *Chest.* 2011;140:290-294.

MacIntyre NR, Sessler CN. Are there benefits or harm from pressure targeting during lung-protective ventilation? *Respir Care.* 2010;55:175-183.

Marini JJ. Point: is pressure assist-control preferred over volume assist-control mode for lung protective ventilation in patients with ARDS? Yes. *Chest.* 2011;140:286-290.

Murata S, Yokoyama K, Sakamoto Y, et al. Effects of inspiratory rise time on triggering work load during pressure-support ventilation: a lung model study. *Respir Care.* 2010;55: 878-884.

Parthasarathy S, Tobin MJ. Effect of ventilator mode on sleep quality in critically ill patients. *Am J Respir Crit Care Med.* 2002;166:1423-1429.

Struik FM, Duiverman ML, Meijer PM, et al. Volume-targeted versus pressure-targeted noninvasive ventilation in patients with chest-wall deformity: a pilot study. *Respir Care.* 2011;56:1522-1525.

Tassaux D, Gainnier M, Battisti A, Jolliet P. Impact of expiratory trigger setting on delayed cycling and inspiratory muscle workload. *Am J Respir Crit Care Med.* 2005;172:1283-1289.

Tassaux D, Michotte JB, Gainnier M, et al. Expiratory trigger setting in pressure support ventilation: from mathematical model to bedside. *Crit Care Med.* 2004;32:1844-1850.

Thille AW, Cabello B, Galia F, et al. Reduction of patient-ventilator asynchrony by reducing tidal volume during pressure-support ventilation. *Intensive Care Med.* 2008;34:1477-1486.

Uchiyama A, Imanaka H, Taenaka N. Relationship between work of breathing provided by a ventilator and patients' inspiratory drive during pressure support ventilation: effects of inspiratory rise time. *Anaesth Intensive Care* 2001;29:349-358.

Yang LY, Huang YC, Macintyre NR. Patient-ventilator synchrony during pressure-targeted versus flow-targeted small tidal volume assisted ventilation. *J Crit Care.* 2007;22:252-257.

Chapter 8
Advanced Modes of Mechanical Ventilation

Introduction

With each generation of ventilators, new modes and variations on previous modes become available. There now exist numerous ventilator modes from a variety of manufacturers. The purpose of this chapter is to describe the technical and clinical aspects of advanced modes of ventilation that have recently become available. Although heavily promoted by their manufacturers, the clinical role of many of these modes remains unproven. Use of these modes is often based upon their availability and clinician's bias, rather than evidence that they are superior to traditional modes.

Dual-Control Modes

With dual-control modes, the ventilator can automatically switch between pressure control and volume control during a single breath. However, it is important to remember that the ventilator is controlling only pressure or volume at any given time, not both at the same time.

The proposed advantage of this mode is a reduced work-of-breathing (WOB) while maintaining a minimum minute volume and tidal volume (V_T). This approach operates during mandatory breaths or pressure-supported breaths to combine the high initial flow of a pressure-controlled breath with the constant volume delivery of a volume-controlled breath. Names for this approach are volume-assured pressure support, pressure augmentation, and machine volume. These modes are not commonly available on the newest generation of ICU ventilators.

The breath is patient or ventilator-triggered. The ventilator then attempts to reach the pressure setting as quickly as possible. This portion of the breath is pressure-controlled and associated with a variable flow. As this pressure is reached, the ventilator determines the volume that has been delivered and determines if the desired V_T will be delivered. If the delivered and set V_T are equal, the breath is a pressure support breath (Figure 8-1). If the patient's inspiratory effort is low, the breath

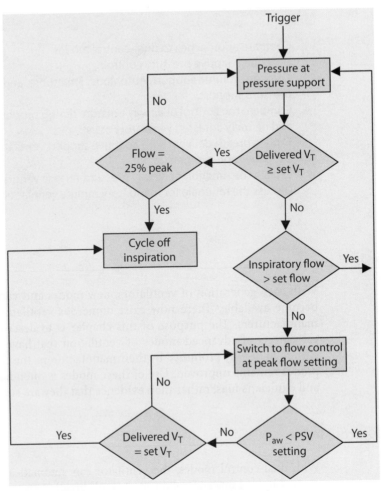

Figure 8-1 Control logic for volume-assured pressure support mode.

changes from a pressure-controlled to a volume-controlled breath. Flow remains constant until the tidal volume has been delivered. During this time the pressure rises above the pressure setting. If pressure reaches the high-pressure alarm setting, the breath is pressure-cycled. The ventilator can allow the patient a V_T larger than that set.

Volume control on the Maquet Servo-i is an example of volume-controlled ventilation (VCV) with a dual-targeting scheme. Each breath begins as VCV, but if the patient makes an inspiratory effort sufficient to decrease airway pressure by 3 cm H_2O, the ventilator switches to pressure-controlled ventilation (PCV) within the breath. This allows the patient's effort to augment the set V_T. Depending on the intensity of the inspiratory effort, the ventilator may switch back to VCV with a volume-cycle criterion or end inspiration with a flow-cycle criterion, similar to a pressure support breath.

Adaptive Pressure Control

Adaptive pressure control is closed-loop PCV. Tidal volume is a feedback control for breath-by-breath adjustment of pressure control (Figure 8-2). All breaths are patient or ventilator-triggered, pressure-controlled, and time-cycled. This mode is available on most current ICU ventilators and has various names, dependent on the manufacturer, such as AutoFlow, pressure-regulated volume control (PRCV), volume control + (VC+), adaptive pressure ventilation, volume-targeted pressure control, and pressure-controlled volume guarantee. The ventilator delivers a test breath and calculates system compliance. A number of breaths are delivered to test the pressure control necessary to achieve the desired tidal volume based on the compliance calculation. The ventilator then increases or decreases the pressure on a breath-by-breath basis to deliver the desired V_T.

Perhaps the most important advantage of this mode is the ability of the ventilator to change inspiratory flow to meet patient's demand while maintaining a constant minute volume (Figure 8-3). An important disadvantage of this mode is that the tidal volume remains constant and peak alveolar pressure increases as the lungs become less compliant (eg, acute respiratory distress syndrome [ARDS]), which could result in alveolar overdistention and acute lung injury. With this mode, breaths can exceed set tidal volume in the presence of strong inspiratory efforts by the patient. When this occurs, the ventilator may excessively reduce the level of support, leading to asynchrony. On some ventilators a low-pressure limit as well as a high-pressure limit can be set.

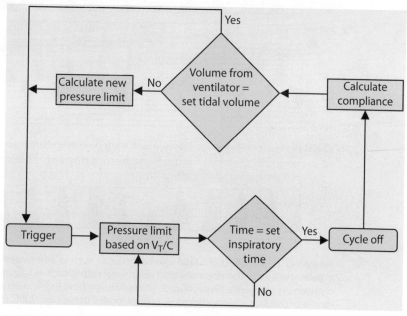

Figure 8-2 Control logic for adaptive pressure control mode.

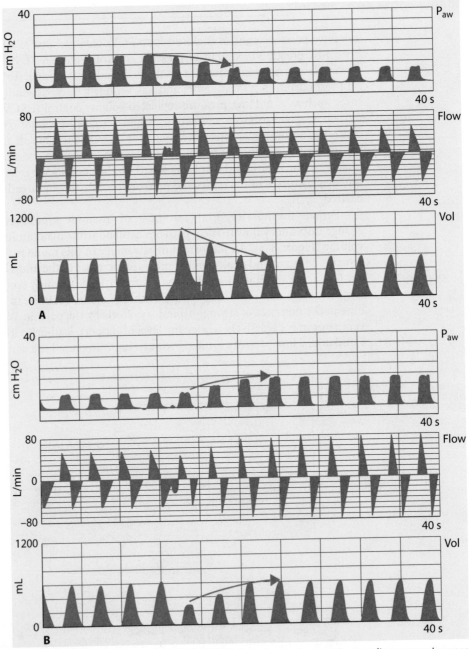

Figure 8-3 (A) The effect of a tidal volume increases, such as an increase in compliance or an increase in patient effort. (B) The effect of a tidal volume decreases, such as a decrease in compliance or a decrease in compliance. (Reproduced with permission from Branson RD, Johannigman JA. The role of ventilator graphics when setting dual-control modes. *Respir Care.* 2005; Feb; 50(2):187-201.)

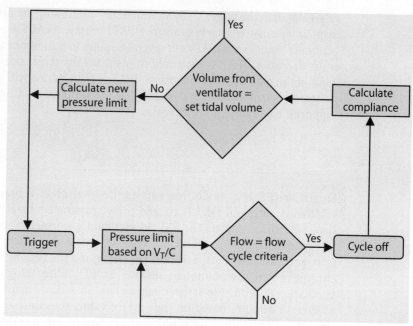

Figure 8-4 Control logic for volume support mode.

Volume Support

Volume support (VS) is closed-loop control of pressure support ventilation (PSV). Tidal volume is used as feedback control to adjust the pressure support level. All breaths are patient-triggered, pressure-limited, and flow-cycled (Figure 8-4). A test breath with a low-pressure is applied. The delivered tidal volume (exiting the ventilator) is measured and compliance is calculated. A number of breaths are then delivered to test the calculated pressure to deliver the set tidal volume. The ventilator then attempts to maintain a constant delivered tidal volume on a breath-to-breath manner. Since VS is a variation on PSV, the breath is flow-cycled.

There are several potential issues with this mode. Auto-positive end-expiratory pressure (auto-PEEP) may occur if the pressure level increases in an attempt to maintain tidal volume in a patient with airflow obstruction. In the patient with a high ventilatory demand, ventilator support will decrease, which could be the opposite of the desired response. This mode of ventilation is available on most current generation ICU ventilators.

AutoMode

AutoMode allows the ventilator to switch between mandatory and spontaneous breathing modes. If the patient is apneic, the ventilator will provide VCV, PCV, or PRVC. If the patient triggers a breath, the ventilator switches from VCV to VS, from PCV to PSV, or from PRVC to VS. If the patient becomes apneic, the ventilator reverts to VCV, PCV, or PRVC.

Average Volume-Assured Pressure Support

Average volume-assured pressure support (AVAPS) is a form of adaptive pressure control available on some ventilators for noninvasive ventilation. It maintains a V_T equal to or greater than the target V_T by automatically controlling the minimum and maximum inspiratory positive airway pressure (IPAP) setting. AVAPS averages V_T over time and gradually changes the IPAP over several minutes to achieve the target V_T. If the patient's effort decreases, IPAP is increased to maintain the target tidal volume. On the other hand, if the patient's effort increases, IPAP is reduced. As with other types of adaptive pressure control, there is a concern that the ventilator will inappropriately decrease support if respiratory drive increases.

SmartCare/PS

SmartCare/PS is a mode that adjusts the level of PSV based on the patient's V_T, respiratory rate, end-tidal Pco_2, and preset parameters based on the patient's condition. SmartCare adjusts the PSV to maintain a normal range of ventilation (called the zone of comfort), defined as $V_T > 300$ mL, a respiratory rate 12 to 30 breaths/min, and end-tidal $Pco_2 < 55$ mm Hg (assuming the patient weighs > 55 kg, without chronic obstructive pulmonary disease [COPD] or neurologic injury). If the patient's ventilation falls outside of these parameters, SmartCare manipulates the PSV as often as every 5 minutes based on the current value, the clinician input parameters, and the patient's historical breathing pattern. SmartCare was designed to automatically wean patients from the ventilator. When the patient is weaned to PSV low enough, a spontaneous breathing trial is performed automatically. If the spontaneous breathing trial (SBT) is successful, the ventilator prompts the clinician to consider extubation.

Adaptive Support Ventilation (ASV)

ASV is based on the minimal work-of-breathing concept, which suggests that the patient will breathe at a tidal volume and respiratory frequency (f_b) that minimizes the elastic and resistive loads while maintaining oxygenation and acid base balance. This is described mathematically as:

$$f_b = (\sqrt{1 + 4\pi^2 \tau ((\dot{V}_E - f_b V_D)/V_D)} - 1)/2\pi^2 \tau$$

where τ is the time constant (product of resistance and compliance), $\dot{V}_E$ is minute ventilation, and V_D is dead space. The ventilator attempts to deliver 100 mL/min/kg of minute ventilation, adjustable from 25% to 350%, which allows the clinician to provide full support or encourage spontaneous breathing.

When connected to the patient, the ventilator delivers a series of test breaths and measures compliance, resistance, and auto-PEEP. Lung mechanics are measured on a breath-to-breath basis and ventilator settings are altered to meet the desired targets (Figure 8-5). The ventilator adjusts the I:E ratio and inspiratory time of the mandatory breaths by calculation of the expiratory time constant (compliance × resistance) to maintain sufficient expiratory time ($3 \times \tau$). The breath types are adaptive pressure control or VS if the patient is triggering).

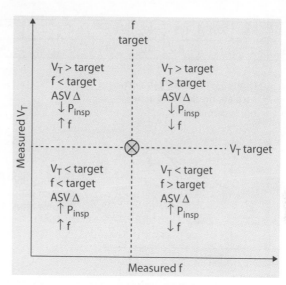

Figure 8-5 Adaptive support ventilation adjusts both the inspiratory pressure of mandatory and/or spontaneous breaths and the mandatory breath rate to maintain the desired breathing pattern. V_T = tidal volume; f = respiratory frequency; Pinsp = inspiratory pressure. (Reproduced with permission from Branson RD. Modes to facilitate ventilator weaning. *Respir Care.* 2012; Oct; 57(10):1635-1648.)

Spontaneous and mandatory breaths can be combined to meet the minute ventilation target (in other words, intermittent mandatory ventilation). If the patient is not triggering, the ventilator determines the respiratory frequency, tidal volume, and pressure required to deliver the tidal volume, inspiratory time, and I:E ratio. If the patient is triggering, the number of mandatory breaths decreases and the ventilator chooses a pressure support that maintains a tidal volume sufficient to ensure alveolar ventilation based on a dead space calculation of 2.2 mL/kg.

Intellivent

Intellivent expands on the concept of ASV by adding closed-loop control of oxygenation to closed-loop control of ventilation. Control of ventilation is primarily based on ASV, but with the option of additional control based on end-tidal Pco_2. End-tidal Pco_2 algorithms for normal lungs, ARDS, head injury, and COPD are available. Oxygenation is based on the ARDSNet PEEP/Fio_2 tables using the Spo_2 to adjust PEEP and Fio_2 (Figure 8-6).

Patient-Controlled Ventilation

This approach to ventilatory support takes control of gas delivery from the clinician and places it on the patient. The two modes of ventilation that fall under the classification of patient-controlled ventilation are proportional-assist ventilation (PAV) and neurally adjusted ventilatory assist (NAVA). With both of these modes, the clinician sets the proportion of work performed by the patient, but they do not force a

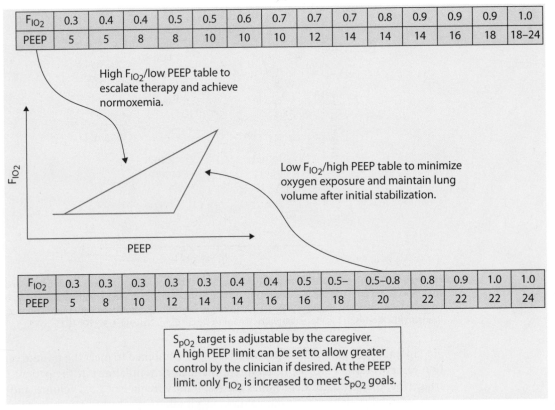

F$_{IO2}$	0.3	0.4	0.4	0.5	0.5	0.6	0.7	0.7	0.7	0.8	0.9	0.9	0.9	1.0
PEEP	5	5	8	8	10	10	10	12	14	14	14	16	18	18–24

High F$_{IO2}$/low PEEP table to escalate therapy and achieve normoxemia.

Low F$_{IO2}$/high PEEP table to minimize oxygen exposure and maintain lung volume after initial stabilization.

F$_{IO2}$	0.3	0.3	0.3	0.3	0.3	0.4	0.4	0.5	0.5–	0.5–0.8	0.8	0.9	1.0	1.0
PEEP	5	8	10	12	14	14	16	16	18	20	22	22	22	24

S$_{pO2}$ target is adjustable by the caregiver. A high PEEP limit can be set to allow greater control by the clinician if desired. At the PEEP limit. only F$_{IO2}$ is increased to meet S$_{pO2}$ goals.

Figure 8-6 Intellivent mode combines adaptive support ventilation (ASV) with closed-loop control of PEEP and F$_{IO2}$. (Reproduced with permission from Branson RD. Modes to facilitate ventilator weaning. *Respir Care.* 2012; Oct; 57(10):1635-1648.)

ventilatory pattern. With these modes, patients can breathe rapid and shallow or slow and deep, based on the patient's breathing pattern. These modes may improve patient-ventilator synchrony and breathing variability.

Proportional-Assist Ventilation

PAV adjusts airway pressure in proportion to patient's effort. This is accomplished by a positive feedback control that amplifies airway pressure proportionally to instantaneous inspiratory flow and volume. With PAV, the amount of support changes with patient's effort, assisting ventilation with a uniform proportionality between ventilator and patient. Because inspiratory effort is a reflection of respiratory drive, this form of support may result in a more physiologic breathing pattern.

PAV is based on the equation of motion:

$$P_{aw} = V/C + R\dot{V}$$

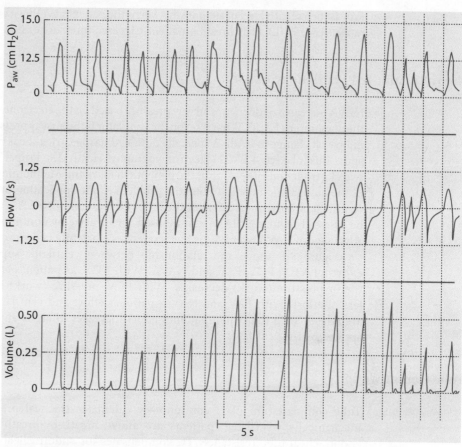

Figure 8-7 Airway pressure, flow, and volume waveforms for proportional-assist ventilation. Note that the airway pressure varies with the inspiratory flow and volume demands of the patient. (Reproduced with permission from Marantz S, et al. Response of ventilator-dependent patients to different levels of proportional assist. *J Appl Physiol.* 1996; Feb; 80(2):397-403.)

where P_{aw} is the total pressure applied at the airway, V is volume, C is compliance, R is resistance, and $\dot{V}$ is flow. Airway pressure is amplified in proportion to the pressure developed by the respiratory muscles. Because flow and volume vary breath-by-breath, the airway pressure during PAV varies breath-by-breath (Figure 8-7). PAV allows the respiratory rate, inspiratory time, and inspiratory pressure to vary.

The newest algorithm for PAV, referred to as PAV+ on the Puritan-Bennett 840, automatically estimates compliance and resistance by performing a 300 milliseconds inspiratory pause every 8 to 15 breaths. Inspiratory $\dot{V}$ is measured and instantaneously integrated to calculate volume. From the measured $\dot{V}$ and pressure calculated from the equation of motion, WOB is calculated:

$$WOB = \int P \times \dot{V} dt$$

PAV is then set at a level of support that keeps the patient's WOB within the normal WOB range (0.3-0.7 J/L). Each breath is patient-triggered (pressure or flow) and flow-cycled.

Neurally Adjusted Ventilatory Assist

NAVA increases or decreases airway pressure based on the electromyographic activity of the diaphragm (EAdi). What is set on the ventilator is the airway pressure applied for each microvolt change in EAdi. A specially designed nasogastric tube is placed in the esophagus. This tube has 4 EMG (Electromyography) electrodes. Proper placement requires two electrodes on either side of the patient's diaphragm. Maintaining proper placement of the nasogastric tube is a potential problem in the application of NAVA. Even a few centimeters' movement can alter the proper operation of NAVA. Tube position should be assessed regularly. NAVA can be used for invasive or noninvasive ventilation. An advantage of NAVA over PAV is that it operates efficiently in the presence of auto-PEEP.

Figure 8-8 shows the relationship between ventilator support and patient's effort for VCV, PCV, PAV, and NAVA. With VCV, as patient's effort increases ventilator pressure (work) decreases. With PCV, pressure (work) is constant regardless of effort. With PAV and NAVA, patient's effort and ventilator pressure (work) are related such that when patient's effort increases, there is an increased pressure applied by the ventilator.

Tube Compensation

Tube compensation (TC) continuously calculates tracheal pressure in intubated mechanically ventilated patients to allow breath-by-breath compensation of endotracheal tube resistance. TC compensates for endotracheal tube resistance via

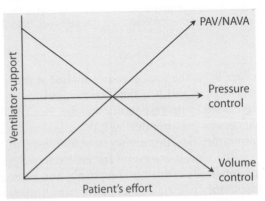

Figure 8-8 Airway pressure with increasing patient's effort for proportional-assist ventilation (PAV) and neurally adjusted ventilatory assist (NAVA), pressure control, and volume control ventilation. Note that the amount of ventilator assist increases with patient's effort for PAV and NAVA, decreases for volume control, and remains constant for pressure control.

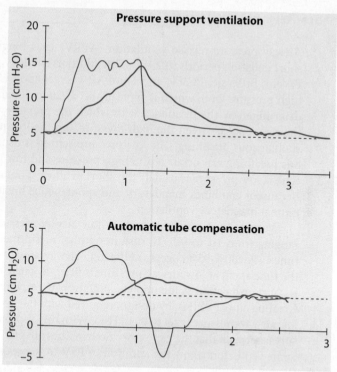

Figure 8-9 Pressure waveforms from the trachea (heavy lines) and the proximal airway (light lines) during pressure support ventilation and tube compensation. Note that the tracheal pressure fluctuated very little during automatic tube compensation. (Reproduced with permission from Fabry B, et al. Breathing pattern and additional work-of-breathing in spontaneously breathing patients with different ventilatory demands during inspiratory pressure support and automatic tube compensation. *Intensive Care Med.* 1997; May; 23(5):545-552.)

closed-loop control of calculated tracheal pressure. It uses the known resistive coefficients of the tracheostomy tube or endotracheal tube and measurement of instantaneous flow to apply pressure proportional to resistance throughout the total respiratory cycle (Figure 8-9).

Incomplete compensation for endotracheal tube resistance may occur because in vivo endotracheal tube resistance is greater than in vitro resistance. Additionally, kinks and accumulation of secretions in the tube change the resistive coefficient and results in incomplete compensation. Whether endotracheal tube resistance poses a clinical concern for increased WOB in adults is controversial. The imposed WOB through the endotracheal tube is modest at a usual minute ventilation for the tube sizes most commonly used for adults. Similar outcomes have been reported when SBTs were conducted with low-level pressure support, TC, or with a T-piece. It has also been reported that the WOB at the conclusion of an SBT is similar to the WOB immediately following extubation. Although prolonged spontaneous breathing through an endotracheal tube is not desirable due to the resistance of the tube, this may not be important during an SBT to assess extubation readiness.

Airway Pressure-Release Ventilation

Airway pressure-release ventilation (APRV) uses long inflation periods (3-5 s) and short deflation periods (0.2-0.8 s). In addition to APRV, it is known as BiLevel, BIPAP, BiVent, BiPhasic, PCV+, and DuoPAP. Oxygenation is determined primarily by the high pressure level, which is typically set at 20 to 30 cm H_2O, and FIO_2. Ventilation is determined by the frequency with which the pressure releases to the lower pressure, the difference between the high pressure and the low pressure, and the magnitude of spontaneous breathing. The low pressure setting is usually 0 to 5 cm H_2O. Spontaneous breathing can occur at the high pressure and low pressure settings, although the time at low pressure is usually too short to allow spontaneous breathing (Figure 8-10). Because it combines mandatory and spontaneous breaths, APRV is technically intermittent mandatory ventilation.

Various time ratios for high-to-low airway pressure have been used with APRV, ranging from 1:1 to 9:1. To sustain optimal recruitment, the greater part of the total time cycle (80%-95%) occurs at the high airway pressure. To minimize de-recruitment, the time spent at low airway pressure is brief. Because the time at low airway pressure is short, exhalation is incomplete and alveolar recruitment due to auto-PEEP results. Creating auto-PEEP is, by design, required with the usual approach to APRV in which low airway pressure is set to 0 cm H_2O. With this approach, the time at low airway pressure is set such that the expiratory flow reaches 50% to 75% of the peak expiratory flow. Some ventilators allow the addition of PSV to the spontaneous breaths during APRV (Figure 8-11).

Spontaneous breathing during the high airway pressure phase of APRV has the potential to generate negative pleural pressures, which may add to the alveolar stretch applied from the ventilator. With APRV, there can also be very high exhaled V_T when the pressure is released from the high pressure to the low pressure. There is concern

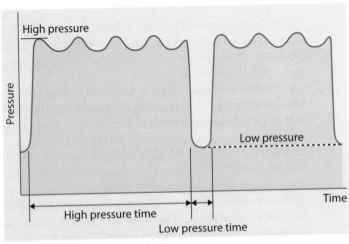

Figure 8-10 Pressure waveform for airway pressure-release ventilation. Note that the patient can breathe at both levels of pressure and that the pressure release is brief.

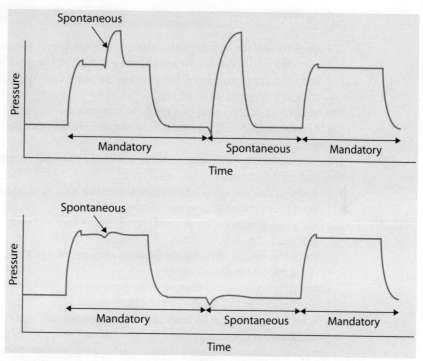

Figure 8-11 Pressure waveforms for BiLevel mode with pressure support (top) and without pressure support (bottom). (Reproduced with permission from Chatburn RL, Primiano FP. A new system for understanding modes of mechanical ventilation. *Respir Care.* 2001; Jun; 46(6):604–621.)

that these relatively large tidal volumes and transpulmonary pressures could contribute to the risk of ventilator-induced lung injury. The improvement in oxygenation that may occur with APRV must be balanced against the potential risk of lung injury.

Mandatory Minute Ventilation

Mandatory minute ventilation (MMV) is a mode intended to guarantee minute ventilation during weaning. If the patient's spontaneous ventilation does not match the target minute ventilation set by the clinician, the ventilator supplies the difference between the patient's minute ventilation and the target minute ventilation. If the patient's spontaneous minute ventilation exceeds the target, no ventilator support is provided. MMV is thus a form of closed-loop ventilation in which the ventilator adjusts its output according to the patient's response. MMV is only available on a few ventilator types used in the United States and its value to facilitate weaning is unclear. MMV can be provided by altering the rate or the tidal volume delivered from the ventilator. Some ventilators increase the mandatory breath rate if the minute ventilation falls below the target level, whereas others increase the level of pressure support when the minute ventilation falls below the target level.

Points to Remember

- Dual-control is a where the ventilator switches from pressure-controlled ventilation to volume-controlled pressure during the breath.
- Adaptive pressure control increases or decreases the pressure limit to maintain a clinician-selected tidal volume.
- Volume support is adaptive pressure support ventilation.
- AutoMode allows the ventilator to switch between mandatory and spontaneous breathing modes.
- SmartCare is a mode that reduces the level of pressure support ventilation to wean the patient from the ventilator.
- Average volume-assured pressure support is a form of adaptive pressure control used during noninvasive ventilation.
- Adaptive support ventilation is based on the minimal work-of-breathing concept.
- Proportional-assist ventilation increases or decreases airway pressure in proportion to patient's effort.
- Neurally adjusted ventilatory assist increases or decreases airway pressure based on changes in the diaphragmatic EMG signal.
- Tube compensation compensates for endotracheal tube resistance via closed-loop control of calculated tracheal pressure.
- Airway pressure-release ventilation uses long inflation periods and short deflation periods.
- Mandatory minute ventilation is a mode intended to guarantee minute ventilation during weaning.

Additional Reading

Alexopoulou C, Kondili E, Vakouti E, et al. Sleep during proportional-assist ventilation with load-adjustable gain factors in critically ill patients. *Intensive Care Med.* 2007;33:1139-1147.

Bosma K, Ferreyra G, Ambrogio C, et al. Patient-ventilator interaction and sleep in mechanically ventilated patients: pressure support versus proportional assist ventilation. *Crit Care Med.* 2007;35:1048-1054.

Branson RD, Chatburn RL. Controversies in the critical care setting. Should adaptive pressure control modes be utilized for virtually all patients receiving mechanical ventilation? *Respir Care.* 2007;52:478-488.

Branson RD, Davis K Jr. Does closed loop control of assist control ventilation reduce ventilator-induced lung injury? *Clin Chest Med.* 2008;29:343-350.

Branson RD, Johannigman JA. Innovations in mechanical ventilation. *Respir Care.* 2009;54:933-947.

Branson RD, Johannigman JA. The role of ventilator graphics when setting dual-control modes. *Respir Care.* 2005;50:187-201.

Branson RD, Johannigman JA. What is the evidence base for the newer-ventilation modes? *Respir Care.* 2004;49:742-760.

Branson RD. Modes to facilitate ventilator weaning. *Respir Care.* 2012;57:1635-1648.

Costa R, Spinazzola G, Cipriani F, et al. A physiologic comparison of proportional assist ventilation with load-adjustable gain factors (PAV+) versus pressure support ventilation (PSV). *Intensive Care Med.* 2011;37:1494-1500.

de la Oliva P, Schüffelmann C, Gómez-Zamora A, et al. Asynchrony, neural drive, ventilatory variability and comfort: NAVA versus pressure support in pediatric patients. A nonrandomized cross-over trial. *Intensive Care Med.* 2012;38:838-846.

Esan A, Hess DR, Raoof S, et al. Severe hypoxemic respiratory failure: part 1—ventilatory strategies. *Chest.* 2010;137:1203-1216.

Kacmarek RM. Proportional assist ventilation and neurally adjusted ventilatory assist. *Respir Care.* 2011;56:140-148.

Morato JB, Sakuma MT, Ferreira JC, Caruso P. Comparison of 3 modes of automated weaning from mechanical ventilation: a bench study. *J Crit Care.* 2012;27:741.e1-e8.

Myers TR, MacIntyre NR. Respiratory controversies in the critical care setting. Does airway pressure release ventilation offer important new advantages in mechanical ventilator support? *Respir Care.* 2007;52:452-460.

Patroniti N, Bellani G, Saccavino E, et al. Respiratory pattern during neurally adjusted ventilatory assist in acute respiratory failure patients. *Intensive Care Med.* 2012;38:230-239.

Piquilloud L, Tassaux D, Bialais E, et al. Neurally adjusted ventilatory assist (NAVA) improves patient-ventilator interaction during noninvasive ventilation delivered by face mask. *Intensive Care Med.* 2012;38:1624-1631.

Randolph AG, Wypij D, Venkataraman ST, et al. Effect of mechanical ventilator weaning protocols on respiratory outcomes in infants and children: a randomized controlled trial. *JAMA.* 2002;288:2561-2568.

Samir J, Delay JM, Matecki S, Sebbane M. Volume-guaranteed pressure-support ventilation facing acute changes in ventilatory demand. *Intensive Care Med.* 2005;31:1181-1188.

Sulemanji DS, Marchese A, Wysocki M, Kacmarek RM. Adaptive support ventilation with and without end-tidal CO_2 closed-loop control versus conventional ventilation. *Intensive Care Med.* 2013;39:703-710.

Xirouchaki N, Kondili E, Vaporidi K, et al. Proportional-assist ventilation with load-adjustable gain factors in critically ill patients: comparison with pressure support. *Intensive Care Med.* 2008;34:2026-2034.

Chapter 9
Flow Waveforms and I:E Ratios

Objectives

1. Apply the concept of time constant to the physiology of mechanical ventilation.
2. Compare constant flow and descending ramp flow patterns during volume-controlled ventilation.
3. Describe the effect of respiratory mechanics on the airway pressure waveform during volume-controlled ventilation.
4. Describe the effect of resistance and compliance on flow during pressure-controlled ventilation.
5. Describe the effect of rise time adjustment during pressure-controlled and pressure support ventilation.
6. Describe the effect of termination flow during pressure support ventilation.
7. Discuss the role of sigh breaths during mechanical ventilation.
8. Discuss the physiologic effects of I:E ratio manipulations.

Introduction

Microprocessor-controlled ventilators allow the clinician to choose among various inspiratory flow waveforms. This chapter describes the technical and physiologic aspects of various inspiratory waveforms during mechanical ventilation.

Time Constant

An important principle for understanding pulmonary mechanics during mechanical ventilation is that of the time constant. The time constant determines the rate of change in the volume of a lung unit that is passively inflated or deflated. It is expressed by the relationship:

$$Vt = Vi \times e^{-t/\tau}$$

where Vt is the volume of a lung unit at time t, Vi is the initial volume of the lung unit, e is the base of the natural logarithm, and τ is the time constant. The relationship between Vt and τ is illustrated in Figure 9-1. Note that the volume change is nearly complete in five time constants.

For respiratory physiology, τ is the product of resistance and compliance. Lung units with a higher resistance and/or a higher compliance will have a longer time constant and require more time to fill and to empty. Conversely, lung units with a lower resistance and/or compliance will have a shorter time constant and thus require less time to fill and to empty. A simple method to measure the expiratory time constant is to divide the expired tidal volume by the peak expiratory flow during passive positive pressure ventilation:

$$\tau = V_T / \dot{V}_{E(peak)}$$

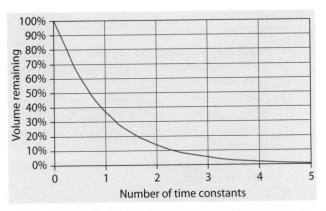

Figure 9-1 The time constant function for lung emptying. After one time constant, 37% of the volume remains in the lungs, 13% remains after two time constants, 5% remains after three time constants, 2% remains after four time constants, and < 1% remains after five time constants.

where V_T is the expired tidal volume and $\dot{V}_{E(peak)}$ is the peak expiratory flow. Although this is a useful index of the global expiratory time constant, it treats the lung as a single compartment and thus does not account for time constant heterogeneity in the lungs.

Flow Waveforms

Volume-Controlled Ventilation

The flow, pressure, and volume waveforms produced with a constant flow pattern are shown in Figure 9-2. This is often called square-wave or rectangular-wave ventilation due to the shape of the flow waveform. With the constant flow pattern, the volume (per unit time) is delivered into the lungs equally throughout inspiration. In other words, volume (per unit time) delivery into the lungs at the beginning of inspiration is the same as that at the end of inspiration. Note that airway pressure increases linearly throughout inspiration, following an initial rapid pressure increase due to the resistance through the endotracheal tube. The effect of resistance and compliance on the airway pressure waveform during constant flow volume ventilation is shown in Figure 9-3.

During volume-controlled ventilation, the inspiratory flow can also be set to a descending ramp. With this pattern, flow is greatest at the beginning of inspiration and decreases to a lower flow at the end of inspiration. Typical flow, pressure, and volume waveforms with a descending ramp are shown in Figure 9-4. Note that most of the tidal volume is delivered early during inspiration and the pressure waveform approaches that of a rectangular shape. A descending ramp flow pattern lengthens the inspiratory time unless the peak flow is increased. The descending ramp flow can be provided in several ways (Figure 9-5). With a complete ramp, flow decreases to 0 at end inspiration. With 50% ramp, the flow at end inspiration is half of the initial flow. Flow can also taper to a fixed, manufacturer-specific level at the end of inspiration (eg, 5 L/min).

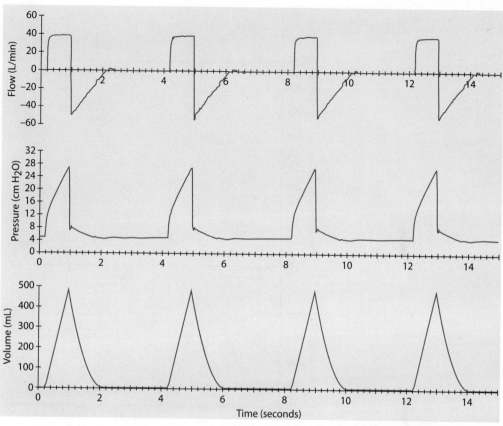

Figure 9-2 Flow, pressure, and volume waveforms with constant flow, volume-controlled ventilation.

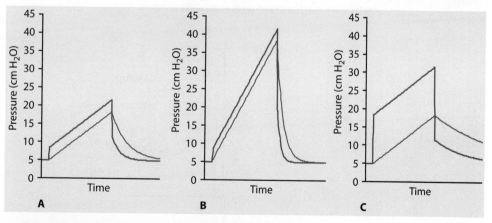

Figure 9-3 Airway pressure waveforms during constant flow volume ventilation. In each case, the tidal volume is 0.675 L, flow is 40 L/min, and PEEP is 5 cm H_2O. The heavy line represents airway pressure and the lighter line represents alveolar pressure. (A) Resistance of 5 cm H_2O/L/s and compliance of 50 mL/cm H_2O. (B) Resistance of 5 cm H_2O/L/s and compliance of 20 mL/cm H_2O. Compared to the left panel, peak inspiratory pressure increases, alveolar pressure increases, but the difference between airway pressure and alveolar pressure does not change. (C) Resistance of 20 cm H_2O/L/s and compliance of 50 mL/cm H_2O. Compared to the left panel, peak inspiratory pressure increases, alveolar pressure is unchanged, and the difference between airway pressure and alveolar pressure is increased.

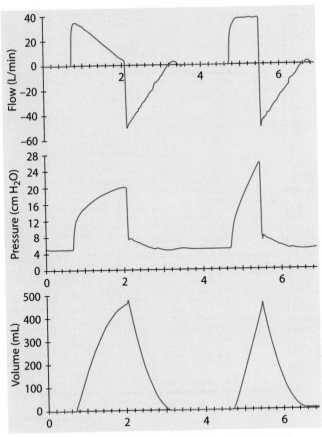

Figure 9-4 Waveforms for descending ramp and constant flows. Note the differences in the shape of the pressure waveform and peak inspiratory pressure.

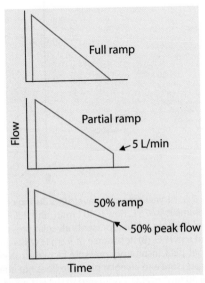

Figure 9-5 Full and partial descending ramp flow with volume-controlled ventilation.

Pressure-Controlled Ventilation

Typical pressure, flow, and volume waveforms during pressure ventilation are shown in Figure 9-6. Note the shape of the pressure waveform and descending (exponential) flow pattern. Also note that most of the tidal volume is delivered early in the inspiratory phase. During pressure-controlled ventilation, flow is determined by the pressure applied to the airway, inspiratory effort, airways resistance, and the time constant (Figure 9-7):

$$\dot{V} = (\Delta P/R) \times (e^{-t/\tau})$$

where ΔP is the transpulmonary pressure (difference between airway pressure and pleural pressure), R is airways resistance, t is the elapsed time after initiation of the inspiratory phase, e is the base of the natural logarithm, and τ is the product of airways resistance and respiratory system compliance (the time constant of the respiratory system). The length of zero flow time at the end of inspiration is determined by the inspiratory time; a longer inspiratory time results in more zero flow time.

With many ventilators, it is possible to adjust the time required to reach the peak inspiratory pressure (rise time). The rise time controls the flow at the beginning of the inspiratory phase (Figure 9-8). With a faster rise time, flow is greater at

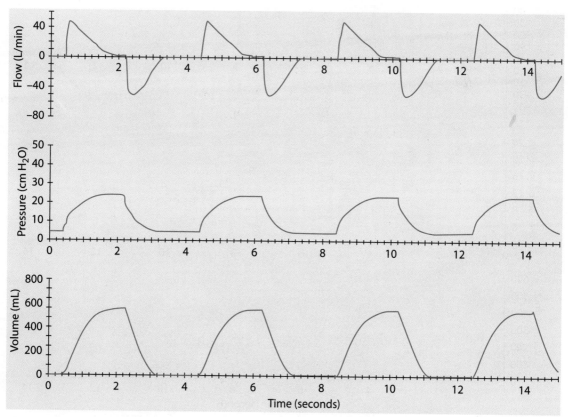

Figure 9-6 Flow, pressure, and volume waveforms during pressure-controlled ventilation.

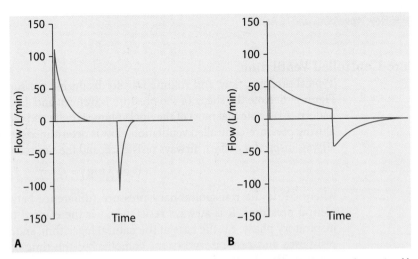

Figure 9-7 During pressure-controlled ventilation, the inspiratory flow pattern is determined by airways resistance and respiratory system compliance. (A) Airways resistance of 10 cm H_2O/L/s and respiratory system compliance of 20 mL/cm H_2O. The inspiratory time is 1.5 seconds and the resulting tidal volume (the area under the flow curve) is 400 mL. (B) Airways resistance of 20 cm H_2O/L/s and respiratory system compliance of 50 mL/cm H_2O. The inspiratory time is 1.5 seconds and the resulting tidal volume (the area under the flow curve) is 775 mL.

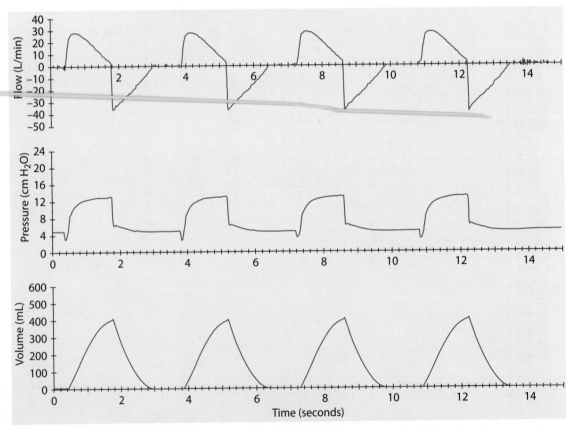

Figure 9-8 Flow, pressure, and volume waveforms for pressure support ventilation.

the beginning of inspiration, which may improve synchrony in patients with a high respiratory drive, but at the cost of a higher V_T.

An inverse ratio can be used in conjunction with pressure-controlled ventilation. This results in pressure-controlled inverse ratio ventilation (PCIRV). This mode has been used in the setting of refractory hypoxemia. Its physiologic effect is to increase mean airway pressure and it is commonly associated with auto-positive end-expiratory pressure (auto-PEEP). The clinical results are determined by the flow pattern, rather than the use of volume-controlled or pressure-controlled ventilation strategies per se. A descending ramp flow pattern with an inspiratory pause can be produced using either pressure-controlled or volume-controlled ventilation. There does not seem to be a benefit from the use of PCIRV on patient outcome.

Despite some clinicians favoring pressure-controlled ventilation in patients with acute respiratory distress syndrome (ARDS), evidence supporting its superiority in this setting is lacking. For the same V_T, the same inspiratory time, and a descending ramp of flow with volume-controlled ventilation, the differences in PaO_2 between pressure-controlled and volume-controlled ventilation are trivial.

Pressure Support Ventilation

The typical waveform for pressure support ventilation (PSV) is shown in Figure 9-9. When the pressure-supported breath is triggered, the ventilator delivers flow sufficient to reach the set pressure (typically, the pressure support is the amount of pressure added to the PEEP). As with pressure-controlled ventilation, all current generation ICU ventilators allow the initial flow (rise time) to be adjusted with PSV, which controls how quickly the pressure reaches the set target.

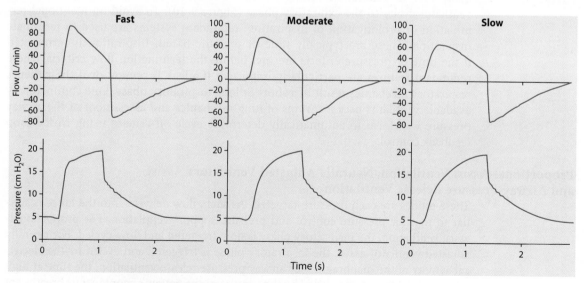

Figure 9-9 Effect of rise time adjustments of waveforms. Note that the faster rise time results in a higher flow at the beginning of inspiration.

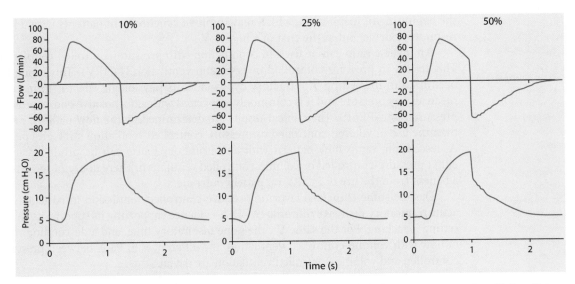

Figure 9-10 Effect of changes in flow termination criteria during pressure support ventilation. Note the effect of a termination flow on inspiratory time.

The pressure-supported breath should terminate when the patient's inspiratory effort ceases. Premature termination may result in double triggering and a prolonged inspiration may result in the patient activating expiratory muscles in an attempt to end the inspiratory phase. The inspiratory phase stops when the flow decreases to a ventilator-determined level (eg, usually 25% of peak flow). To improve synchrony, many current generation ventilators allow adjustment of the flow at which the ventilator cycles to the expiratory phase (Figure 9-10). To avoid unintentional termination or prolongation of inspiration, redundant systems are used to terminate inspiration. These are typically time or pressure-based. Inspiration is terminated if the time or pressure criteria are met before the termination flow criteria. These redundant features are particularly important if a leak is present or if the patient's respiratory mechanics result in a short or long inspiratory phase. One commercially available ventilator uses measures of lung mechanics and assessment of the airway pressure waveform to automatically determine cycle off criteria using closed-loop feedback control.

Proportional-Assist Ventilation, Neurally Adjusted Ventilatory Assist, and Airway-Pressure Release Ventilation

These modes are each pressure-targeted. As such, flow delivery into the lungs is similar to that for pressure control and pressure support ventilation. For proportional-assist ventilation, the inspiratory phase is flow-triggered and flow-cycled. For neurally adjusted ventilator assist, the inspiratory phase is triggered and cycled by the electrical activity of the diaphragm. For airway pressure release ventilation, the time at high pressure is triggered and cycled by the ventilator; the patient's spontaneous breaths are flow-triggered and flow-cycled.

Expiratory Flow

Expiratory flow is normally passive (ie, it does not require expiratory muscle activation) and determined by alveolar driving pressure (Palv), airways resistance, the elapsed expiratory time, and the time constant of the respiratory system:

$$\dot{V} = - (Palv/R) \times (e^{-t/\tau})$$

By convention, expiratory flow is displayed on the flow-time graphic in the direction negative and inspiratory flow is displayed in the positive direction. Also note that end-expiratory flow is present if Palv is greater than the proximal airway pressure. This indicates air-trapping (intrinsic PEEP; auto-PEEP).

Physiologic Effects of Waveform Manipulations

The clinical usefulness of inspiratory flow waveform manipulations is controversial. Evidence is lacking that manipulation of the flow waveform affects patient outcome. The choice of waveform is usually one of clinician bias, rather than the desire to achieve a specific therapeutic goal. The following generalizations can be made regarding inspiratory waveform manipulations.

- Mean airway pressure is higher with descending ramp of flow and lower with constant flow.
- Peak inspiratory pressure is lower with descending ramp flow and higher with constant flow.
- For the same respiratory mechanics and tidal volume, peak alveolar pressure (plateau pressure) will be the same regardless of the inspiratory flow waveform.
- Gas distribution is improved with descending ramp flow. This often improves gas exchange, but only to a small degree.
- Mean airway pressure is increased with an end-inspiratory pause. An end-inspiratory pause may improve distribution of ventilation. During the period of no flow, gas from areas of the lungs with low airway resistance (short time constants) may be redistributed to areas of the lungs with high airway resistance (long time constants); this is called pendelluft.
- Asynchrony may be affected by the inspiratory flow waveform. Some patients are more asynchronous on one flow waveform compared to another, but inter-patient differences do not allow one waveform to be recommended over another as always associated with better synchrony.

Effect of Flow Patterns on I:E Ratio

When the inspiratory flow pattern is changed from constant flow to descending ramp flow during volume-controlled ventilation, the ventilator must adjust either the peak flow or inspiratory time to maintain the delivered tidal volume (Figure 9-11). If peak

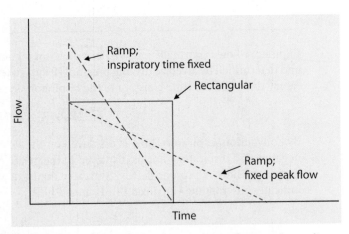

Figure 9-11 When the flow pattern is changed from a constant flow to a descending ramp flow, either the inspiratory time or the peak inspiratory flow must increase.

flow is adjusted, then inspiratory time and I:E ratio are constant. For a descending ramp flow pattern, the peak flow ($\dot{V}_{pk}$) is determined by the inspiratory time (T_I) and the flow at the end of inspiration ($\dot{V}_f$):

$$\dot{V}_{pk} = [V_T - (0.5)\,(\dot{V}_f)\,(T_I)]/[(0.5)\,(T_I)]$$

For example, if V_T is 0.75 L, T_I is 1.5 seconds, and $\dot{V}_f$ is 5 L/min (0.083 L/s), then $\dot{V}_{pk}$ will need to be 55 L/min (0.92 L/s).

If inspiratory time is adjusted when the flow pattern is changed, then the peak flow set on the ventilator is maintained at the initial flow. For a descending ramp flow pattern, the increase in inspiratory time will be determined by the peak flow and the flow at the end of inspiration:

$$T_I = (V_T)/(0.5)\,(\dot{V}_{pk} + \dot{V}_f)$$

For example, if V_T is 0.75 L, $\dot{V}_{pk}$ is 90 L/min (1.5 L/s), and $\dot{V}_f$ is 5 L/min (0.083 L/s), then T_I will be 0.95 second. For full deceleration (ie, $\dot{V}_f = 0$), either the inspiratory time or the peak flow must double.

Sigh Volume

The sigh breath is a deliberate increase in tidal volume for one or more breaths at regular intervals. Sighs during mechanical ventilation were commonly used in the 1970s, but have been rarely used since. There is again interest in the use of sighs during mechanical ventilation as a recruitment maneuver, but the value of this is yet to be determined. One way of producing a sigh during pressure support ventilation is to set an inspiratory pressure of 20 to 30 cm H_2O, for 1 to 3 seconds, 2 to 4 times/min, using a ventilator with an active exhalation valve (Figure 9-12).

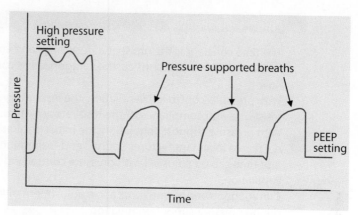

Figure 9-12 Pressure waveform illustrating the use of a sigh with pressure support ventilation.

I:E Ratio

The relationship between inspiratory time and expiratory time (I:E ratio) is an important consideration during mechanical ventilation. A longer inspiratory time (and a shorter expiratory time) increases the mean airway pressure, which may increase arterial oxygenation but may also decrease cardiac output. A longer inspiratory time may also result in air trapping (auto-PEEP), particularly if inspiratory time is greater than the expiratory time (inverse I:E ratio). Normally, expiratory time is longer than inspiratory time. An inspiratory time of 0.5 to 1.5 second is usually appropriate during adult mechanical ventilation. A shorter inspiratory time is desirable for patients who are ventilated with a rapid respiratory rate. In patients who are triggering the ventilator, the inspiratory time should be set to match the patient's neural inspiratory time to avoid asynchrony.

Several approaches can be used by ventilators to set the I:E ratio.

- I:E ratio and rate. For example, at an I:E ratio of 1:3 and a rate of 15/min (cycle time of 4 seconds), the inspiratory time is 1 second and the expiratory time is 3 seconds.
- Flow, tidal volume, and rate. For example, suppose there is a constant inspiratory flow of 30 L/min, tidal volume of 0.35 L, and rate of 12/min. The inspiratory time is therefore 0.7 second, the expiratory time is 4.3 seconds, and the I:E ratio is 1:6.
- Inspiratory time and respiratory rate. With an inspiratory time of 1 second and a rate of 10/min, the expiratory time is 5 seconds and the I:E ratio is 1:5. Note that some ventilators adjust inspiratory time and flow independently during volume-controlled ventilation. If the volume is delivered before the set inspiratory time is reached, the additional time is an end-inspiratory pause. For example, if the flow is set at 60 L/min constant flow, the tidal volume at 500 mL, and inspiratory time is set at 1 second, there will be 0.5 second inspiratory hold after the tidal volume is delivered.
- Percent inspiratory time and rate. At a rate of 15/min and 25% inspiratory time, the inspiratory time is 1 second (25% of the total cycle time of 4 seconds), the expiratory time is 3 seconds, and the I:E ratio is 1:3.

Points to Remember

- The time constant is the product of resistance and compliance.
- Inspiratory flow waveforms can be categorized as constant or descending ramp flow.
- With pressure-controlled ventilation, the inspiratory flow is determined by the resistance and compliance of the respiratory system.
- With pressure support ventilation, the initial inspiratory flow is high and then decreases to a manufacturer-specific end-inspiration cycle flow.
- Rise time can be adjusted with pressure control and pressure support ventilation.
- Current generation ventilators allow adjustment of the termination flow criteria during pressure support ventilation.
- A descending ramp flow pattern generates higher mean airway pressures, lower peak airway pressure, and may improve gas distribution.
- An end-inspiratory pause increases mean airway pressure.
- When an inspiratory flow pattern other than constant flow is chosen during volume-controlled ventilation, the ventilator must adjust either the peak flow or inspiratory time to maintain a constant delivered tidal volume.
- The I:E ratio affects mean airway pressure and in that way affects oxygenation and cardiac output.

Additional Reading

Calderini E, Confalonieri M, Puccio PG, Francavilla N, Stella L, Gregoretti C. Patient-ventilator asynchrony during noninvasive ventilation: the role of expiratory trigger. *Intensive Care Med.* 1999;25:662-667.

Chatmongkolchart S, Williams P, Hess DR, Kacmarek RM. Evaluation of inspiratory rise time and inspiration termination criteria in new-generation mechanical ventilators: a lung model study. *Respir Care.* 2001;46:666-677.

Chiumello D, Pelosi P, Croci M, et al. The effects of pressurization rate on breathing pattern, work-of-breathing, gas exchange, and patient comfort in pressure support ventilation. *Eur Respir J.* 2001;18:107-114.

Chiumello D, Pelosi P, Taccone P, Slutsky A, Gattinoni L. Effect of different inspiratory rise time and cycling off criteria during pressure support ventilation in patients recovering from acute lung injury. *Crit Care Med.* 2003;31:2604-2610.

Du HL, Amato MB, Yamada Y. Automation of expiratory trigger sensitivity in pressure support ventilation. *Respir Care Clin N Am.* 2001;7:503-517.

Hess DR. Ventilator waveforms and the physiology of pressure support ventilation. *Respir Care.* 2005;50:166-186.

Patrioniti N, Foti G, Cortihovis B, et al. Sigh improves gas exchange and lung volume in patients with acute respiratory distress syndrome undergoing pressure support ventilation. *Anesthesiology.* 2002;96:788-794.

Tassaux D, Gainnier M, Battisti A, Jolliet P. Impact of expiratory trigger setting on delayed cycling and inspiratory muscle workload. *Am J Respir Crit Care Med.* 2005;172:1283-1289.

Tassaux D, Michotte JB, Gainnier M, Gratadour P, Fonseca S, Jolliet P. Expiratory trigger setting in pressure support ventilation: from mathematical model to bedside. *Crit Care Med.* 2004;32:1844-1850.

Tokioka H, Tanaka T, Ishizu T, et al. The effect of breath termination criterion on breathing patterns and the work of breathing during pressure support ventilation. *Anesth Analg.* 2001;92:161-165.

Uchiyama A, Imanaka H, Taenaka N. Relationship between work of breathing provided by a ventilator and patients' inspiratory drive during pressure support ventilation; effects of inspiratory time. *Anaesth Intensive Care.* 2001;29:349-358.

Chapter 10
High Frequency Ventilation

- Introduction
- Approaches Available
- Factors Affecting Gas Exchange
- Rationale for Use
- Indications for Use
- Points to Remember
- Additional Reading

Introduction

High frequency ventilation (HFV) has been available since the late 1960s, but was not an accepted approach to ventilatory support in adults until the late 20th century. The primary reason is a lack of definitive evidence indicating HFV's superiority over conventional ventilation. Although there have been many animal studies demonstrating a physiologic benefit for HFV, evidence is lacking for a survival benefit in adults with high frequency oscillation (HFO). Equivalence has become even more pronounced with the use of lung protective approaches to conventional ventilatory support. Recent evidence indicates that HFV may be detrimental when used with high airway pressures, similar to established concerns with conventional ventilation.

Approaches Available

Conventional mechanical ventilation is provided at respiratory rates < 1 Hz (1 Hz = 60 breaths/min). HFV uses respiratory rates at 2 to 15 Hz. The frequency range is determined by the specific technique and the size of the patient. Regardless of technique, adults are generally ventilated toward the lower end of the respiratory rate spectrum and neonates toward the high end of the spectrum.

There are four techniques for HFV: high frequency positive pressure ventilation (HFPPV), high frequency jet ventilation (HFJV), high frequency oscillatory ventilation (HFOV), and high frequency percussive ventilation (HFPV) (Table 10-1).

Table 10-1 **Types of HFV**

Type	Frequency range
HFPPV	2-4 Hz
HFJV	2-8 Hz
HFO	2-15 Hz
HFPV	2-8 Hz

Abbreviations: HFJV, high frequency jet ventilation; HFO, high frequency oscillation; HFPV, high frequency percussive ventilation; HFPVV, high frequency positive pressure ventilation; HFV, high frequency ventilation.

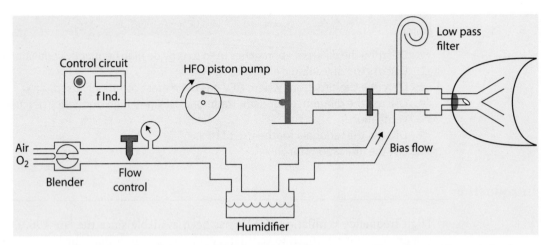

Figure 10-1 Essential parts of a high frequency oscillatory system. (Reproduced with permission from Chatburn RL, Branson RD. High frequency ventilators. In: Branson RD, Hess DR, Chatburn RL. *Respiratory Care Equipment*. Philadelphia: Lippincott, Williams & Wilkins; 1995:458-469.)

With HFPPV, conventional ventilators are used to provide rates at the low end of the HFV spectrum. With HFPPV rates slightly above, conventional rates are used and gas flow is provided by the same gas delivery mechanism as in conventional ventilation. This form of HFV is not commonly used. During HFJV, gas under high pressure is injected into the airway while a secondary gas source is entrained to provide the tidal volume. This approach uses respiratory rates in the low to middle part of the HFV rate spectrum. With HFJV, a jet ventilator in tandem with a conventional ventilator may be needed. HFOV has an active inspiratory and expiratory phase. HFOV establishes gas flow into the airway by the rapid movement of a diaphragm or piston (Figure 10-1). With HFOV, respiratory rates at 3 to 8 Hz are used with adults, at the highest rate that allows an adequate $PaCO_2$. The most commonly used high frequency technique is HFOV. With HFPV, small tidal volume oscillations are superimposed on conventional pressure-controlled ventilation (Figure 10-2) at rates in the 2 to 8 Hz range.

Factors Affecting Gas Exchange

At the rates provided with HFJV and HFOV, tidal volumes are often smaller than those with conventional ventilation. Generally speaking, the higher the respiratory rate, the lower the tidal volume. At moderate to high rates (≥ 8 Hz), tidal volumes can be less than anatomic dead space.

Although numerous mechanisms are active during HFV to establish gas exchange (Figure 10-3), normal convection and molecular diffusion are the primary mechanisms affecting gas exchange. Other principles enhance molecule diffusion and the

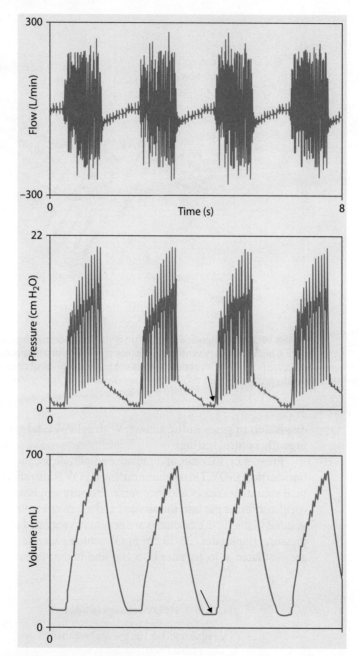

Figure 10-2 Eight-second graph of high-frequency flow, high frequency pressure, and high frequency volume during high frequency percussive ventilation. The graphs demonstrate an accumulation in high-frequency flow and pressure over the duration of a set inspiratory time to achieve a low-frequency tidal volume and flow. The end-expiratory point is indicated by the arrow. (Reproduced with permission from Allan PF. High-frequency percussive ventilation: pneumotachograph validation and tidal volume analysis. *Respir Care.* 2005; Jun; 55(6):734-740.)

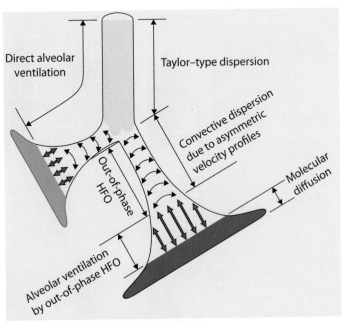

Figure 10-3 More than one mechanism of gas transport may operate in various regions of the lung during high-frequency ventilation. Moreover, mechanisms may act synergistically. Gas velocities decrease from the airway opening to alveolus. (Chang HF. Mechanisms of gas-transport during ventilation by high-frequency oscillation. *J Appl Physiol Respir Environ Exerc Physiol.* 1984; Mar; 56(3):553-563.)

dispersion of gases in the airway. With HFPV, tidal volume is also dependent on the pressure control setting.

Frequency, I:E ratio, and pressure amplitude are the three variables affecting ventilation during HFOV. Tidal volume during HFOV is also affected by rate. As rate is decreased, tidal volume increases and vice versa. Pressure amplitude (the pressure developed as the oscillator forces gas into the airway) and a longer inspiratory time also increase the tidal volume (Table 10-2). Neonates are generally ventilated at high rates (10-15 Hz) and low-pressure amplitudes (20-30 cm H_2O), which generate very small tidal volumes. Adults are ventilated at lower rates (3-8 Hz) and higher pressure amplitudes (60-90 cm H_2O).

Table 10-2 HFOV settings in adults

- Frequency: 3-8 Hz; the highest that allows acceptable $Paco_2$
- Pressure amplitude: 60-90 cm H_2O
- I:E ratio: 1:2
- Bias flow: 30 L/min
- Mean airway pressure: 25-35 cm H_2O

Abbreviation: HFOV, high frequency oscillatory ventilation.

With neonates, the bias flow in the circuit is about 10 L/min, whereas with adults the bias flow is about 30 L/min range. In adults, tidal volumes approaching those delivered by conventional mechanical ventilation (3-4 mL/kg) are possible at 3 Hz and 90 cm H_2O pressure amplitude. During HFOV, it is not possible for the patient to trigger the ventilator; heavy sedation, and sometimes paralysis, is needed to ensure patient-ventilator synchrony. In the setting of a high $PaCO_2$ and maximal ventilator settings, the cuff may be deflated, which clears CO_2 from the central airway and endotracheal tube. Oxygenation with HFOV is determined by FIO_2 and mean airway pressure ($\overline{P}aw$). $\overline{P}aw$ is similar to positive end-expiratory pressure (PEEP) in its effect on oxygenation, since at the alveolar level there is minimal pressure change during HFOV (particularly at high rates).

It is estimated that as little as 15% of the inspiratory pressure amplitude is transmitted to the alveolar level through an 8-mm internal diameter endotracheal tube at 8 Hz. With smaller tubes and more rapid rates, less pressure is transmitted. With a pressure amplitude of 60 cm H_2O (30 cm H_2O above and 30 cm H_2O below $\overline{P}aw$ during inhalation and exhalation, respectively) at 8 Hz with an 8-mm internal diameter tube, the alveolar pressure would fluctuates 4.5 cm H_2O above and below the $\overline{P}aw$. A lung recruitment maneuver is often performed when HFOV is initiated, by increasing $\overline{P}aw$ for a short time and then decreasing it to the lowest level that maintains oxygenation. In adults, $\overline{P}aw$ during HFO are generally set at 25 and 35 cm H_2O.

With HFJV the tidal volume is affected by the gas that is entrained via the conventional ventilator. Estimation of tidal is currently not possible during HFOV and HFPV. With HFJV and HFPV, oxygenation is controlled in the same manner as during conventional ventilation. PEEP and FIO_2 are set to achieve the desired oxygenation status.

Rationale for Use

With HFOV, overdistending peak airway pressures and $\overline{P}aw$ airway pressure applied tends to be much higher than what is used during conventional ventilation. In addition, if low respiratory rates are used (3-6 Hz), the attenuation of the pressure amplitude at the alveolus may not be as great as expected and alveolar pressures may greatly exceed 30 cm H_2O, particularly if the $\overline{P}aw$ is $\geq$ 30 cm H_2O. With HFJV and HFPV, it is difficult to estimate the peak alveolar pressure. During jet ventilation, the higher the pressure generating the jet flow, the higher is the potential peak airway pressure. HFPV has been proposed as a mechanism to move secretions more effectively along the tracheobronchial tree.

Indications for Use

HFOV is used in adults with severe acute respiratory distress syndrome (ARDS) and refractory hypoxemia. However, evidence is lacking for the superiority of HFOV to conventional ventilation, and there is some evidence that survival with HFOV may be worse than with conventional ventilation. Thus, the improved oxygenation with HFOV does not translate to better outcomes. Issues with the use of HFOV are the high cost of current devices, that patients receiving HFOV must be heavily sedated and sometimes paralyzed, and that most clinicians lack familiarity with HFOV. In addition, during HFOV, there is no mechanism to monitor peak alveolar pressure or tidal volume. The available devices in the United States may require a significantly greater number of arterial blood gases than with conventional ventilation. Other than the treatment of severe ARDS, there is no role for HFOV in the management of adults.

In adults, HFJV has been reserved for intraoperative use and for percutaneous transtracheal ventilation when an airway cannot be established. HFJV can be used as a method of providing ventilatory support during tracheal or bronchial surgery. HFJV may also be used in a trauma setting where tracheal intubation is difficult or impossible. The use of transtracheal jet ventilation via the cricothyroid membrane is part of the difficult airway algorithm.

HFPV has found a niche in some burn centers for the management of patients with ARDS. Some believe the addition of oscillations on top of the pressure control facilitates movement of secretions to the larger airways, allowing for their suctioning. However, there is no convincing evidence that the use of HFPV improves outcome over conventional ventilation.

Points to Remember

- High frequency ventilation (HFV) refers to respiratory rates between 2 and 15 Hz.
- High frequency oscillatory ventilation (HFOV) is the most commonly used approach to high frequency ventilation.
- During HFOV, the higher the rate, the smaller the tidal volume.
- Most of the pressure amplitude during HFOV is dissipated before reaching the alveolar level.
- HFOV used for acute respiratory distress syndrome (ARDS) in adults may result in poorer outcomes than conventional ventilation.
- Use of high frequency jet ventilation in adults is primarily in the operating room and for management of the difficult airway.
- High frequency percussive ventilation is primarily used in the management of patients with ARDS in burn centers.
- With all forms of HFV, care should be exercised to ensure that the delivered pressure and tidal volume is lung protective.

Additional Reading

Ahmad Y, Turner MW. Transtracheal jet ventilation in patients with severe airway compromise and stridor. *Br J Anaesth.* 2011;106:602.

Ali S, Ferguson ND. High-frequency oscillatory ventilation in ALI/ARDS. *Crit Care Clin.* 2011;27:487-499.

Allan PF, Osborn EC, Chung KK, Wanek SM. High-frequency percussive ventilation revisited. *J Burn Care Res.* 2010 Jul-Aug;31:510-520.

Allan PF. High-frequency percussive ventilation: pneumotachograph validation and tidal volume analysis. *Respir Care.* 2010;55:734-740.

Chung KK, Wolf SE, Renz EM, et al. High-frequency percussive ventilation and low tidal volume ventilation in burns: a randomized controlled trial. *Crit Care Med.* 2010;38: 1970-1977.

Derdak S. Lung-protective higher frequency oscillatory ventilation. *Crit Care Med.* 2008;36: 1358-1360.

Esan A, Hess DR, Raoof S, et al. Severe hypoxemic respiratory failure: part 1—ventilatory strategies. *Chest.* 2010;137:1203-1216.

Ferguson ND, Cook DJ, Guyatt GH, et al. High-frequency oscillation in early acute respiratory distress syndrome. *N Engl J Med.* 2013;368:795-805.

Fessler HE, Hess DR. Respiratory controversies in the critical care setting. Does high-frequency ventilation offer benefits over conventional ventilation in adult patients with acute respiratory distress syndrome? *Respir Care.* 2007;52:595-608.

Goffi A, Ferguson ND. High-frequency oscillatory ventilation for early acute respiratory distress syndrome in adults. *Curr Opin Crit Care.* 2014;20:77-85.

Hess D, Mason S, Branson R. High-frequency ventilation design and equipment issues. *Respir Care Clin N Am.* 2001;7:577-598.

Ip T, Mehta S. The role of high-frequency oscillatory ventilation in the treatment of acute respiratory failure in adults. *Curr Opin Crit Care.* 2012;18:70-79.

Kuluz MA, Smith PB, Mears SP, et al. Preliminary observations of the use of high-frequency jet ventilation as rescue therapy in infants with congenital diaphragmatic hernia. *J Pediatr Surg.* 2010;45:698-702.

Leiter R, Aliverti A, Priori R, et al. Comparison of superimposed high-frequency jet ventilation with conventional jet ventilation for laryngeal surgery. *Br J Anaesth.* 2012;10:690-907.

Norfolk SG, Hollingsworth CL, Wolfe CR, et al. Rescue therapy in adult and pediatric patients with pH1N1 influenza infection: a tertiary center intensive care unit experience from April to October 2009. *Crit Care Med.* 2010;38:2103-2107.

Pawlowski J. Anesthetic considerations for interventional pulmonary procedures. *Curr Opin Anaesthesiol.* 2013;26:6-12.

Starnes-Roubaud M, Bales EA, Williams-Resnick A, et al. High frequency percussive ventilation and low F_{IO_2}. *Burns.* 2012;38:984-991.

Young D, Lamb SE, Shah S, et al. High-frequency oscillation for acute respiratory distress syndrome. *N Engl J Med.* 2013;368:806-813.

Chapter 11
Noninvasive Ventilation

Objectives

1. Discuss patient selection for noninvasive ventilation (NIV).
2. Compare interfaces for NIV.
3. List advantages and disadvantages of various ventilator types for NIV.
4. List the steps in the initiation of NIV.

Introduction

One of the significant advances in respiratory critical care over the past 20 years has been the emergence of noninvasive ventilation (NIV). NIV is used increasingly in patients with acute respiratory failure. In appropriately selected patients, need for intubation is reduced with the use of NIV. Because an artificial airway increases the risk of nosocomial pneumonia, it is not surprising that use of NIV decreases the incidence of ventilator-associated pneumonia. In some clinical settings, such as chronic obstructive pulmonary disease (COPD) exacerbation or acute cardiogenic pulmonary edema, the use of NIV affords a survival benefit. This chapter covers clinical and technical issues related to use of NIV.

Patient Factors

Patient Selection

The strength of evidence for the use of NIV for various causes of acute respiratory failure is summarized in Table 11-1. High-level evidence supports the effectiveness of NIV for COPD exacerbation. Equally strong evidence supports the use of NIV for acute cardiogenic pulmonary edema. There is also evidence to support the use of NIV in patients with respiratory failure following solid organ transplantation and those who are immunosuppressed. Although some evidence supports the use of NIV for acute asthma, the evidence in this setting is weak. The use of NIV as an alternative to invasive ventilation in severely hypoxemic patients with acute respiratory distress syndrome is not recommended.

NIV can be used to allow earlier extubation in selected patients who do not successfully complete a spontaneous breathing trial (SBT), but its use in this setting should be restricted to patients who are intubated for COPD exacerbation or patients with neuromuscular disease. In patients who successfully complete an SBT, but are at risk for extubation failure, NIV should be used to prevent extubation failure. These patients are extubated directly to NIV. NIV should be used cautiously in patients who successfully complete an SBT, but develop respiratory failure after extubation. In this setting, NIV is indicated only in patients with hypercapnic respiratory failure.

When to Start and When to Stop

A two-step process is used to identify patients likely to benefit from NIV (Table 11-2). In appropriately selected patients, NIV reduces, but does not eliminate, the need for intubation. Thus, it is important to promptly recognize when patients are failing NIV.

Table 11-1 Strength of evidence supporting use of noninvasive ventilation for acute respiratory failure

COPD exacerbation	Many randomized controlled trials support lower rate of intubation and improved survival
Cardiogenic pulmonary edema	Many randomized controlled trials support lower rate of intubation and improved survival
Prevent extubation/ decannulation failure	A few randomized controlled trials and observational studies support the use of NIV in patients at risk for postextubation respiratory failure
Transplantation and immunocompromise	A few randomized controlled trials and observational studies support the use of NIV
Respiratory failure following lung resection surgery	A few randomized controlled trials and observational studies support the use of NIV
Neuromuscular disease	A few randomized controlled trials and observational studies support the use of NIV
Obesity hypoventilation syndrome	Observational studies support the use of NIV
Asthma	A few randomized controlled trials and observational studies support the use of NIV
Do not intubate/do not resuscitate	Observational studies support NIV in patients with COPD exacerbation or cardiogenic pulmonary edema
Acute respiratory distress syndrome	Evidence does not support use in most patients
Failed extubation	Beneficial only for postextubation respiratory failure with hypercapnia

Abbreviations: COPD, chronic obstructive pulmonary disease; NIV, noninvasive ventilation.

Table 11-2 Selection of appropriate patients for noninvasive ventilation

- **Step 1: Patient needs mechanical ventilation**
  - Respiratory distress with dyspnea, use of accessory muscles, abdominal paradox
  - Respiratory acidosis; pH < 7.35 with $Paco_2$ > 45 mm Hg
  - Tachypnea; respiratory rate > 25 breaths/min
  - Diagnosis that responds well to NIV (eg, COPD exacerbation, cardiogenic pulmonary edema)
- **Step 2: No exclusions for NIV**
  - Airway protection: respiratory arrest, unstable hemodynamics, aspiration risk, copious secretions
  - Unable to fit mask: facial surgery, craniofacial trauma or burns, anatomic lesion of upper airway
  - Uncooperative patient; anxiety
  - Patient wishes

Abbreviations: COPD, chronic obstructive pulmonary disease; NIV, noninvasive ventilation.

Table 11-3 **Patient's response to NIV**[a]

- **Assessment shortly after initiation of NIV**
  - Is NIV being used in lieu of intubation?
  - Does the patient have hypoxemic respiratory failure (not related to cardiogenic edema or immunocompromise)?
  - Will the patient be intubated if NIV fails?
  - Are relative contraindications for NIV present (airway protection, aspiration risk, copious secretions)?
  - Is patient tolerating NIV poorly/appears uncomfortable?
  - Is much coaching required for patient to tolerate NIV?
  - Will frequent titration of settings be required?
  - Is patient hemodynamically unstable?
  - Does patient remain hypoxemic (Spo_2 < 92% or Fio_2 > 0.6)?
  - **A "Yes" response to any of the above should prompt transfer to the ICU.**

- **Assessment after 2 hours of NIV**
  - Has gas exchange and dyspnea improved in past 2 h?
  - Is the goal of NIV being met?
  - Does patient tolerate removal of the mask for 30-60 min?
  - Is patient tolerating NIV well/comfortable?
  - Is Spo_2 > 92% and Fio_2 < 0.6?
  - Is patient hemodynamically stable?
  - Does patient tolerate NIV without excessive coaching?
  - Is patient stable on IPAP ≤ 15 cm H_2O?
  - **A "No" response to any of the above should prompt transfer to the ICU.**

Abbreviations: NIV, noninvasive ventilation; ICU, intensive care unit; IPAP, inspiratory positive airway pressure.
[a]Patient assessment shortly after the initiation of NIV and after 2 hours can be used to determine if a patient should be continued on NIV and admitted to an intensive care unit.

A more rapid decrease in $Paco_2$ occurs when NIV is successful. NIV failure has been associated with greater severity of illness, greater mouth leak, and difficulty acclimating to NIV. NIV success is greater for patients with higher baseline pH levels, perhaps because low pH is considered a marker of more severe illness. A good level of consciousness also has been associated with successful responses to NIV for patients with COPD and acute hypercapnic respiratory failure. Other factors that contribute to NIV failure include poor patient selection, progression of the underlying disease process, clinician's inexperience, and lack of appropriate equipment. If a patient does not improve on NIV within 1 to 2 hours of initiation, alternative therapy such as intubation should be considered. Patients receiving NIV for acute respiratory failure should be transferred to a unit where patients are well monitored, such as an intensive care unit (ICU) (Table 11-3).

Technical Factors

Patient Interface

The interface distinguishes NIV from invasive ventilation. Unlike invasive ventilation, where the airway is sealed, leaks of variable degree occur with NIV. A variety of interfaces

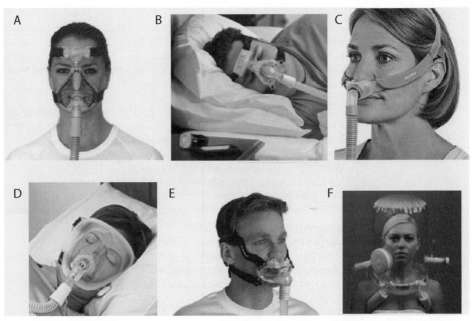

Figure 11-1 Interfaces used for noninvasive ventilation. (A) Oronasal mask (ResMed, San Diego, CA). (B) Nasal mask (Philips Respironics, Murraysville, PA). (C) Nasal pillows (ResMed, San Diego, CA). (D) Total facemask (Philips Respironics, Murraysville, PA). (E) Hybrid mask (ResMed, San Diego, CA). (F) Helmet (StarMed, Mirandola, Italy).

are available and these have improved in variety and quality in recent years. The patient interface has a major impact on patient's comfort and compliance during NIV. Common interfaces for NIV in patients with acute respiratory failure are the oronasal mask, nasal mask, and total facemask (Figure 11-1). The nasal pillows and mouthpieces are more commonly used during NIV for chronic respiratory failure and continuous positive airway pressure (CPAP) used to treat obstructive sleep apnea. The oronasal mask and total facemask are more commonly used for acute respiratory failure. Outside of North America, the helmet is used for NIV and CPAP. There are advantages and disadvantages of each type of interface (Table 11-4).

Selecting the correct mask size is critical. The nasal mask should fit just above the junction of the nasal bone and cartilage, directly at the sides of both nares, and just below the nose above the upper lip. The oronasal mask should fit from just above the junction of the nasal bone and cartilage to just below the lower lip. A common mistake is to choose a mask that is too large. This results in leaks, decreased effectiveness, and patient's discomfort. Leaks through the mouth are not uncommon when using a nasal mask. When mouth leak interferes with the effectiveness of ventilation, an oronasal mask can be used. For acute respiratory failure, an oronasal mask or total facemask is better tolerated and more effective than a nasal interface. Upper airway dryness is greater with use of a nasal mask because of mouth leak, which can be addressed by using heated humidification or an oronasal mask. A humidifier should be used for NIV and set to patient's comfort.

Table 11-4 Advantages and disadvantages of the interfaces for noninvasive ventilation

Interface	Advantages	Disadvantages
Nasal mask	Less risk for aspiration Easier secretion clearance Less claustrophobia Easier speech May be able to eat Easy to fit and secure Less dead space	Mouth leak Higher resistance through nasal passages Less effective with nasal obstruction Nasal irritation and rhinorrhea Mouth dryness
Nasal pillows	Lower profile allows wearing eye glasses Less facial skin breakdown Simple headgear Easy to fit	Mouth leak Higher resistance through nasal passages Less effective with nasal obstruction Nasal irritation and rhinorrhea Mouth dryness
Oronasal mask	Better oral leak control More effective in mouth breathers	Increased dead space Claustrophobia Increased aspiration risk Increased difficulty speaking and eating Asphyxiation with ventilator malfunction
Mouthpiece	Less interference with speech Very little dead space May not require headgear	Less effective if patient cannot maintain mouth seal Usually requires nasal or oronasal interface at night Nasal leak Potential for orthodontic injury
Hybrid	Eliminates mouth leak Lower profile allows wearing eye glasses Less facial skin breakdown	Increased aspiration risk Increased difficulty speaking and eating Asphyxiation with ventilator malfunction
Total face mask	May be more comfortable for some patients Easier to fit (one size fits all) Less facial skin breakdown	Potentially greater dead space Potential for drying of the eyes Cannot deliver aerosolized medications
Helmet	May be more comfortable for some patients Easier to fit (one size fits all) Less facial skin breakdown	Rebreathing Poorer patient-ventilator synchrony Less respiratory muscle unloading Ear damage from noise Cannot deliver aerosolized medications

A common mistake is to fit the headgear too tightly. It should be possible to pass one or two fingers between the headgear and the face. Fitting the headgear too tightly usually will not improve the fit and always decreases patient's comfort and compliance. The design of most masks for NIV is such that the top of the mask is secured on the forehead rather than at the bridge of the nose. Forehead spacers and an adjustable bridge on the mask are important to fill the gap between the forehead and the mask, thus reducing pressure on the bridge of the nose. This improves comfort and decreases the likelihood of pressure sores.

Aerophagia commonly occurs with noninvasive ventilation, but this is usually benign because the airway pressures are less than the esophageal opening pressure. Thus, a gastric tube is not routinely necessary for mask ventilation. In fact, a gastric tube may interfere with the effectiveness of mask ventilation in several ways. It may be more difficult to achieve a mask seal if a gastric tube is present. The gastric tube forced against the face by the mask cushion increases the likelihood of facial skin breakdown. A nasogastric tube also increases resistance to gas flow through the nose, which may decrease the effectiveness of mask ventilation—particularly nasal ventilation.

Pressure sores on the bridge of the nose can occur during NIV. Fortunately, ulceration and skin breakdown can be avoided in most patients. Correct mask fit and size should be reassessed. The tension of the headgear should be reduced. A different mask style may be tried. A hydrocolloid dressing or commercially available nasal pad may also be helpful.

Ventilators for NIV

Leaks during NIV can be a significant contributor to patient-ventilator asynchrony. Large leaks can also compromise inspiratory and expiratory pressures, and tidal volume delivery. Thus, an important consideration in the selection of a ventilator for NIV is leak compensation.

Three categories of ventilators can be used for NIV: critical care ventilators, bilevel ventilators, and intermediate ventilators. Bilevel ventilators use a single limb circuit with a passive exhalation port. Critical care ventilators have separate inspiratory and expiratory limbs, with an active exhalation valve. Intermediate ventilators are typically used for patient transport or home ventilation; they may have a passive exhalation port or an active exhalation valve. Ventilators that use an active exhalation valve have traditionally been leak-intolerant. However, the newer-generation of critical care ventilators features NIV modes that compensate for leaks. With bilevel ventilators, leak is composed of the intentional leak through the passive exhalation port as well as unintentional leaks that may be present in the circuit or at the interface.

Bilevel ventilators compensate well for leaks. They are blower devices that vary inspiratory and expiratory pressures in response to patient's demand. These ventilators provide pressure-controlled or pressure support ventilation. None provides volume-controlled ventilation, although some provide volume-targeted adaptive pressure ventilation. Some bilevel ventilators automatically adjust the inspiratory trigger and expiratory cycle by tracking the patient's inspiratory and expiratory flows. Others allow the clinician to adjust the trigger and/or cycle. Rise time can be adjusted on some bilevel ventilators to improve patient-ventilator synchrony. To minimize CO_2 rebreathing, bilevel ventilators cannot be used without positive end-expiratory pressure ([PEEP] ≥ 4 cm H_2O). Modern bilevel ventilators use a blender to provide a precise FIO_2.

With a critical care ventilator, the level of pressure support is the pressure above the baseline level of PEEP. The approach is different with bilevel ventilators, where an inspiratory positive airway pressure (IPAP) and expiratory positive airway pressure (EPAP) are set. Here the difference between the IPAP and EPAP is the level of pressure support (Figure 11-2).

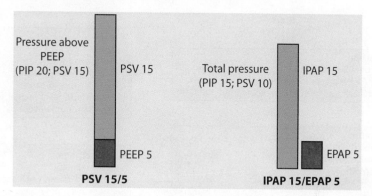

Figure 11-2 Comparison of pressure support with a critical care ventilator and inspiratory positive airway pressure (IPAP) with a bilevel ventilator. Note that the IPAP is the peak inspiratory pressure (PIP) and includes the expiratory positive airway pressure (EPAP), whereas pressure support is provided on top of the positive end-expiratory pressure (PEEP); thus, PIP is the pressure support setting plus the PEEP setting.

Caregiver Issues

If NIV is to be successful, those caring for the patient (physicians, nurses, respiratory therapists) must be committed to this approach. This is usually achieved by familiarizing these persons with the accumulated evidence suggesting that NIV improves outcome in selected patients. Physicians must appreciate selection criteria, respiratory therapists must understand the issues related to ventilator management and selection of an appropriate interface, and nursing personnel must appreciate issues related to mask fit and skin care. Some clinicians are reluctant to initiate NIV due to concerns related to time requirements and difficulties encountered when NIV is initiated. Fitting the mask, selection of appropriate ventilator settings, and patient coaching are labor-intensive for the first hours of NIV.

Clinical Application

The application of NIV (Figure 11-3) requires caregiver's patience and skills with both the technical aspects of mechanical ventilation and the ability to coach patients to adapt to the mask and ventilator. The primary goal when initiating NIV is patient's comfort and not an improvement in arterial blood gases per se (an improvement in blood gases will usually follow if patient comfort and respiratory muscle unloading is achieved). Important steps in the clinical application of NIV are as follows: (1) choose a ventilator capable of meeting patient's needs (usually pressure ventilation), (2) choose the correct interface and avoid a mask that is too large, (3) explain therapy to the patient, (4) silence alarms and choose low settings, (5) initiate NIV while holding the mask in place, (6) secure the mask, avoiding a tight fit, (7) titrate pressure to patient's comfort, (8) titrate F_{IO_2} to SpO_2 > 90%, (9) avoid peak pressure > 20 cm H_2O (which increases

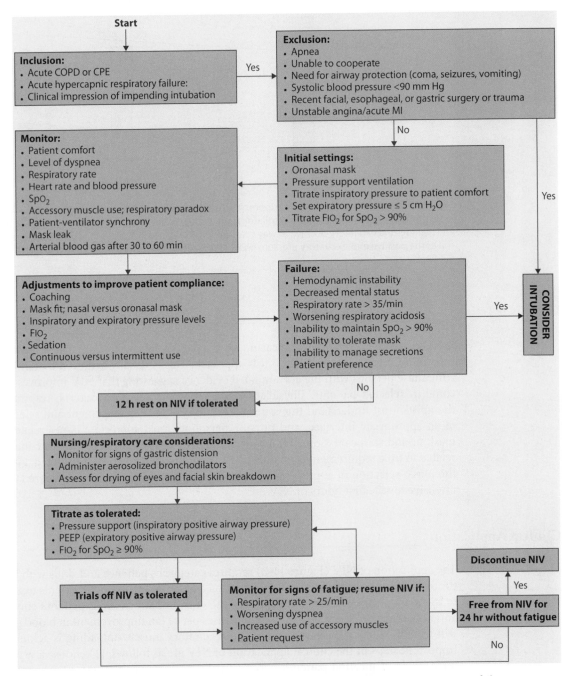

Figure 11-3 Algorithm for initiation of noninvasive ventilation for acute respiratory failure.

the risk of gastric insufflation), (10) titrate PEEP per trigger effort and SpO_2, and (11) continue to coach and reassure patient, and make adjustments to improve patient's compliance. Complications of NIV (usually minor) include leaks, mask discomfort, facial skin breakdown, oropharyngeal drying, eye irritation, sinus congestion, patient-ventilator asynchrony, gastric insufflation, and hemodynamic compromise.

> ### Points to Remember
>
> - The use of noninvasive ventilation (NIV) in appropriately selected patients decreases the need for endotracheal intubation and affords a survival benefit.
> - Patients in whom the success of NIV is the greatest are those with chronic obstructive pulmonary disease exacerbation or cardiogenic pulmonary edema.
> - An interface should be selected that is comfortable for the patient and minimizes leaks.
> - The ventilator selected for NIV should have good leak compensation.
> - Bilevel ventilators compensate for leaks.
> - The initiation of NIV is time-consuming but cost-effective.

Additional Reading

Agarwal R, Aggarwal AN, Gupta D, Jindal SK. Role of noninvasive positive-pressure ventilation in postextubation respiratory failure: a meta-analysis. *Respir Care.* 2007;52:1472-1479.

Agarwal R, Aggarwal AN, Gupta D. Role of noninvasive ventilation in acute lung injury/acute respiratory distress syndrome: a proportion meta-analysis. *Respir Care.* 2010;55:1653-1660.

Azoulay E, Demoule A, Jaber S, et al. Palliative noninvasive ventilation in patients with acute respiratory failure. *Intensive Care Med.* 2011;37:1250-1257.

Bello G, De Pascale G, Antonelli M. Noninvasive ventilation for the immunocompromised patient: always appropriate? *Curr Opin Crit Care.* 2012;18:54-60.

Boldrini R, Fasano L, Nava S. Noninvasive mechanical ventilation. *Curr Opin Crit Care.* 2012;18:48-53.

Burns KE, Adhikari NK, Meade MO. A meta-analysis of noninvasive weaning to facilitate liberation from mechanical ventilation. *Can J Anaesth.* 2006;53:305-315.

Chiumello D, Chevallard G, Gregoretti C. Non-invasive ventilation in postoperative patients: a systematic review. *Intensive Care Med.* 2011;37:918-929.

Curtis JR, Cook DJ, Sinuff T, et al. Noninvasive positive pressure ventilation in critical and palliative care settings: understanding the goals of therapy. *Crit Care Med.* 2007;35:932-939.

Hess DR. How to initiate a noninvasive ventilation program: bringing the evidence to the bedside. *Respir Care.* 2009;54:232-245.

Hess DR. Noninvasive positive-pressure ventilation and ventilator-associated pneumonia. *Respir Care.* 2005;50:924-931.

Hess DR. Patient-ventilator interaction during noninvasive ventilation. *Respir Care.* 2011;56: 153-167.

Hess DR. Noninvasive ventilation for acute respiratory failure. *Respir Care.* 2013;58:950-972.

Jaber S, Chanques G, Jung B. Postoperative noninvasive ventilation. *Anesthesiology.* 2010;112:453-461.

Keenan SP, Mehta S. Noninvasive ventilation for patients presenting with acute respiratory failure: the randomized controlled trials. *Respir Care*. 2009;54:116-126.

Keenan SP, Sinuff T, Burns KE, et al. Clinical practice guidelines for the use of noninvasive positive-pressure ventilation and noninvasive continuous positive airway pressure in the acute care setting. *CMAJ*. 2011;183:E195-E214.

Mehta S, Al-Hashim AH, Keenan SP. Noninvasive ventilation in patients with acute cardiogenic pulmonary edema. *Respir Care*. 2009;54(2):186-197.

Nava S, Hill N. Non-invasive ventilation in acute respiratory failure. *Lancet*. 2009;374:250-259.

Nava S, Schreiber A, Domenighetti G. Noninvasive ventilation for patients with acute lung injury or acute respiratory distress syndrome. *Respir Care*. 2011;56:1583-1588.

Ram FS, Picot J, Lightowler J, Wedzicha JA. Non-invasive positive pressure ventilation for treatment of respiratory failure due to exacerbations of chronic obstructive pulmonary disease. *Cochrane Database Syst Rev*. 2004:CD004104.

Soroksky A, Klinowski E, Ilgyev E, et al. Noninvasive positive pressure ventilation in acute asthmatic attack. *Eur Respir Rev*. 2010;19:39-45.

Vital FM, Saconato H, Ladeira MT, et al. Non-invasive positive pressure ventilation (CPAP or bilevel NPPV) for cardiogenic pulmonary edema. *Cochrane Database Syst Rev*. 2008:CD005351.

Chapter 12
Humidification and the Ventilator Circuit

Objectives

1. Explain why humidification of the inspired gas is necessary during mechanical ventilation.
2. Compare and passive humidification.
3. Discuss issues related to the ventilator circuit and gas delivery to the patient.
4. Describe why circuit compressible volume is an important consideration during mechanical ventilation.
5. Discuss the appropriate role of alarms during mechanical ventilation.

Introduction

Care of mechanically ventilated patients requires attention to both physiologic and technical issues. To deliver an adequate tidal volume, the patient-ventilator circuit and interface must be unobstructed, leak-free, and have minimal compliance and compressible volume. This chapter discusses issues related to humidification and the ventilator circuit.

Humidification

Physiologic Principles

Inspired gases are conditioned in the airway so that they are fully saturated with water at body temperature when they reach the alveoli (37°C, 100% relative humidity, 44 mg/L absolute humidity, 47 mm Hg water vapor pressure). The point in the airway at which the inspired gases reach body temperature and humidity is the isothermic saturation boundary (ISB). Distal to this point, there is no fluctuation of temperature and humidity. The ISB is normally just distal to the carina. Proximal to the ISB, heat and humidity are added to the inspired gases, and heat and humidity are extracted from the expired gases. This portion of the airway acts as a heat and moisture exchanger. Much of this portion of the airway is bypassed in patients with an endotracheal or tracheostomy tube, necessitating the use of an external humidifying apparatus in the breathing circuit. Under normal conditions, there is about 250 mL of insensible water lost from the lungs each day to humidify the inspired gases.

Inadequate and Excessive Humidity

Gases delivered from ventilators are typically dry and the upper airways of such patients are functionally bypassed by artificial airways. The physiologic effects of inadequate humidity can be due to heat loss or moisture loss. Heat loss from the respiratory tract occurs due to humidification of the inspired gases. However, heat loss due to mechanisms other than breathing is usually more important for temperature homeostasis. Moisture loss from the respiratory tract, and subsequent dehydration of the respiratory tract, results in epithelial damage, particularly of the trachea and upper bronchi.

The result of this is an alteration in pulmonary function such as decreased compliance and decreased surfactant activity. Clinically, drying of secretions, atelectasis, and hypoxemia can occur.

Overhumidification is possible only if the temperature and humidity of the inspired gases is greater than physiologic conditions. This can occur in the setting of therapeutic hypothermia, as is commonly used in patients following cardiac arrest. In this setting, the inspired gas should be conditioned to the patient's core temperature and 100% relative humidity at that temperature. Although it is difficult to produce excessive humidification with a heated humidifier, complete humidification of the inspired gases (during mechanical ventilation) eliminates the insensible water loss that normally occurs during breathing. Failure to consider this could result in a positive water balance (250 mL/day).

With active humidification systems, significant heat gain is unlikely and tracheal injury due to high temperature output of a humidifier is rare. Because the specific heat of gases is low, it is difficult to transfer significant amounts of heat without the presence of aerosol particles to cause tracheal burns. In hypothermic patients, superwarming of inspired gases has little effect in the facilitation of core rewarming. Breathing gases warmed and humidified to normal body conditions, however, complements other rewarming techniques because it prevents further heat loss from the respiratory tract.

Problems of excessive humidity are more likely when aerosols are administered. Bland aerosol therapy has the potential to contribute to a positive water balance, particularly in patients with renal failure. Aerosols have also been associated with contamination of the lower respiratory tract. Cool aerosols can increase airway resistance by increasing the volume of secretions and by irritation of airways. Molecular humidity, rather than aerosolized water, should be used for humidification for patients with reactive airways, and all patients requiring mechanical ventilation.

Techniques of Humidification of Inspired Gases

Conditioning of the inspired gas with heat and humidity should match the normal conditions at that point of entry into the respiratory system (Figure 12-1). If the temperature and humidity are less than this, a humidity deficit is produced. If the temperature and humidity are greater than this, overhumidification may occur. Inspired gases that bypass the upper respiratory tract (eg, endotracheal tubes and tracheostomy tubes) should usually be 37°C and 100% relative humidity.

Active Humidification

Humidifiers produce molecular water (water vapor). High-flow heated humidifiers are capable of providing a relative humidity of 100% at body temperature. The specific devices used during mechanical ventilation are usually a passover designs. Many heated humidifier systems are servocontrolled with a thermistor at the proximal airway to maintain the desired gas delivery temperature.

The circuit that carries gas from the humidifier to the patient is usually heated. This prevents a temperature drop in the circuit and a more precise temperature of gas

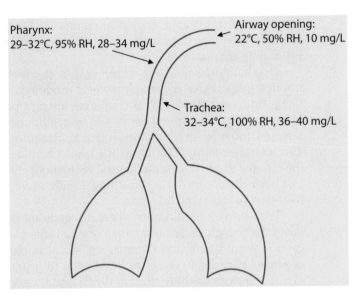

Pharynx:
29–32°C, 95% RH, 28–34 mg/L

Airway opening:
22°C, 50% RH, 10 mg/L

Trachea:
32–34°C, 100% RH, 36–40 mg/L

Figure 12-1 Normal temperature, relative humidity, and absolute humidity levels at three sites in the respiratory tract. The output of any therapeutic gas delivery system should match the normal conditions at that point of entry into the respiratory system.

delivered to the patient. By heating the inspiratory and expiratory limbs, a heated circuit also decreases the amount of condensation in the circuit. If the temperature of the circuit is less than the temperature of the gas leaving the humidifier, condensation will occur in the circuit. On the other hand, if the temperature of the circuit is greater than the temperature of the gas leaving the humidifier, the relative humidity of the gas will drop. This decrease in relative humidity, which can occur with heated circuits, might produce drying of secretions (Figure 12-2). Water condensation in the inspiratory limb of the ventilator circuit near the patient, or in the proximal endotracheal tube, indicates 100% relative humidity of the inspired gas.

Another issue related to the use of humidifiers in ventilator circuits relates to flow resistance. Depending on the point where the ventilator senses patient's effort, this may affect the ability of the ventilator to adequately respond to patient's effort. If the humidifier is between the patient and the point at which the ventilator is triggered, patient work-of-breathing will increase. However, the flow resistance through the humidifier may be less important if trigger pressure is measured at the proximal airway of the patient, which is the most common configuration.

Passive Humidification

A heat and moisture exchanger (HME), colloquially called an artificial nose, passively humidifies the inspired gases by collecting the patient's expired heat and moisture and returning it during the following inspiration (Figure 12-3). These devices are attractive alternatives to active heated humidifiers because of their passive operation (they do not require electricity or heating) and their relatively low cost.

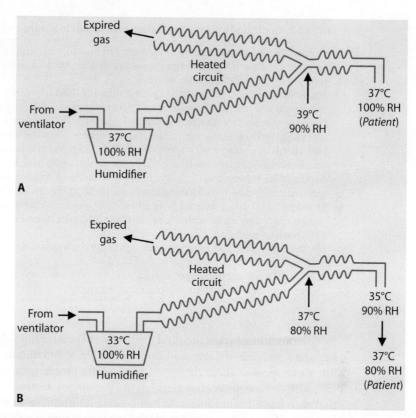

Figure 12-2 (A) Properly set humidifier with heated wire circuit that delivers 100% body humidity to the patient. (B) Heated wire circuit with setting too low, delivering inadequate humidity to the patient.

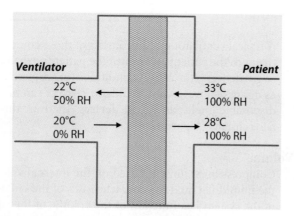

Figure 12-3 Schematic diagram of a heat and moisture exchanger showing the temperature and relative humidity on the patient and ventilator sides of the device during inhalation and exhalation.

Table 12-1 Contraindications for the use of heat and moisture exchanger

- Copious secretions. Secretions in the heat and moisture exchanger will significantly increase resistance to flow. If a patient has copious secretions, the lack of therapeutic humidity may result in thickening of secretions.
- Small tidal volumes. With small tidal volumes, the dead space of the device may compromise ventilation and lead to retention of CO_2. This is an issue with lung-protective ventilation.
- High spontaneous minute ventilation (> 10 L/min). The resistance through heat and moisture exchangers increases with time, and this may make spontaneous breathing difficult.
- Low ventilatory reserve with spontaneous breathing. The resistance through these devices may result in decreased breathing ability for patients who have low ventilatory reserves.
- Expired tidal volume less than 70% of the inspired tidal volume. To function properly, both inspired gases and expired gases must travel through the artificial nose. Patients with a bronchopleural fistula will not have an adequate expired volume through the device. A similar effect may occur with a nasal interface and exhalation through the mouth during noninvasive ventilation.
- Hypothermia. heat and moisture exchangers are contraindicated with a body temperature < 32°C.
- A heat and moisture exchanger should be removed from the ventilator circuit during aerosol treatments when the nebulizer is placed in the circuit.

The additional resistance and dead space of passive humidifiers can be problematic because it increases the imposed work-of-breathing and minute ventilation requirement. The dead space of these devices is particularly problematic when the tidal volume is low, such as lung-protective ventilation. The output of passive humidifiers is less than that with heated humidifiers. When passive humidification is used during prolonged mechanical ventilation, the patient must be frequently assessed for signs of inadequate humidification (eg, thick secretions, bronchial casts, mucus plugging). If signs of inadequate humidification are present, heated humidification should be initiated. There are several clinical conditions that contraindicate the use of an artificial nose (Table 12-1).

The Ventilator Circuit

A typical ventilator circuit consists of those components that deliver gas from the ventilator to the patient and return the patient's exhaled gas to the atmosphere. In addition to gas delivery, the circuit conditions the inspired gases by filtering and humidification as discussed previously. Ventilator circuits can be sterilized and reused, but many are disposable single patient-use devices. There are three common configurations of ventilator circuits (Figure 12-4).

Compression Volume

Compression volume is based on the internal volume of the ventilator, the volume of the humidifier, and the characteristics of the circuit tubing. The compression volume of the system is a function of the volume of the circuit, the compliance (elasticity) of the tubing material, and the ventilation pressure. The volume of gas compressed in the circuit is not delivered to the patient, which becomes clinically important with high

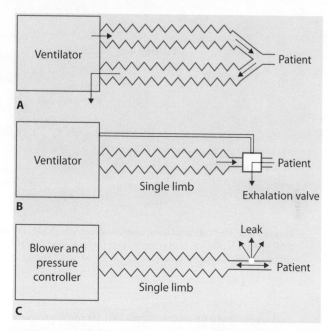

Figure 12-4 (A) Dual-limb circuit with separation on inspired and expired gases. This configuration is most commonly used with critical care ventilators. (B) Single-limb circuit with exhalation valve near the patient. This configuration is most commonly used with portable ventilators. (C) Single-limb circuit with a passive exhalation port. This configuration is used with noninvasive ventilations. With this configuration, flow through the circuit during exhalation must be sufficient to prevent rebreathing.

pressures and low tidal volumes. The volume that leaves the exhalation valve of the ventilator includes the exhaled volume from the patient as well as the volume of gas compressed in the ventilator circuit. Unless volume is measured directly at the patient's airway, the exhaled volume displayed by the ventilator may overestimate the patient's actual tidal volume by the amount of the compressible volume. Most current generation ventilators correct volume for circuit compression volume, so that the displayed tidal volume is an estimate of the volume delivered to the patient.

The compressible volume is often expressed as the compression factor, which is calculated by dividing the compression volume by the corresponding ventilation pressure. If the compression factor is known, the compressible volume can be calculated by multiplying it by the ventilating pressure. The delivered tidal volume is the volume leaving the exhalation valve minus the compression volume:

$$V_T = V_T exh - (factor \times [PIP - PEEP])$$

where $V_T exh$ is the volume leaving the exhalation valve and V_T is the tidal volume corrected for compression volume (Figure 12-5).

Consideration of compression volume is important for several reasons. Most importantly, it decreases the delivered tidal volume to the patient. Failure to consider compression volume results in overestimation of lung compliance. Auto-positive

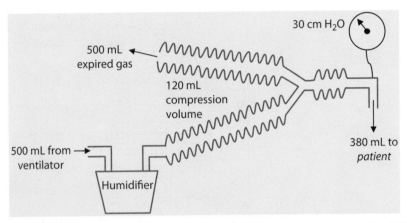

Figure 12-5 Illustration of compression volume. In this example, if airway pressure is 30 cm H_2O, set tidal volume is 500 mL, and compression factor is 4 mL/cm H_2O, then the actual tidal volume delivered to the patient is only 380 mL.

end-expiratory pressure (auto-PEEP) measurements are also affected by circuit compression volume:

$$\text{auto-PEEP} = (\text{Crs} + \text{Cpc})/\text{Crs} \times \text{estimated auto-PEEP}$$

where Crs is the compliance of the respiratory system, Cpc is the compliance of the patient circuit, and estimated auto-PEEP is the value that is measured. Compression volume also affects the measurement of mixed exhaled P_{CO_2}, and the following correction can be used:

$$\bar{PE}_{CO_2} = \text{Pexh}_{CO_2} \times (V_T\text{exh}/V_T)$$

where $\bar{PE}_{CO_2}$ is the true mixed exhaled P_{CO_2} and Pexh_{CO_2} is measured mixed exhaled P_{CO_2} (including gas compressed in the ventilator circuit). To avoid the effect of compression volume on $\bar{PE}_{CO_2}$, mainstream volumetric capnography can be used.

Resistance

Ventilator circuits and endotracheal tubes increase the imposed work-of-breathing for the patient. Circuit resistance adds to the resistance of the endotracheal tube. Circuit resistance increases with the addition of a passive humidifier. The resistance through the expiratory limb of the circuit is primarily due to the exhalation valve and PEEP devices. Current generation ventilators use an exhalation valve with a large diaphragm that is electrically controlled, and thus produces a more consistent circuit pressure regardless of flow. Most ventilators use an active exhalation valve during pressure-controlled ventilation, reducing the risk of circuit overpressurization. An active exhalation valve opens and closes to keep pressure in the circuit at the target level set on the ventilator.

Dead Space

The circuit dead space is the volume of the circuit through which rebreathing occurs. It is called mechanical dead space and is functionally an extension of the patient's anatomic dead space. Mechanical dead space is the volume of tubing between the Y-piece and the artificial airway. It becomes particularly important when the patient is ventilated with a small tidal volume. During low tidal volume ventilation, such as is used as part of a lung-protective strategy, the volume of mechanical dead space should be minimized. Dead space is increased with the use of an HME.

Bias Flow

Many current generation ventilators pass a bias flow of gas through the circuit during the expiratory phase. The purpose of this bias flow is to improve triggering during flow-triggered ventilation. Due to this bias flow, it is not possible to accurately measure tidal volume or exhaled gas concentrations by attaching flow and gas measuring sensors distal to the exhalation outlet on the ventilator.

Nosocomial Pneumonia

Intubated mechanically ventilated patients are at risk for nosocomial pneumonia. In the past, the ventilator circuit has been implicated in the risk of ventilator-associated pneumonia. However, the source of contamination of the lower respiratory tract is usually aspiration of upper airway secretions from around the cuff. Ventilator-associated pneumonia (VAP) might be better called endotracheal tube-associated pneumonia. Ventilator circuits do not need to be changed on a scheduled basis. Circuit changes are only necessary between patients, if the circuit malfunctions, or when the circuit is visibly soiled. There is no strong evidence that the use of a heated wire circuits or an HME decreases the risk of VAP.

Troubleshooting

The patient-ventilator system should be evaluated periodically related to the technical aspects of the ventilator system and the pathophysiology of the patient. The patient-ventilator system check is a documented evaluation of a ventilator and the patient's response to mechanical ventilatory support. It should be performed at regular intervals and more frequently if the patient becomes unstable or requires ventilator adjustments. A flow sheet is typically used to record these assessments.

Perhaps the most troublesome aspect of ventilator troubleshooting is the detection and correction of circuit leaks. These must be corrected promptly to prevent patient harm due to hypoventilation. To avoid patient injury due to hypoxia (and possibly death), a disconnect alarm must be set at all times. The disconnect alarm is usually low exhaled volume or low airway pressure. A manual resuscitator should be at the bedside of all mechanically ventilated patients to allow ventilation in the event of a ventilator failure.

Between patients, all ventilators should be calibrated and an operational verification procedure should be conducted as recommended by the manufacturer. With current generation microprocessor ventilators, sophisticated integral computerized self-test diagnostics are used. At manufacturer-determined intervals, more complete ventilator preventive maintenance is required.

Alarms

All critical care ventilators feature a variety of alarms to warn of events. These events may be malfunctions of the ventilator (eg, circuit leak), malfunctions of the patient-ventilator interface (eg, disconnect), or pathologic changes affecting the patient (eg, high airway pressure). Alarms can be classified as immediately life-threatening, potentially life-threatening, and those that are not life-threatening but a possible source of patient harm. Although ventilator alarms are necessary, they contribute to noise pollution in the critical care unit. Alarms should be set sensitive enough to detect critical events without producing false alarms. If false alarms occur frequently, desensitization of the clinical staff can occur, with potentially disastrous results if a true alarm situation occurs.

Points to Remember

- Inadequate humidification of the inspired gases can result in drying of secretions and atelectasis.
- The temperature and humidity output of any therapeutic gas delivery device should match the normal conditions at that point of entry into the respiratory system.
- Heated humidifiers produce molecular water vapor.
- Heat and moisture exchangers passively heat and humidify the inspired gases.
- Compression volume is the gas compressed in the ventilator circuit during inspiration, and thus not delivered to the patient.
- Ventilator-associated pneumonia is usually not circuit-related.
- Ventilator circuits do not need to be changed on a scheduled basis.
- Ventilator alarms should be set sensitive enough to detect critical events without producing false alarms.

Additional Reading

Doyle A, Joshi M, Frank P, et al. A change in humidification system can eliminate endotracheal tube occlusion. *J Crit Care.* 2011;26:637.e1-4.

Gross JL, Park GR. Han J, Liu Y. Effect of ventilator circuit changes on ventilator-associated pneumonia: a systematic review and meta-analysis. *Respir Care.* 2010;55:467-474.

Hess D. Prolonged use of heat and moisture exchangers: why do we keep changing things? *Crit Care Med.* 2000;28:1667-1668.

Hess DR, Kallstrom TJ, Mottram CD, et al. Care of the ventilator circuit and its relation to ventilator-associated pneumonia. *Respir Care.* 2003;48:869-879.

Gross JL, Park GR. Humidification of inspired gases during mechanical ventilation. *Minerva Anestesiol.* 2012;78:496-502.

Kelly M, Gillies D, Todd DA, Lockwood C. Heated humidification versus heat and moisture exchangers for ventilated adults and children. *Cochrane Database Syst Rev.* 2010;CD004711.

Kola A, Eckmanns T, Gastmeier P. Efficacy of heat and moisture exchangers in preventing ventilator-associated pneumonia: meta-analysis of randomized controlled trials. *Intensive Care Med.* 2005;31:5-11.

Lacherade JC, Auburtin M, Cerf C, et al. Impact of humidification systems on ventilator-associated pneumonia: a randomized multicenter trial. *Am J Respir Crit Care Med.* 2005;172:1276-1282.

Lellouche F, Pignataro C, Maggiore SM, et al. Short-term effects of humidification devices on respiratory pattern and arterial blood gases during noninvasive ventilation. *Respir Care.* 2012;57:1879-1886.

Morán I, Cabello B, Manero E, Mancebo J. Comparison of the effects of two humidifier systems on endotracheal tube resistance. *Intensive Care Med.* 2011;37:1773-1779.

Nishida T, Nishimura M, Fujino Y, Mashimo T. Performance of heated humidifiers with a heated wire according to ventilatory settings. *J Aerosol Med.* 2001;14:43-51.

Pelosi P, Chiumello D, Severgnini P, et al. Performance of heated wire humidifiers: an in vitro study. *J Crit Care.* 2007;22:258-264.

Restrepo RD, Walsh BK. Humidification during invasive and noninvasive mechanical ventilation: 2012. *Respir Care.* 2012;57:782-788.

Sottiaux TM. Consequences of under- and over-humidification. *Respir Care Clin N Am.* 2006;12:233-252.

Chapter 13
F_{IO_2}, Positive End-Expiratory Pressure, and Mean Airway Pressure

---

Objectives

1. Discuss the pathophysiology of hypoxemia.
2. Discuss the physiologic effects of positive end-expiratory pressure (PEEP).
3. Discuss the indications for the application of PEEP.
4. Discuss the application, monitoring, and withdrawal of PEEP in acute respiratory distress syndrome.
5. Discuss the overall management of oxygenation in critically ill patients.

Introduction

The principles associated with management of oxygenation are more complex than those associated with ventilation. Provided that cardiovascular function and $\dot{V}CO_2$ are constant, increases in alveolar ventilation generally result in decreases in $Paco_2$ and vice versa. Oxygenation status, although dependent on F_{IO_2}, is also affected by cardiopulmonary disease, positive end-expiratory pressure (PEEP), and mean airway pressure ($\overline{P}aw$). In this chapter, the aspects of mechanical ventilation that affect oxygenation are discussed, as well as approaches to these techniques during patient management.

Pathophysiology of Hypoxemia

Normal Pao_2 is 80 to 100 mm Hg when breathing room air at sea level, with hypoxemia defined as a Pao_2 of < 80 mm Hg. To maintain normal tissue oxygenation it is necessary to provide an adequate F_{IO_2}, appropriate matching of ventilation and perfusion ($\dot{V}/\dot{Q}$), sufficient hemoglobin, adequate cardiac output, and appropriate O_2 unloading to the tissue. A breakdown at any stage in this process may result in tissue hypoxia. At sea level, hypoxemia results from one of a number of alterations in cardiopulmonary function. Specifically, hypoxemia is caused by shunt, $\dot{V}/\dot{Q}$ mismatch, diffusion defect, and hypoventilation. Hypoxemia is also worsened by cardiovascular compromise. A reasonable target Pao_2 in mechanically ventilated patients is 55 to 80 mm Hg (Spo_2 88%-95%).

Shunt

Shunt is perfusion without ventilation. When present, venous blood (shunted blood) mixes with arterialized blood in the pulmonary veins or left heart causing a decrease in Pao_2 of blood leaving the left heart. Because the majority of O_2 is carried by hemoglobin, even a small shunt (Figure 13-1) can result in significant hypoxemia. Increasing F_{IO_2} improves oxygenation only in the settings of small shunt. A large shunt is unresponsive to an F_{IO_2} increase. Improvement in oxygenation in the setting of a large shunt is usually focused on resolution of the shunt (eg, decompression of a pneumothorax, resolution of a pneumonia, re-expansion of atelectasis, diuresis). The use of PEEP,

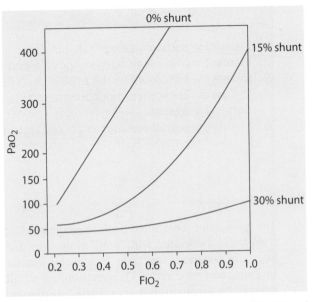

Figure 13-1 Comparison of the theoretical F_{IO_2} – Pa_{O_2} relationships with 0%, 15% and 30% shunts. These relationships were calculated assuming normal ventilation, hemoglobin of 15 g, $C(a - \bar{v})O_2$ difference of 5 vol %, and normal cardiac output, metabolic rate, pH and P_{CO_2}. Note that as shunt increases, the Pa_{O_2} at a given F_{IO_2} decreases substantially. (Reproduced with permission from Shapiro BA, et al. *Clinical Application of Blood Gases*. 4th ed. Chicago, IL: Mosby-Year Book; 1994.)

recruitment maneuvers, and maneuvers to elevate $\overline{Paw}$ might improve oxygenation in this setting. A common, but often unrecognized, cause of shunt in mechanically ventilated patients is a patent foramen ovale. A functionally closed foramen ovale may open during mechanical ventilation and acute respiratory failure.

$\dot{V}/\dot{Q}$ Mismatch

The normal $\dot{V}/\dot{Q}$ is 0.8. Hypoxemia results when this ratio is low (Figure 13-2). The most effective methods of altering Pa_{O_2} in the presence of $\dot{V}/\dot{Q}$ mismatch are to improve distribution of ventilation and increase in F_{IO_2}. This is particularly true for patients with chronic obstructive lung disease, where gross mismatching of $\dot{V}/\dot{Q}$ is present. As illustrated in Figure 13-2, in some settings, minor increases in F_{IO_2} can markedly increase Pa_{O_2}. In many ventilated patients, hypoxemia is caused by both shunt and $\dot{V}/\dot{Q}$ mismatch. In these patients, management of oxygenation may require increasing F_{IO_2}, PEEP, and $\overline{Paw}$.

Diffusion Defect

Hypoxemia in this setting is due to the increased time for equilibration of O_2 across the alveolar capillary membrane. This is the result of thickening of the alveolar-capillary membrane or a decrease in surface area available for diffusion. Interstitial fluid, fibrotic changes of the alveolar-capillary membrane, and emphysematous changes of the lung parenchyma are the primary causes of a diffusion defect. Increasing F_{IO_2} improves oxygenation with a diffusion defect.

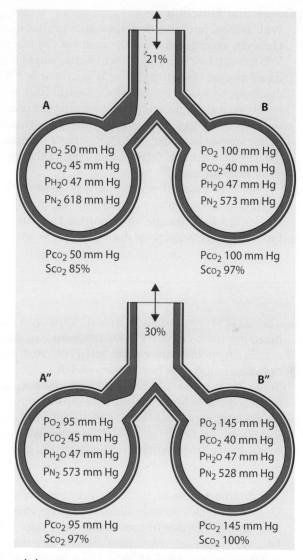

Figure 13-2 Effect of V̇/Q̇ mismatch on oxygenation. In alveolus A (A″), V̇/Q̇ is < 0.8. As a result, less O$_2$ reaches the lung unit than is removed by circulation causing the alveolar P$_{O_2}$ to decrease and the alveolar P$_{CO_2}$ to increase. In alveolus B (B″), the normal V̇/Q̇ is maintained. Increasing the F$_{IO_2}$ from 0.21 to 0.30 (A″ and B″) markedly diminishes the effect that the low V̇/Q̇ has on oxygenation. (From Shapiro BA, et al. *Clinical Application of Blood Gases.* 4th ed. Chicago, IL: Mosby-Year Book; 1994.)

Hypoventilation

Elevation of alveolar P$_{CO_2}$ decreases the alveolar P$_{O_2}$, as predicted by the alveolar gas equation. The elevated Pa$_{CO_2}$ causes the oxyhemoglobin dissociation curve to shift to the right, decreasing Sa$_{O_2}$ but increasing the unloading of O$_2$ at tissues. Improvement in ventilation is the best treatment for hypoxemia caused by hypoventilation, although this cause of hypoxemia also responds to O$_2$ administration.

Decreased Cardiovascular Function

With normal lung function, decreased cardiac output does not result in hypoxemia. However, altered cardiovascular function can magnify the hypoxemic effects of either $\dot{V}/\dot{Q}$ mismatch or shunting. When cardiac output is low, tissue O_2 extraction is high and mixed venous O_2 content is low. When shunt or $\dot{V}/\dot{Q}$ mismatch is present with low cardiac output, blood with a lower O_2 content from shunted areas mixes with blood from nonshunted areas, resulting in a greater degree of hypoxemia than if the cardiac output were higher. Management of hypoxemia due to cardiovascular dysfunction is corrected by appropriate hemodynamic management. Although increasing F_{IO_2} is appropriate in this setting, there are certain settings (eg, cardiogenic pulmonary) where moderate levels of PEEP are useful.

Since mechanical ventilation may cause $\dot{V}/\dot{Q}$ mismatch, even patients without marked cardiopulmonary dysfunction (eg, postoperative, drug overdose) may require an elevated F_{IO_2} to maintain a normal Pa_{O_2}. In these settings, however, rarely is an $F_{IO_2} > 0.40$ necessary except during specific procedures (eg, suctioning, bronchoscopy).

F_{IO_2}

O_2 Toxicity

The role of oxygen toxicity in critically ill patients is controversial. In healthy mammals, breathing 100% O_2 for 24 hours results in structural changes at the alveolar-capillary membrane, pulmonary edema, atelectasis, and decreased Pa_{O_2}. In healthy humans, the same process has been observed, but requires a longer period of time. Thus, the lowest F_{IO_2} necessary to maintain the target Pa_{O_2} should always be used. However, in severely diseased lungs, antioxidants capable of minimizing the effect of high F_{IO_2} may be induced, allowing tolerance to a high F_{IO_2}. For patients with acute lung injury, $F_{IO_2} > 0.60$ is generally avoided. However, it is less dangerous to increase the F_{IO_2} than to expose the lungs to the damaging effects of high alveolar pressure (> 30 cm H_2O).

100% O_2

The continuous use of 100% O_2 should be avoided. In addition to the potential for O_2 toxicity, high F_{IO_2} may cause absorption atelectasis in poorly ventilated, unstable lung units due to denitrogenation. But this does not mean that 100% O_2 should never be used. Whenever oxygenation status is in question or generalized cardiopulmonary instability occurs, 100% O_2 should be administered, but should be reduced as rapidly as possible to more appropriate levels when the acute issue has resolved. Use of 100% O_2 during procedures such as bronchoscopy is recommended. In addition, 100% O_2 is usually administered during initial ventilator setup and quickly reduced when appropriate Pa_{O_2} and Sp_{O_2} are established.

Positive End-Expiratory Pressure (PEEP)

PEEP is the application of pressures greater than atmospheric to the airway during the expiratory phase. The term continuous positive airway pressure (CPAP) is usually reserved for constant pressures greater than atmospheric applied to the airway of a spontaneously breathing patient. With CPAP, the patient is responsible for ventilation (no additional pressure during inhalation), whereas inspiratory assistance is provided with PEEP.

Physiologic Effects

PEEP increases $\bar{P}aw$ and mean intrathoracic pressure. This has effects on many physiologic functions (Table 13-1). When applied to appropriate levels for the clinical setting, PEEP improves pulmonary mechanics and gas exchange, and may have varying effects on the cardiovascular system.

Pulmonary mechanics Since pressure and volume in the lungs are related, the application of PEEP increases the functional residual capacity (FRC). In the setting of alveolar collapse, PEEP maintains alveolar recruitment. With recruitment of collapsed lung units, lung compliance improves. The increase in lung volume with PEEP can be the result of alveolar recruitment or an increased volume of already open alveoli. If PEEP overdistends already open alveoli, compliance will decrease. Depending on the overall balance between recruitment and overdistention, the application of PEEP may increase, decrease, or not affect tidal compliance. However, the appropriate application of PEEP in a patient with lung injury generally improves lung compliance. An appropriate level

Table 13-1 Potential Physiologic Effects of Appropriately and Excessively Applied PEEP

	Appropriate level	*Excessive level*
Intrathoracic pressure	Increased	Increased
FRC	Increased	Increased
Lung compliance	Increased	Decreased
$Paco_2$	Decreased	Increased
Q_S/Q_T	Decreased	Increased
$P\bar{v}o_2$	Normal	Decreased
$Paco_2 - Petco_2$	Decreased	Increased
V_D/V_T	Decreased	Increased
Work-of-breathing	Decreased	Increased
Pulmonary vascular resistance	Normal	Increased
Cardiac output	Normal	Decreased
Left ventricular afterload	Decreased	Decreased
Arterial blood pressure	Normal	Decreased
Intracranial pressure	Normal	Increased
Urine output	Normal	Decreased

Abbreviations: FRC, functional residual capacity; Q_S/Q_T, shunt fraction; $P\bar{v}o_2$, mixed venous O_2 pressure; $Petco_2$, end-tidal Pco_2; V_D/V_T, dead space/tidal volume ratio.

of PEEP also decreases work-of-breathing in spontaneously breathing patients. Excessive PEEP places the lung on the upper flat portion of the pressure-volume curve, thus decreasing compliance and increasing work-of-breathing.

Gas exchange In most clinical applications, PEEP is applied to improve Pao_2. This is accomplished through alveolar recruitment and decreasing intrapulmonary shunt. Appropriate PEEP may also improve $Paco_2 - Petco_2$ (end-tidal CO_2) and $Paco_2$ by decreasing dead space. Excessive PEEP can decrease perfusion to well-ventilated areas of the lungs, causing an increase in dead space and $Paco_2$. For patients with unilateral lung disease, PEEP may result in overdistension of healthy lung units with shunting of blood to the diseased lung units, worsening hypoxemia.

Cardiovascular function The effect of PEEP on the cardiovascular system is dependent on the level of PEEP, the compliance of the respiratory system, and the cardiovascular status. Because PEEP increases $\bar{P}aw$ and mean intrathoracic pressure, venous return and cardiac output may decrease as PEEP is applied. PEEP has the greatest effect on cardiac output in a setting where lung compliance is high, chest wall compliance is low and cardiovascular reserve is low. High levels of PEEP decrease right ventricular preload, increases right ventricular afterload (increased pulmonary vascular resistance), and may shift the interventricular septum to the left. This, along with a reduction in pericardial pressure gradient, limits left ventricular distensibility, reducing left ventricular end-diastolic volume and stroke volume. Thus, both pulmonary and systemic vascular pressures are affected by PEEP. Because PEEP increases pressure outside of the heart, it decreases left ventricular afterload. The net result may be a decreased cardiac output, arterial blood pressure, urine output, and tissue oxygenation. Thus, PEEP may increase arterial oxygenation but decrease tissue oxygenation.

Intracranial pressure As PEEP decreases venous return, intracranial pressure may increase with the application of PEEP. This is usually not an issue unless intracranial pressure is already increased. The effect of PEEP is decreased by elevating the head, which is commonly applied in the care of these patients. PEEP should be used cautiously in any patient where increased intracranial pressure is a concern, but levels less than or equal to 10 cm H_2O are usually not a problem.

Barotrauma The amount of overdistention produced with PEEP determines the probability of barotrauma. As lung injury is often heterogeneous, overdistention of an individual lung unit may be achieved at any PEEP level. However, barotrauma occurs due to a high end-inspiratory pressure and, thus, PEEP increases the risk of barotrauma only to the extent that it promotes end-inspiratory overdistention.

Indications

Indications for PEEP are shown in Table 13-2.

Acute respiratory distress syndrome Application of 10 to 20 cm H_2O PEEP is standard practice in patients with early acute respiratory distress syndrome (ARDS) to maintain alveolar recruitment. In later stages of ARDS, however, fibroproliferation is observed and generally 5 to 10 cm H_2O PEEP is used in this setting.

Table 13-2 **Indications for PEEP**

- Acute respiratory distress syndrome
- Chest trauma
- Postoperative atelectasis
- Cardiogenic edema
- Acute artificial airway
- Auto-PEEP

Abbreviation: PEEP, positive end-expiratory pressure.

Chest trauma PEEP is used to stabilize the chest wall and prevent paradoxical movement in the setting of flail chest. If ARDS is not present, 5 to 10 cm H$_2$O PEEP is indicated, provided no pulmonary air leak is present and the patient is hemodynamically stable.

Postoperative atelectasis Use of CPAP by facemask may be beneficial to treat postoperative atelectasis. CPAP can be administered continuously or applied for 15 to 30 minutes every 2 to 6 hours at levels of 5 to 10 cm H$_2$O.

Cardiogenic pulmonary edema PEEP decreases preload and afterload. The use of PEEP or CPAP at 5 to 10 cm H$_2$O improves oxygenation, decreases work-of-breathing, increases left-ventricular performance, and improves cardiac output.

Artificial airways Insertion of an artificial airway decreases FRC and may compromise gas exchange. Application of 5 cm H$_2$O PEEP is typically used with intubated patients unless otherwise contraindicated. However, most patients with long-term tracheostomy do not need PEEP or CPAP.

Auto-PEEP The magnitude of auto-PEEP is dependent on the time constant (resistance and compliance), expiratory time, and tidal volume (V$_T$). Auto-PEEP is not observed on the ventilator unless an end-expiratory hold is used. The first indication of auto-PEEP may be inability to trigger the ventilator. Applying PEEP in this setting counterbalances auto-PEEP, decreases the effort needed to trigger, and may not affect end-expiratory alveolar pressure. For the patient who is having difficulty triggering the ventilator, PEEP can be slowly increasing until patient is able to comfortably trigger each breath. At the appropriate level of applied PEEP, patient rate decreases and signs of cardiopulmonary stress subside. PEEP counterbalances auto-PEEP with flow limitation (dynamic airway closure). However, PEEP does not affect auto-PEEP when auto-PEEP is due to high minute ventilation. In volume-controlled ventilation (VCV), if the applied PEEP increases end-expiratory alveolar pressure, peak inspiratory pressure (PIP) and plateau pressure (Pplat) increase. If changes in applied PEEP does not affect PIP with VCV, or tidal volume with PCV (and constant PIP), then auto-PEEP is present.

Ventilator-associated pneumonia Because PEEP raises intratracheal pressure, it decreases the amount of microaspiration around the cuff of the artificial airway. In that way, it decreases contamination of lower respiratory tract and decreases the risk of ventilator-associated pneumonia.

PEEP in ARDS

The primary indication for PEEP is ARDS. The goal of PEEP in this setting is prevention of de-recruitment and maintenance of tissue oxygenation. PEEP improves shunt, reverses hypoxemia, and decreases the work-of-breathing. Further, this is accomplished without adversely affecting cardiac output.

The goal is to set PEEP at a level that maximizes alveolar recruitment and avoids overdistention. Higher levels of PEEP may be appropriate for moderate to severe ARDS and modest levels of PEEP may be appropriate for mild ARDS. Because the potential for recruitment is variable among patients with ARDS, it must be titrated for the individual patient. Arterial blood pressure and pulse oximetry are monitored when PEEP is applied. The specific approach used to titrate PEEP is one of the most contentious subjects related to mechanical ventilation. PEEP can be titrated after a recruitment maneuver. Using this approach, PEEP is set higher than necessary to maintain alveolar recruitment and then slowly decreased until the lowest PEEP maintaining the best compliance is identified. Alternatively, PEEP is increased stepwise while monitoring Spo_2, Pplat, compliance, and blood pressure. A decrease in Spo_2, decrease in compliance, decrease in blood pressure, and Pplat more than 30 cm H_2O suggests overdistention. In the setting of a stiff chest wall, PEEP is set to counterbalance the alveolar collapsing effect of the chest wall, and an esophageal balloon may be useful in this setting to estimate pleural pressure. Another approach is to use PEEP/Fio_2 combinations as have been used in the ARDS network studies. PEEP for ARDS is generally set between 10 and 20 cm H_2O. Hemodynamic monitoring is necessary during PEEP titration due to the potential to adversely affect cardiovascular function.

PEEP should not be abruptly withdrawn. If PEEP is reevaluated on a regular basis, there is usually no need to make large changes in PEEP. Of concern is alveolar de-recruitment and hemodynamic instability with the withdrawal of PEEP. If the Spo_2 decreases when PEEP is decreased, the prior level should be re-established rather than increasing the Fio_2.

Mean Airway Pressure

$\overline{Paw}$ is the average pressure applied over the entire respiratory cycle. $\overline{Paw}$ is dependent on all of the factors that effect ventilation (Table 13-3). Increasing the inspiratory time increases $\overline{Paw}$ without elevating peak alveolar pressure and maintains a

---

Table 13-3 Factors Affecting Mean Airway Pressure

- Inspiratory pressure
- PEEP
- I:E ratio (inspiratory time and rate)
- Inspiratory pressure waveform

Abbreviation: PEEP, positive end-expiratory pressure.

constant level of ventilation, provided that auto-PEEP does not occur. If auto-PEEP occurs, either peak alveolar pressure or tidal volume is compromised. With VCV, auto-PEEP increases peak alveolar pressure because V$_T$ is constant. With PCV, tidal volume decreases as auto-PEEP develops. If inspiratory time is increased, it should be limited to the level that does not create auto-PEEP. Auto-PEEP causes a less uniform distribution of PEEP and FRC than applied PEEP. That is, as a result of heterogeneous lung disease, pulmonary time constants can vary considerably from one lung unit to another. With auto-PEEP, FRC and total PEEP will be largest in the most compliant lung units (longest expiratory time constant) and lowest in the least compliant lung unit (shortest expiratory time constant).

Management of Oxygenation

Assuming appropriate treatment of the underlying condition, optimization of oxygenation requires the use of PEEP, administration of O$_2$, and the assurance of adequate cardiovascular function. Management of oxygenation should always be based on the underlying pathophysiology. In diffuse ARDS, high levels of PEEP may be needed, whereas in localized pneumonia, high PEEP may compromise oxygenation. PEEP should be set to balance recruitment against overdistention. F$_{IO_2}$, PEEP, and $\overline{P}$aw should target Pao$_2$ of 55 to 80 mm Hg (Spo$_2$ 88%-95%).

Points to Remember

- Normal tissue oxygenation requires an adequate Pao$_2$, sufficient hemoglobin, and adequate cardiac output.
- Hypoxemia often results from shunt, $\dot{V}/\dot{Q}$ mismatch, diffusion defect, hypoventilation, and cardiovascular compromise.
- Use the lowest F$_{IO_2}$ to maintain the target Pao$_2$.
- Use 100% O$_2$ during initiation of mechanical ventilation, with cardiopulmonary instability, and whenever stressful procedures are performed.
- Positive end-expiratory pressure (PEEP) increases functional residual capacity and maintains recruitment of unstable lung units.
- Alveolar recruitment resulting from PEEP decreases shunt and improves oxygenation.
- The effect of PEEP on hemodynamic function is dependent on the level of PEEP, the compliance of the respiratory system, and cardiovascular status.
- Indications for PEEP are acute respiratory distress syndrome (ARDS), chest trauma, postoperative atelectasis, cardiogenic pulmonary edema, and counterbalancing auto-PEEP.
- Monitoring of blood gases, pulse oximetry and hemodynamics are necessary during the application of PEEP.
- In ARDS, PEEP is applied at the lowest level that prevents derecruitment (10-20 cm H$_2$O).
- F$_{IO_2}$, PEEP, and $\overline{P}$aw should target Pao$_2$ of 55 to 80 mm Hg (Spo$_2$ 88%-95%).

Additional Reading

Briel M, Meade M, Mercat A, et al. Higher vs lower positive end-expiratory pressure in patients with acute lung injury and acute respiratory distress syndrome: systematic review and meta-analysis. *JAMA.* 2010;303:865-873.

Brower RG, Lanken PN, MacIntyre N, et al. Higher versus lower positive end-expiratory pressures in patients with the acute respiratory distress syndrome. *N Engl J Med.* 2004;351: 327-336.

Dasenbrook EC, Needham DM, Brower RG, Fan E. Higher PEEP in patients with acute lung injury: a systematic review and meta-analysis. *Respir Care.* 2011;56:568-575.

Di Marco F, Devaquet J, Lyazidi A, et al. Positive end-expiratory pressure-induced functional recruitment in patients with acute respiratory distress syndrome. *Crit Care Med.* 2010;38:127-132.

Gordo-Vidal F, Gómez-Tello V, Palencia-Herrejón E, et al. High PEEP vs. conventional PEEP in the acute respiratory distress syndrome: a systematic review and meta-analysis. *Med Intensiva.* 2007;31:491-501

Hess DR. Approaches to conventional mechanical ventilation of the patient with acute respiratory distress syndrome. *Respir Care.* 2011;56:1555-1572.

Hess DR. How much PEEP? Do we need another meta-analysis? *Respir Care.* 2011;56:710-713.

Koutsoukou A, Bekos B, Sotiropoulou C, et al. Effects of positive end-expiratory pressure on gas exchange and expiratory flow limitation in adult respiratory distress syndrome. *Crit Care Med.* 2002;30:1941-1949.

Meade MO, Cook DJ, Guyatt GH, et al. Ventilation strategy using low tidal volumes, recruitment maneuvers, and high positive end-expiratory pressure for acute lung injury and acute respiratory distress syndrome: a randomized controlled trial. *JAMA.* 2008;299:637-645.

Mercat A, Richard JC, Vielle B, et al. Positive end-expiratory pressure setting in adults with acute lung injury and acute respiratory distress syndrome: a randomized controlled trial. *JAMA.* 2008;299:646-655.

Miller RR, Macintyre NR, Hite RD, et al. Point: should positive end-expiratory pressure in patients with ARDS be set on oxygenation? Yes. *Chest.* 2012;141:1379-1382.

Oba Y, Thameem DM, Zaza T. High levels of PEEP may improve survival in acute respiratory distress syndrome: A meta-analysis. *Respir Med.* 2009;103:1174-1181.

Putensen C, Theuerkauf N, Zinserling J, et al. Meta-analysis: ventilation strategies and outcomes of the acute respiratory distress syndrome and acute lung injury. *Ann Intern Med.* 2009;151:566-576

Schmidt GA. Counterpoint: should positive end-expiratory pressure in patients with ARDS be set based on oxygenation? No. *Chest.* 2012;141:1382-1387.

Villar J, Kacmarek RM, Pérez-Méndez L, Aguirre-Jaime A. A high positive end-expiratory pressure, low tidal volume ventilatory strategy improves outcome in persistent acute respiratory distress syndrome: a randomized, controlled trial. *Crit Care Med.* 2006;34: 1311-1318.

Chapter 14
Initial Settings for Mechanical Ventilation

Objectives

1. Discuss the difference between hypercapnic and hypoxemic respiratory failure and list the causes of each.
2. Describe the indications for mechanical ventilation.
3. Discuss concerns and approaches to the initiation of mechanical ventilation.
4. Discuss the criteria used to initially set the mechanical ventilator for patients with normal lungs, and with obstructive and restrictive diseases.
5. Discuss the ethical considerations related to initiation of mechanical ventilation.

Introduction

Ventilatory support should be instituted when a patient's ability to maintain gas exchange has failed to the level that death is imminent if support is not provided. Respiratory failure is categorized as hypercapnic or hypoxemic. Once the decision is made to initiate mechanical ventilation, selection of the initial ventilator settings is based on the patient's physiologic status and the best available evidence. Whenever mechanical ventilation is considered, the ethical consequences of the decision must also be addressed.

Hypercapnic Versus Hypoxemic Respiratory Failure

Hypoxemic respiratory failure is characterized by a failure to oxygenate. Hypercapnic respiratory failure is a failure of the ventilatory pump (ventilatory muscles). Frequently, respiratory failure is a result of both hypoxemic and hypercapnic failure, and can be classified as compensated or uncompensated.

Hypercapnic Respiratory Failure

The ventilatory pump comprises the diaphragm and chest wall muscles, as well as the neural control of them. This is responsible for ensuring adequate alveolar ventilation. Four aspects of the ventilatory pump, either alone or in combination, can result in pump failure: weak muscles, excessive load, impaired neuromuscular transmission, motor neuron disease, or decreased respiratory drive (Table 14-1). Hypercapnic respiratory failure results in an elevated $Paco_2$.

Weak respiratory muscles may occur as a result of inherited myopathies and muscular dystrophies malnutrition, electrolyte imbalance, inadequate peripheral nerve function, or compromised substrate delivery. Long term use of corticosteroids and aminoglycoside antibiotics or calcium channel blockers can impair neuromuscular transmission. Chronic pulmonary disease and neuromuscular disease may precipitate pump failure because of a decrease in the force-velocity relationship of the muscle, decreasing maximal muscular contraction. Ventilatory muscle force may also be decreased by the mechanical disadvantage caused by a flattening of the diaphragm as in severe chronic obstructive pulmonary disease or a deformed thoracic cage as in

Table 14-1 Causes of Hypercapnic Respiratory Failure

Inadequate ventilatory muscle function	**Excessive ventilatory load**

• Electrolyte imbalance
  – Magnesium
  – Potassium
  – Phosphate
• Malnutrition
• Pharmacologic agents
  – Long-term corticosteroids
  – Aminoglycoside antibiotics
  – Calcium channel blocking agents
• Inherited myopathies and muscular dystrophies
• Mechanical disadvantage
  – Flattened diaphragm
  – Thoracic deformity
• Atrophy
• Fatigue
	• Secretions
	• Mucosal edema
	• Bronchospasm
	• Increased dead space
	• Increased carbon dioxide production
	• Dynamic hyperinflation (auto-PEEP)
	
	Decreased central ventilatory drive
	• Pharmacologic agents (sedatives and narcotics)
	• Hypothyroidism
	• Idiopathic central alveolar hyperventilation
	• Severe medullary brainstem injury

Impaired neural transmission • Spinal cord injury • Motor neuron disease • Neuromuscular blockade	

kyphoscoliosis. Patients in the ICU who are mechanically ventilated, especially those paralyzed and receiving steroids, may develop critical illness myopathies. In addition, chronic pulmonary disease or neuromuscular disease may lead to detraining, atrophy, or fatigue of ventilatory muscles, all leading to a reduced efficiency of ventilation and carbon dioxide retention.

Excessive load may cause hypercapnic failure, but it is usually associated with other factors that compromise pump function. For patients with chronic pulmonary or neuromuscular disease, the increased load resulting from secretion accumulation, mucosal edema, or bronchospasm may precipitate failure. For patients with thoracic deformities, increased ventilatory load is a chronic problem. Any factor that elevates minute ventilation requirements increasing ventilatory load may precipitate failure when associated with reduced neuromuscular capability.

Depressed respiratory drive may be caused by drugs, hypothyroidism, or diseases affecting the respiratory center. Increased respiratory drive may also precipitate acute respiratory failure, especially when coupled with compromised pump function and increased ventilatory load. For example, metabolic acidosis, increased carbon dioxide production, and dyspnea-related anxiety may result in an intolerable increase in ventilatory drive.

Hypoxemic Respiratory Failure

Failure of the lungs to maintain arterial oxygenation is hypoxemic respiratory failure (Table 14-2). Hypoxemic respiratory failure usually does not result in carbon dioxide retention unless acute or chronic pump failure is also present. Hypoxemic respiratory

Table 14-2 **Causes of Hypoxemic Respiratory Failure**

- Ventilation–perfusion imbalance
- Right to left shunt
- Alveolar hypoventilation
- Diffusion deficit
- Inadequate F_{IO_2}

failure can usually be treated with oxygen, but mechanical ventilation may be necessary in severe cases of acute respiratory distress syndrome (ARDS), heart failure, or pneumonia.

Indications for Mechanical Ventilation

From a physiologic perspective, indications for mechanical ventilation are listed in Table 14-3. Acute respiratory failure requires mechanical ventilation when the Pa_{CO_2} is elevated sufficiently to cause an acute acidosis (pH < 7.30), although the precise limits on pH and Pa_{CO_2} must be individually evaluated in each patient.

Impending ventilatory failure is an indication for mechanical ventilation when the patient's clinical course indicates deterioration despite maximum treatment. Examples include the patient with neuromuscular disease, or the patient with asthma who demonstrates increasingly compromised respiratory function in the presence of maximum therapy.

Oxygenation deficit is the least likely indication for mechanical ventilation. However, the severe hypoxemia caused by ARDS or pneumonia may require mechanical ventilation. When a high F_{IO_2} (> 0.80) is required, mechanical ventilation should be considered. Unloading the work of the ventilatory pump with mechanical support frequently improves oxygenation status because of the reduced oxygen cost of breathing, and also due to the higher mean airway pressure.

Initiation of Mechanical Ventilation

Hemodynamic compromise is common when mechanical ventilation is started. Mean intrathoracic pressure transitions from negative to positive when mechanical ventilation is begun. Adequate ventilation and oxygenation may result in decreased autonomic tone. Sedation is frequently provided at the initiation of mechanical ventilation,

Table 14-3 **Indications for Mechanical Ventilation**

- Apnea
- Acute ventilatory failure
- Impending acute ventilatory failure
- Severe oxygenation deficit

which can lead to hypotension. The hemodynamic compromise associated with the initiation of mechanical ventilation may need to be treated with fluid administration and vasoactive drugs.

Initial Ventilator Settings

Actual ventilator settings depend on the level of patient interaction with the ventilator, the underlying pathophysiology, and the respiratory mechanics. Patients of similar size and age, one presenting with a drug overdose and the other with severe asthma, should not be ventilated in the same manner.

Mode

There is much controversy over the best mode and little evidence to direct the choice of mode. More importantly, during the initial phases of mechanical ventilation, full support should usually be provided. This may be accomplished with continuous mandatory ventilation (assist/control) applied as either volume-controlled ventilation (VCV) or pressure-controlled ventilation (PCV). The key is to set the rate high enough to ensure little if any spontaneous effort is required by the patient.

Volume and Pressure Levels

Because of concern regarding ventilator-induced lung injury, plateau pressure should not exceed 30 cm H_2O unless chest wall compliance is reduced. The V_T should be 4 to 8 mL/kg ideal body weight (IBW). Patients with normal lungs (eg, overdose, postoperative) should have the V_T set at 6 to 8 mL/kg IBW and those with lung disease should receive a V_T of 4 to 8 mL/kg (Table 14-4). The IBW used to set the absolute tidal volume is calculated as:

$$\text{Male} = 50 + 2.3 \, (\text{ht [in]} - 60) \text{ kg}$$
$$\text{Female} = 45.5 + 2.3 \, (\text{ht [in]} - 60) \text{ kg}$$

Table 14-4 Initial V_T and Rate

- Normal pulmonary mechanics
  - V_T 6-8 mL/kg
  - Rate 15-20 breaths/min
- Acute lung injury
  - V_T 4-8 mL/kg
  - Rate 20-25/min
- Obstructive lung disease
  - V_T 4-8 mL/kg
  - Rate 8-12 breaths/min

Note: Keep plateau pressure less than 30 cm H_2O unless chest wall compliance is decreased.

Setting of pressure control is determined by the tidal volume (V_T) delivered. Pressure levels should be set to achieve a V_T similar that that with VCV. Regardless of approach used to deliver V_T, the actual volume delivered to a patient's lungs should be small (4-8 mL/kg) in patients with lung disease, and may be moderate (6-8 mL/kg IBW) in patients with normal lungs.

Flow Pattern, Peak Flow, and Inspiratory Time

With VCV, the peak flow and flow pattern are set on the ventilator. Although a descending ramp flow pattern may potentially improve V_T distribution, a rectangular flow pattern may be equally acceptable during the initiation of mechanical ventilation. Peak flow should be set initially to produce an inspiratory time less than or equal to 1 second. For patients triggering the ventilator, flow and inspiratory time should be set according to inspiratory demand. Inspiratory time should be set so that it is less than the expiratory time to avoid air trapping and hemodynamic compromise.

Rate

The rate chosen depends on tidal volume, pulmonary mechanics, and $Paco_2$ (Table 14-4). For patients with obstructive lung disease, lower rate in the range of 8 to 12/min, as well as lower minute ventilation, are set low to avoid the development of auto-positive end-expiratory pressure (auto-PEEP). For patients with acute lung injury, an initial rate of 20 to 25/min is generally adequate to produce an acceptable minute ventilation. Patients with normal lungs usually tolerate an initial rate set at 15 to 20/min. Adjustments to rate are made after monitoring the effect of mechanical ventilation.

Fio_2 and PEEP

At initiation of mechanical ventilation, Fio_2 of 1.0 is recommended and then titrated to 88% to 95% oxygen saturation measured with pulse oximetry, for a Pao_2 of 55 to 80 mm Hg. An initial PEEP of 5 cm H_2O is set to maintain functional residual capacity and prevent atelectasis. In the setting of acute lung injury, higher levels of PEEP are appropriate.

Ethical Considerations

Before committing a patient to mechanical ventilatory support, consideration should be given to the reversibility of the disease process. If there is little likelihood of reversing the acute disease process, the potential for long-term ventilation must be weighed against the result of not providing ventilatory support. Noninvasive ventilation may be appropriate while discussions regarding the advisability of intubation and long-term support can be evaluated. In some patients, such as those with progressive neuromuscular disease, either full time noninvasive ventilation or tracheostomy with long-term ventilation initiated as per patient wishes.

Points to Remember

- Respiratory failure may occur as a result of respiratory muscle weakness, excessive ventilatory load, a compromised central ventilatory drive, or a combination of these.
- Respiratory drive may be depressed by drugs, hypothyroidism, or neurologic lesions.
- Physiologic indications for mechanical ventilation are apnea, acute respiratory failure, impeding respiratory failure, and severe oxygenation deficit.
- During initial selection of ventilatory mode, continuous mandatory ventilation (CMV) (assist/control) with either volume-controlled ventilation (VCV) or pressure-controlled ventilation is recommended, provided that rate is set to ensure full ventilatory support.
- The tidal volume and pressure levels should be set based on pulmonary mechanics, pathophysiology, and a maximum plateau pressure of 30 cm H_2O.
- Set V_T at 6 to 8 mL/kg ideal body weight (IBW) in patients with normal lungs, and 4 to 8 mL/kg IBW in patients with lung disease.
- Initial inspiratory flow pattern with VCV should be set to ensure an inspiratory time less than or equal to 1 second.
- Respiratory rate is set based on V_T, pulmonary mechanics, and targeted Pa_{CO_2}.
- Initial F_{IO_2} should be set at 1 and then adjusted based on pulse oximetry.
- Ventilatory support should not be initiated unless the acute process necessitating ventilation is reversible.
- Tracheostomy and long-term ventilation may be initiated in some cases based on patient's wishes.

Additional Reading

Fuller BM, Mohr NM, Drewry AM, Carpenter CR. Lower tidal volume at initiation of mechanical ventilation may reduce progression to acute respiratory distress syndrome—a systematic review. *Crit Care.* 2013;18;17:R11.

Gattinoni L. Counterpoint: is low tidal volume mechanical ventilation preferred for all patients on ventilation? No. *Chest.* 2011;140:11-13.

Gattinoni L, Carlesso E, Langer T. Towards ultraprotective mechanical ventilation. *Curr Opin Anaesthesiol.* 2012;25:141-147.

Hubmayr RD. Point: is low tidal volume mechanical ventilation preferred for all patients on ventilation? Yes. *Chest.* 2011;140:9-11.

Lipes J, Bojmehrani A, Lellouche F. Low tidal volume ventilation in patients without acute respiratory distress syndrome: a paradigm shift in mechanical ventilation. *Crit Care Res Pract.* 2012;2012:416862.

Mohr NM, Fuller BM. Low tidal volume ventilation should be the routine ventilation strategy of choice for all emergency department patients. *Ann Emerg Med.* 2012;60:215-216.

Nyquist P, Stevens RD, Mirski MA. Neurologic injury and mechanical ventilation. *Neurocrit Care.* 2008;9:400-408.

Papadakos PJ, Karcz M, Lachmann B. Mechanical ventilation in trauma. *Curr Opin Anaesthesiol.* 2010;23:228-32.

Ramsey CD, Funk D, Miller RR, Kumar A. Ventilator management for hypoxemic respiratory failure attributable to H1N1 novel swine origin influenza virus. *Crit Care Med.* 2010; 38(4 Suppl):e58-e65.

Rose L. Clinical application of ventilator modes: ventilatory strategies for lung protection. *Aust Crit Care.* 2010;23:71-80.

Chapter 15
Patient-Ventilator Asynchrony

Introduction

Asynchrony is a mismatch between the neural respiratory drive of the patient and the ventilator response. It is relatively common and has been associated with a longer stay on mechanical ventilation, although cause and effect has not been established. To the extent that asynchrony is stressful for the patient, it is generally agreed that good patient-ventilator synchrony is desirable. How a patient interacts with the ventilator is determined by many factors (Figure 15-1). These include the underlying disease process, the effects of therapeutic interventions, ventilator performance, and how the

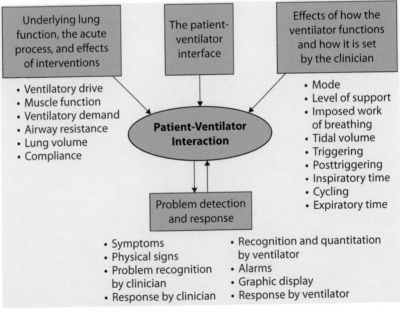

Figure 15-1 Schematic representation of factors that influence patient-ventilator interaction. (Reproduced with permission from Pierson DJ. Patient-ventilator interaction. *Respir Care.* 2011; Feb; 56(2):214-228.)

clinician sets the ventilator. In this chapter, the causes of asynchrony and appropriate clinical responses are described.

Trigger Asynchrony

Trigger asynchrony occurs when the initiation of the inspiratory phase does not occur with the onset of the patient's inspiratory effort. In other words, there is a lack of synchrony between the onset of neural inspiration and the response of the ventilator. It can occur either because the ventilator autotriggers or because the patient has difficulty triggering the ventilator. The ventilator trigger sensitivity should be set as sensitive as possible without causing autotriggering. Although flow triggering is commonly used, there is little difference between flow triggering and pressure triggering on modern ventilators.

Autotriggering causes the ventilator to trigger in response to an artifact. One such artifact is cardiac oscillations, in which the heart beating against the lungs produces sufficient flow or pressure change at the proximal airway to trigger the ventilator (Figure 15-2). This is addressed by adjusting the trigger sensitivity. Other causes of autotriggering include excessive water condensation in the ventilator circuit and leaks in the circuit. This is addressed by draining water from the circuit and correcting the leak. Leak compensation is useful during noninvasive ventilation to minimize autotriggering.

Inability of the patient to trigger can be caused by an insensitive trigger setting on the ventilator. It can also be due to respiratory muscle weakness. But perhaps the most common cause of failure to trigger is auto-positive end-expiratory pressure (auto-PEEP or intrinsic PEEP) in patients with obstructive airways disease. If the patient's inspiratory effort is not sufficient to counterbalance the auto-PEEP, the result is a missed trigger (Figure 15-3). Using PEEP to counterbalance auto-PEEP can be effective for patients with chronic obstructive pulmonary disease (COPD) (Figure 15-4), but this is only effective in the setting of flow limitation. When PEEP is used to counterbalance auto-PEEP, care must be taken to avoid additional hyperinflation with the addition of PEEP. If the peak inspiratory pressure increases when PEEP is added (during volume-controlled ventilation [VCV]), overdistention should be suspected. Triggering will also be improved by reduction of auto-PEEP through lowering minute ventilation, shortening the I:E ratio, or reducing airway obstruction through administration of bronchodilators and clearing of secretions. Note that, in the presence of auto-PEEP, flow triggering is no better than pressure triggering because the patient must generate enough effort to overcome auto-PEEP before either the pressure or the flow changes at the proximal airway.

Neural efforts triggered by the ventilator are called reverse-triggered breaths. They occur at the transition from the ventilator inspiration to expiration (Figure 15-5). Of concern is that, reverse triggering can result in breath stacking and overdistention.

Flow Asynchrony

Flow asynchrony occurs when the ventilator does not meet the inspiratory flow demand of the patient. This can be seen on the airway pressure waveform. With asynchrony,

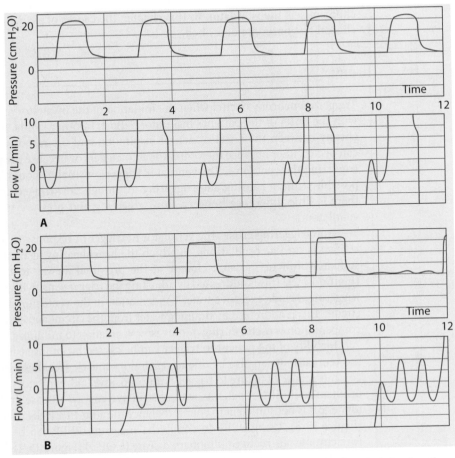

Figure 15-2 (A) Cardiac oscillations triggering the ventilator at a rate of 24 breaths/min when the flow trigger is set at 2 L/min. (B) After changing the flow trigger to 8 L/min, the ventilator rate is 16 breaths/min, which is what is set on the ventilator. The cardiac oscillations are producing a flow of 4 to 6 L/min at the proximal airway.

the pressure waveform with each breath differs from every other, and there is breath-to-breath variability in the peak airway pressure (Figure 15-6). Clinical signs of flow asynchrony include tachypnea, retractions, and chest-abdominal paradox. Strategies to address flow asynchrony include increasing the flow setting or changing the inspiratory flow pattern during VCV, by changing from VCV to pressure-controlled ventilation (PCV), or by increasing in the pressure setting or the rise time setting during PCV or pressure support ventilation (PSV).

Whether synchrony is better with PCV than VCV is debatable. Some have reported better synchrony with PCV, but others have not been able to confirm this. Some clinicians favor PCV because it allows the patient to increase flow if respiratory drive increases. However, with pressure-targeted modes such as PCV and PSV, inspiratory

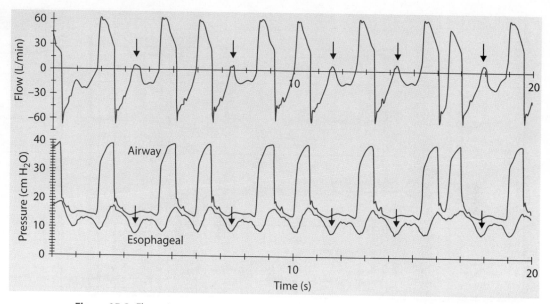

Figure 15-3 Flow, airway pressure, and esophageal pressure waveforms of a patient with chronic obstructive pulmonary disease and auto-positive end-expiratory pressure. The arrows indicate missed trigger efforts.

flow and tidal volume are determined by the difference between airway pressure and pleural pressure. Although pressure-targeted modes maintain a constant pressure applied to the airway, any additional effort from the patient will lower the pleural pressure and the transpulmonary pressure will increase (Figure 15-7). This may make it

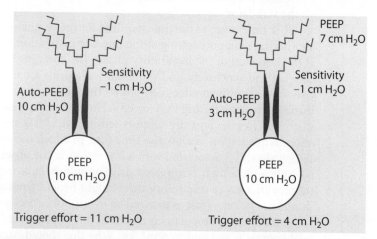

Figure 15-4 With an auto-positive end-expiratory pressure (auto-PEEP) of 10 cm H_2O and a trigger sensitivity of −1 cm H_2O, the patient must generate an inspiratory effort of 11 cm H_2O to trigger the ventilator. When the PEEP is increased to 7 cm H_2O, the inspiratory effort of the patient required to trigger the ventilator is only 4 cm H_2O. With flow limitation, PEEP set counterbalances the auto-PEEP.

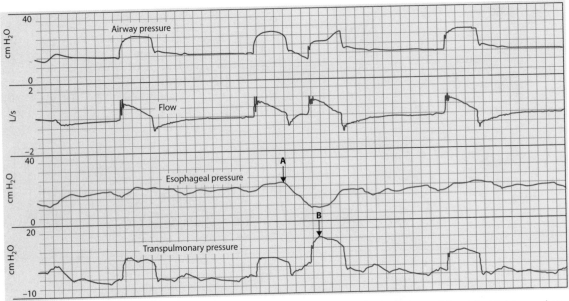

Figure 15-5 An example of reverse triggered breaths. The neural effort of the patient is triggered at the end of the ventilator inspiratory phase (A). This results in breath stacking and a greater transpulmonary pressure (B).

difficult to avoid alveolar overdistention with pressure-targeted modes in the setting of a vigorous inspiratory drive. In the hands of a skilled clinician, either VCV or PCV can be used effectively; what is most important is limitation of tidal volume and alveolar distending pressure in a manner that promotes synchrony, regardless of the mode set on the ventilator.

Rise time refers to the time required for the ventilator to reach the pressure control and pressure support setting at the onset of inspiration. It is the rate of pressurization at the initiation of the inspiratory phase. The rise time should be adjusted to patient's comfort and synchrony, and ventilator waveforms are useful to guide this setting. The rise-time adjustment effectively allows the clinician to set the flow at the onset of the inspiratory phase during PCV or PSV. Note that a fast rise time (one in which the ventilator reaches the pressure support setting quickly) is associated with high flow at the onset of inspiration. A slow rise time (one in which the ventilator reaches the pressure setting slowly) is associated with a lower flow at the onset of inhalation. Theoretically, patients with a high respiratory drive should benefit from a fast rise time, whereas those with a lower respiratory drive might benefit from a slower rise time. Rise time should not be set so fast as to avoid an overshoot of pressure at the onset of inspiration.

It is the perception of many clinicians that patient-ventilator asynchrony occurs when tidal volume is reduced to 6 mL/kg. Why this should occur is unclear. A normal tidal volume is 6 to 8 mL/kg, so it would seem that this tidal volume should be comfortable during mechanical ventilation. There are several potential reasons why a tidal volume of 6 to 8 mL/kg might not be comfortable in patients with acute respiratory disease syndrome

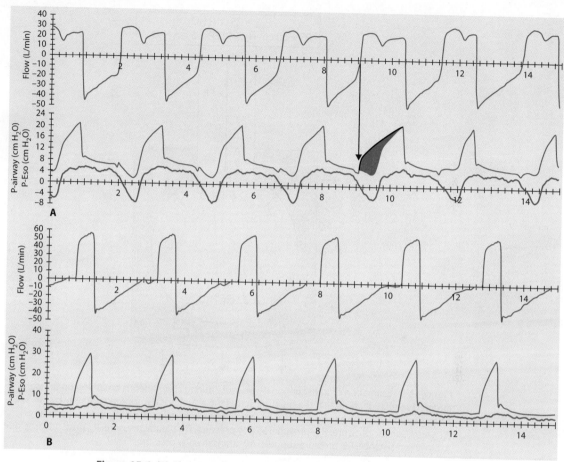

Figure 15-6 (A) Flow asynchrony in which the inspiratory effort of the patient is not met by the fixed flow from the ventilator during volume-controlled ventilation. The dashed line represents the airway pressure curve that would result from passive inflation, and the shaded area represents the work done by the patient against the insufficient flow from the ventilator. (B) When the flow setting of the ventilator is increased, the patient is synchronous with the ventilator.

(ARDS). First, dead space is increased with ARDS and, thus, respiratory acidosis will occur unless minute ventilation is increased. Respiratory rates up to 35 breaths/min are used in an attempt to avoid acidosis. Another potential reason for asynchrony is pain and anxiety due to endotracheal intubation and the disease process. Thus, adequate attention should be given to address these discomforts. A number of strategies can be used to improve patient-ventilator synchrony during lung-protective ventilation (Table 15-1).

Cycle Asynchrony

The ventilator should cycle to exhalation at the end of the neural inspiratory time. If the breath terminates before the end of neural inhalation, the patient may double-trigger

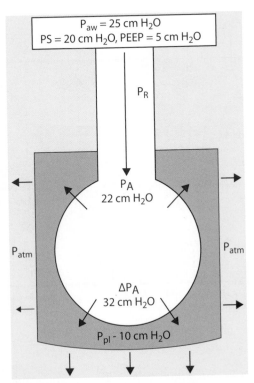

Figure 15-7 Estimation of transpulmonary pressure during spontaneous breathing on pressure-targeted ventilation. Note that the pressure across the alveolus is determined not only by the pressure applied to the airway, but also by the change in pleural pressure. P_A, alveolar pressure; P_{atm}, atmospheric pressure; P_{aw}, proximal airway pressure; P_{pl}, pleural pressure; P_R, pressure drop due to airways resistance; PS, pressure support; ΔP_A, transalveolar pressure.

the ventilator. Even if the patient does not double-trigger, a distinctive flow waveform suggests that the ventilator cycled prematurely (Figure 15-8). If breath delivery continues into neural exhalation, the patient may actively exhale causing the ventilator to pressure-cycle.

During VCV, double triggering can cause breath stacking, such that the patient is effectively receiving a tidal volume twice what is set. For a set tidal volume, the inspiratory time is determined primarily by the peak flow and flow pattern. In the setting of double triggering, decreasing the peak flow setting or switching from constant flow to a descending ramp of flow will lengthen the inspiratory time. Inspiratory time is also lengthened by adding pause time. With PCV, the inspiratory time is either set directly or by the I:E ratio. If double triggering occurs and the inspiratory time is lengthened with PCV, this may also result in an end-inspiratory pause.

During PSV, the ventilator is normally flow-cycled at a fraction of the peak flow. Secondary cycle criteria are pressure (if the pressure exceeds the pressure support target) and time (if the inspiratory phase is prolonged). The inspiratory time during PSV is determined by lung mechanics and the flow cycle criteria. With decreased

---

Table 15-1 Approaches to Patient-Ventilator Asynchrony.

1. Sedation, analgesia, paralysis: Adequate sedation and analgesia are necessary during mechanical ventilation regardless of tidal volume. Factors such as agitation, delirium, metabolic acidosis, drug withdrawal, septic encephalopathy, and pain need to be considered. Neuromuscular blocking agents should be considered in the 48 h following intubation in patients with severe lung injury, otherwise, paralysis should only be used to achieve patient-ventilator synchrony if sedation and analgesia are insufficient and when other methods described here have been exhausted.

2. Respiratory rate: An increase in respiratory rate setting on the ventilator may match the breathing pattern of the patient to the ventilator, thereby enhancing synchrony. Increasing the respiratory rate setting decreases work-of-breathing and increases patient's comfort. During transition to lower tidal volume ventilation, the respiratory rate should be increased as tidal volume is decreased to maintain constant minute ventilation.

3. Tidal volume: An increase in V_T, if accompanied by an increase in alveolar ventilation, decreases respiratory drive. The ARDSNet protocol allows tidal volume to be increased to 8 mL/kg IBW in the case of asynchrony and severe dyspnea, provided plateau pressure is ≤ 30 cm H_2O.

4. Trigger sensitivity: Set trigger as sensitive as possible without causing autotriggering.

5. Auto-PEEP: Minimize auto-PEEP.

6. Inspiratory flow: An increase in inspiratory flow may better meet the flow demand of the patient and improve patient's comfort. A higher inspiratory flow also decreases neural inspiratory time, which results in a greater spontaneous breathing frequency and may further contribute to asynchrony.

7. Inspiratory time: A shorter inspiratory time (higher inspiratory flow during VCV) may improve patient-ventilator synchrony. If the inspiratory time setting on the ventilator is less than the neural inspiratory time, however, double triggering and worsening asynchrony may occur. In this case, a longer inspiratory time may be appropriate.

8. Flow waveform: Asynchrony may improve with a descending flow waveform in some patients. For the same peak flow, inspiratory time is longer with a descending flow, which may achieve the goal of better synchrony because of the higher flow while avoiding double triggering secondary to an inspiratory time that is too short.

9. PCV: PCV achieves the goals of a descending flow waveform and an adjustable inspiratory time independent of flow. PCV may result in better synchrony in some patients. A limitation of PCV is the possibility that transpulmonary pressure (an important determinant of volutrauma) may increase because of the generation of high negative intrapleural pressure swings, consequently increasing delivered tidal volume. For the same tidal volume and inspiratory flow, work-of-breathing is likely the same for PCV and VCV.

10. Pressure rise time: With PCV, the clinician can adjust the rate of rise in pressure at the onset of the inspiratory phase. If the pressure rises more quickly, flow is higher at the beginning of inhalation, which might affect work-of-breathing and patient's comfort.

Abbreviations: IBW, ideal body weight; PCV, pressure-controlled ventilation; PEEP, positive end-expiratory pressure; VCV, volume-controlled ventilation.

compliance, the flow cycle is reached earlier in the inspiratory phase, and the result is early inspiratory termination and the potential for double triggering. With an increased compliance and increased resistance, as occurs with COPD, there is a slow descent in flow, meaning that the flow cycle criteria will be reached later and the inspiratory phase will be prolonged. Prolongation of the inspiratory phase can result in air-trapping and

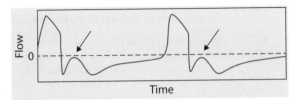

Figure 15-8 Flow waveform when the patient's neural inspiratory time is greater than the inspiratory time set on the ventilator. The arrows represent the patient's continued inspiratory effort after the ventilator cycles to exhalation.

dynamic hyperinflation. This can also result in activation of the expiratory muscles, which can be detected clinically by palpation of the patient's abdomen or observing the pressure waveform for a pressure increase at the end of the inspiratory phase (Figure 15-9). Prolonged inspiration causing cycle asynchrony during PSV can be corrected by lowering the pressure support level, by an increase in the termination

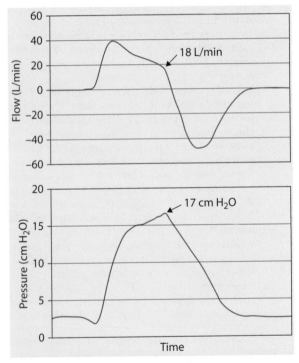

Figure 15-9 An example of delayed termination of inhalation during pressure support ventilation in a patient with chronic obstructive pulmonary disease. The pressure support is 12 cm H_2O and positive end-expiratory pressure is 3 cm H_2O, so the inspiratory pressure target is 15 cm H_2O. Note that the ventilator cycles at a flow of 18 L/min, despite the flow termination criteria being set at 25% of the peak flow. The pressure increase above the set level of pressure support causes the ventilator to pressure-cycle in response to the patient's active exhalation. (Reproduced with permission from Branson RD, Campbell RS. Pressure support ventilation, patient ventilator synchrony, and ventilator algorithms (editorial). *Respir Care.* 1998; Dec; 43(12):1045-1047).

flow setting, or by use of pressure control instead of pressure support (pressure control causes inspiration to be time-cycled rather than flow-cycled).

Mode Asynchrony

Although asynchrony can occur with any mode, the potential is greater for some modes. With synchronized intermittent mandatory ventilation, for example, asynchrony can occur because of the different mandatory and spontaneous breath types. This is because the patient's inspiratory effort is often no different for the mandatory and spontaneous breaths (Figure 15-10). With volume-targeted adaptive pressure modes (eg, pressure-regulated volume control, volume support), asynchrony can occur because the ventilator reduces support if the tidal volume exceeds the target. There are also modes that enhance synchrony, specifically proportional assist ventilation (PAV) and neurally adjusted ventilatory assist (NAVA). These modes vary ventilator support according to respiratory drive, provided that the patient does not have neuromuscular disease.

Due to lack of a backup rate, periodic breathing (Figure 15-11) and sleep fragmentation can occur with PSV. This is due to hyperventilation when awake and loss of wakefulness drive to breathe during sleep. It can be corrected by reducing the level of

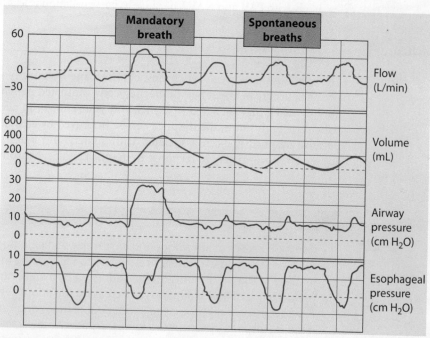

Figure 15-10 Synchronized intermittent mandatory ventilation. Note that the esophageal pressure change for the mandatory breath is nearly as great as that for the spontaneous breaths.

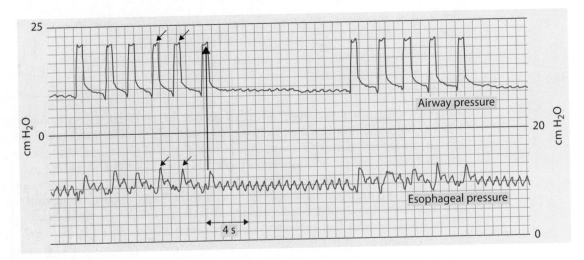

Figure 15-11 Periodic breathing in a patient receiving pressure support ventilation. Note the period of apnea interspersed with triggered breaths. Also note the asynchrony due to forced exhalation to cycle the breath (arrows).

pressure support (making hyperventilation less likely) or using a mode with a backup rate (continuous mandatory ventilation). Periodic breathing and sleep fragmentation is less likely with PAV and NAVA because hyperventilation is less likely with these modes.

Synchrony Versus Comfort Versus Dyspnea

The relationship between synchrony, comfort, and dyspnea has not been well studied. Dyspnea occurs in about half of mechanically ventilated patients who are not sedated, but how often that is related to asynchrony is unknown. In about a third of ventilated patients with dyspnea, the dyspnea can be improved by changes in ventilator settings. Because dyspnea is often associated with anxiety and pain, these factors should be addressed appropriately in response to dyspnea and asynchrony.

Points to Remember

- Common causes of autotriggering are cardiac oscillations and leaks.
- Auto-positive end-expiratory pressure (auto-PEEP) is the most common cause of inability to trigger, and this can be addressed by increasing the PEEP setting in the presence of flow limitation or decreasing the minute ventilation.
- If the set inspiratory time is too short, double triggering can occur.
- If the set inspiratory time is too long, the patient may actively exhale in an attempt to terminate the inspiratory phase.

- The flow cycle criteria can be adjusted during pressure support ventilation to address cycle asynchrony.
- Some ventilator modes increase the potential for asynchrony, whereas others improve patient-ventilator interaction.
- Dyspnea occurs commonly during mechanical ventilation, but it is unclear whether it is associated with asynchrony.

Additional Reading

Akoumianaki E, Lyazidi A, Rey N, et al. Mechanical ventilation-induced reverse-triggered breaths: a frequently unrecognized form of neuromechanical coupling. *Chest.* 2013;143:927-938.

Branson RD. Patient-ventilator interaction: the last 40 years. *Respir Care.* 2011;56:15-24.

Branson RD, Blakeman TC, Robinson BR. Asynchrony and dyspnea. *Respir Care.* 2013;58: 973-989.

de Wit M. Monitoring of patient-ventilator interaction at the bedside. *Respir Care.* 2011;56:61-72.

Epstein SK. How often does patient-ventilator asynchrony occur and what are the consequences? *Respir Care.* 2011;56:25-38.

Gentile MA. Cycling of the mechanical ventilator breath. *Respir Care.* 2011;56:52-60.

Hess DR, Thompson BT. Patient-ventilator dyssynchrony during lung protective ventilation: what's a clinician to do? *Crit Care Med.* 2006;34:231-233.

Hess DR. Patient-ventilator interaction during noninvasive ventilation. *Respir Care.* 2011;56:153-167.

Kacmarek RM. Proportional assist ventilation and neurally adjusted ventilatory assist. *Respir Care.* 2011;56:140-152.

MacIntyre NR. Patient-ventilator interactions: optimizing conventional ventilation modes. *Respir Care.* 2011;56:73-84.

Pierson DJ. Patient-ventilator interaction. *Respir Care.* 2011;56:214-228.

Robinson BR, Blakeman TC, Toth P, et al. Patient-ventilator asynchrony in a traumatically injured population. *Respir Care.* 2013;58:1847-1855.

Sassoon CSH. Triggering of the ventilator in patient-ventilator interactions. *Respir Care.* 2011;56:39-51.

Schmidt M, Demoule A, Polito A, et al. Dyspnea in mechanically ventilated critically ill patients. *Crit Care Med.* 2011;39:2059-2065.

Chapter 16
Ventilator Liberation

> ### Objectives
>
> 1. Identify patients ready for ventilator discontinuation.
> 2. Discuss the important role of the spontaneous breathing trial (SBT) to determine extubation readiness.
> 3. Contrast the approaches used to wean patients from ventilatory support.
> 4. List causes of a failed SBT.
> 5. Discuss the role of sedation in the ventilator discontinuation process.
> 6. Discuss the use of ventilator discontinuation protocols.
> 7. Discuss criteria used to indicate readiness for extubation.
> 8. Discuss issues related to prolonged mechanical ventilation and chronic critical illness.

Introduction

The ultimate goal of mechanical ventilation is ventilator discontinuation. Most patients can be liberated from the ventilator when the physiologic reason for ventilatory support is reversed. In others, this may be a more prolonged process and associated with chronic critical illness. Because of their underlying disease process, some patients may become chronically ventilator-dependent (eg, those with neuromuscular disease). This chapter addresses issues defining readiness for ventilator discontinuation, assessments that predict readiness for ventilator liberation, approaches to liberation from ventilator support, use of protocols, automated weaning, and assessment for extubation. The content of this chapter is written to be consistent with evidence-based clinical practice guidelines (Table 16-1).

Assessing Readiness for Ventilator Discontinuation

There are four commonsense factors to be assessed to determine readiness for ventilator discontinuation: (1) reversal of the indication for ventilator support, (2) adequate gas exchange, (3) ability to initiate a breath, and (4) hemodynamic stability.

Reversal of Indication for Ventilator Support

The most important indicator of readiness for discontinuation of ventilatory support is some reversal of the indication for ventilatory support. In addition to respiratory failure, this includes consideration of fever, nutrition, and electrolyte balance. Renal, liver, or gastrointestinal dysfunction may adversely impact the ability to liberate the patient from the ventilator and, thus, attention should be given to correcting these abnormalities.

Gas Exchange

There should be acceptable gas exchange before initiation of the ventilator discontinuation process. From an oxygenation perspective, this typically means a Pao_2 more than

Table 16-1 ACCP-SCCM-AARC Evidence-Based Ventilator Weaning/Discontinuation Guidelines[a]

1. In patients requiring mechanical ventilation for more than 24 h, a search for all causes that may be contributing to ventilator dependence should be undertaken. Reversing all possible ventilatory and nonventilatory issues should be an integral part of the ventilator discontinuation process.

2. Patients receiving mechanical ventilation for respiratory failure should undergo a formal assessment of discontinuation potential if the following criteria are satisfied: evidence for some reversal of the underlying cause for respiratory failure, adequate oxygenation and pH, hemodynamic stability, and capability to initiate an inspiratory effort.

3. Formal discontinuation assessments for patients receiving mechanical ventilation for respiratory failure should be done during spontaneous breathing rather than while the patient is still receiving substantial ventilatory support.

4. Removal of the artificial airway from a patient who has successfully been discontinued from ventilatory support should be based upon assessments of airway patency and the ability of the patient to protect the airway.

5. Patients receiving mechanical ventilation for respiratory failure who fail an SBT should have the cause for the failed SBT determined. Once reversible causes for failure are corrected, subsequent SBTs should be performed every 24 h.

6. Patients receiving mechanical ventilation for respiratory failure who fail an SBT should receive a stable, nonfatiguing, comfortable form of ventilatory support.

7. Anesthesia/sedation strategies and ventilator management aimed at early extubation should be used in postsurgical patients.

8. Weaning/discontinuation protocols designed for nonphysician health care professionals should be developed and implemented by ICUs. Protocols aimed at optimizing sedation should also be developed and implemented.

9. Tracheostomy should be considered after an initial period of stabilization on the ventilator when it becomes apparent that the patient will require prolonged ventilator assistance.

10. Unless there is evidence for clearly irreversible disease (eg, high spinal cord injury, advanced amyotrophic lateral sclerosis), a patient requiring prolonged mechanical ventilatory support for respiratory failure should not be considered permanently ventilator-dependent until 3 months of weaning attempts have failed.

11. When medically stable for transfer, patients who have failed ventilator discontinuation attempts in the ICU should be transferred to those facilities that have demonstrated success and safety in accomplishing ventilator discontinuation.

12. Weaning strategy in the prolonged mechanically ventilated patient should be slow-paced, and should include gradually lengthening self-breathing trials.

Abbreviations: ICU, intensive care unit; SBT, spontaneous breathing trial.
[a]See MacIntyre NR, Cook DJ, Ely EW, et al. Evidence-based guidelines for weaning and discontinuing ventilator support. *Chest.* 2001;120:375S-395S for the complete text.

60 mm Hg with an F_{IO_2} less than or equal to 0.50 and positive end-expiratory pressure (PEEP) less than or equal to 8 cm H_2O. A high ventilation requirement for a pH more than 7.25 decreases the likelihood of successful liberation. A dead space to tidal volume ratio (V_D/V_T) less than 60% and a minute ventilation less than 12 L/min is associated with a greater potential for ventilator liberation.

Ability to Initiate a Breath

To be liberated from mechanical ventilation, the patient must be able to initiate a breath. This means that there are no central ventilatory drive issues. The principal reason for ventilatory drive suppression is excessive sedation. For this reason, a spontaneous awakening trial (SAT) in which sedation is stopped is an important step in the ventilator liberation process. A daily SAT safety screen should be performed, which consists of the following: not receiving a sedative infusion except for active seizures or alcohol withdrawal, not receiving escalating sedative doses due to ongoing agitation, not receiving neuromuscular blockers, no evidence of active myocardial ischemia in the past 24 hours, and no evidence of increased intracranial pressure. Patients passing the screen should receive an SAT, during which time all sedatives and analgesics used for sedation are stopped for up to 4 hours, but analgesics needed for active pain are continued. Patients are deemed to have passed the SAT if they open their eyes to verbal stimuli. Patients are deemed to have failed the SAT if they develop sustained anxiety, agitation, or pain; respiratory rate more than 35 breaths/min for 5 minutes or longer; Spo_2 less than 88% for 5 minutes or longer; acute cardiac dysrhythmia; or two or more signs of respiratory distress including tachycardia, bradycardia, use of accessory muscles, abdominal paradox, diaphoresis, or marked dyspnea. For a failed SAT, sedatives are started at half the previous dose and then titrated to achieve patient's comfort.

The choice of sedative agent may also affect the ventilator liberation process. Benzodiazepine administration is associated with the development of delirium, and delirium has been associated with a longer period of ventilator dependence. On the other hand, when compared with a benzodiazepine, use of dexmedetomidine resulted in less time on the ventilator and less delirium.

Hemodynamic Stability

Cardiovascular function should be optimized before initiation of the ventilator discontinuation process. Arrhythmias, fluid overload, and myocardial contractility should be managed appropriately. The patient should be hemodynamically stable with minimal cardiovascular support, no cardiac ischemia, and no unstable arrhythmia.

Weaning Parameters

A number of so-called weaning parameters have been introduced, the intent of which is to identify extubation readiness. Most predictors of weaning outcome focus on the ability to achieve or sustain a specific ventilatory parameter. Unfortunately, no predictive parameter is 100% accurate in identifying individuals who will successfully be liberated from the ventilator. In fact, the best predictor of successful ventilator liberation

Table 16-2 **Weaning Parameters Used to Predict Potential for Successful Ventilator Liberation**

Predictor	Value
• Evaluation of ventilatory drive	
– $P_{0.1}$	< 6 cm H_2O
• Ventilatory muscle capabilities	
– Vital capacity	> 10 mL/kg
– Maximum inspiratory pressure	< -30 cm H_2O
• Ventilatory performance	
– Minute ventilation	< 10 L/min
– Maximum voluntary ventilation	< 3 times $\dot{V}E$
– Rapid shallow breathing index	< 105
– Respiratory rate	< 30/min

is the patient's response to an SBT. High-level evidence supporting the use of weaning parameters is lacking.

The most commonly used predictors of weaning success are listed in Table 16-2. They are grouped into indices that evaluate ventilatory drive, ventilatory muscle capability, and ventilatory performance. The most accurate predictor of weaning success is the rapid-shallow breathing index (RSBI). This index is determined by dividing the respiratory rate by the tidal volume in liters, determined 1 minute after removing the patient from the ventilator. If the RSBI is less than or equal to 105, the probability of successful weaning is high and if it is more than 105, the probability of failure is high. However, more recent reports have shown that the RSBI may not be as highly predictive of ventilator liberation as originally reported.

Spontaneous Breathing Trials

The spontaneous breathing trial (SBT) is the best way to determine readiness for ventilator liberation. Patients who tolerate an SBT for 30 to 120 minutes should be considered liberated from ventilatory support and candidates for extubation. The traditional way of performing an SBT is with a T-piece connected to the endotracheal tube, providing humidified oxygen. Many clinicians use the ventilator for SBTs, which has the advantage of maintaining a precise FIO_2 and patient monitoring during the SBT. Moreover, if the SBT fails, ventilatory support can be quickly reestablished. If the SBT is to simulate a T-piece trial, the pressure support and PEEP should both be set at 0.

It is the practice of some clinicians to perform the SBT using low levels of pressure support (5-10 cm H_2O), PEEP (5 cm H_2O), or tube compensation. Most patients do equally well on T-piece trials, pressure support and PEEP set at 0, or low levels of pressure support and PEEP. The intent of using a low level of pressure support or tube compensation is to overcome the resistive load of the endotracheal tube. However, the resistive load of the endotracheal tube is usually not excessive unless the tube size is small. Patients with small endotracheal tubes or nasal intubation may benefit from

Table 16-3 Criteria for Failure of a Spontaneous Breathing Trial
• Respiratory rate > 35/min
• Use of accessory muscles
• Dyspnea
• Thoracoabdominal paradox
• Spo_2 < 90%
• Heart rate > 140/min or sustained 20% increase in heart rate
• Systolic BP > 180 mm Hg, diastolic > 90 mm Hg
• Anxiety
• Diaphoresis

the application of low levels of pressure support (5-10 cm H_2O). Otherwise, breathing through the endotracheal tube with no support from the ventilator closely simulates the resistance through the upper airway after extubation.

Use of low levels of PEEP during the SBT is discouraged. In patients with chronic obstructive pulmonary disease (COPD), the application of 5 cm H_2O PEEP during the SBT may counterbalance auto-PEEP. In patients with poor cardiac function, a low level of PEEP during the SBT may be sufficient to keep the patient out of failure. In patients with COPD or poor cardiac failure, the use of PEEP during the SBT might predict success, only to have the patient develop respiratory failure soon after extubation.

Patients successfully completing an SBT of 30 to 120 minutes are considered for extubation (Table 16-3). If the patient does not tolerate the SBT, the ventilator is set to provide a comfortable level of support. Once a comfortable level of support is provided, evidence is lacking for reducing the level of support before the next SBT. Before the next SBT, usually on the following day, an attempt should be made to identify and correct all potential causes of the failed SBT.

Approaches to a Failed Spontaneous Breathing Trial

A common reason for a failed SBT is an imbalance between the capacity of the respiratory muscles (weakness) and the load that is placed on them (Table 16-4). Causes of respiratory muscles weakness include critical illness weakness, electrolyte imbalance, malnutrition, and primary neuromuscular disease. An excessive respiratory muscle load can be the result of high airways resistance, as in the patient with COPD, or a low compliance, as in a patient with pneumonia or pulmonary edema. Auto-PEEP and a high minute ventilation requirement also increase the load on the respiratory muscles.

The maximal inspiratory pressure (Pi_{max}) is used to measure respiratory muscle strength. To ensure the best results, measurement of Pi_{max} should be performed at residual volume. To achieve this, a one-way valve as illustrated in Figure 16-1 is used. This allows exhalation but not inspiration. Thus the lung volume at which Pi_{max} is measured decreases with each breathing attempt. The Pi_{max} measurement should be performed for about 20 seconds provided no arrhythmias or desaturation occurs.

There is increasing evidence supporting the role of early mobility of critically ill mechanically ventilated patients. This improves skeletal muscle conditioning, including

Table 16-4 A Failed Spontaneous Breathing Trial is Often the Result of a Mismatch Between the Load on the Respiratory Muscles and the Capability of the Respiratory Muscles.

Respiratory muscle load	*Respiratory muscle capacity*
• **Minute ventilation**	• **Depressed respiratory drive**
– Pain and anxiety	– Sedative drugs
– Sepsis	– Brain stem lesion
– Increased dead space	• **Respiratory muscle weakness**
– Excessive feeding	– Primary neuromuscular disease
• **Increased resistance**	– Cervical spine or phrenic nerve injury
– Bronchospasm	– Critical illness polyneuropathy
– Secretions	– Hyperinflation
– Small endotracheal tube	– Malnutrition
• **Decreased Compliance**	– Electrolyte disturbance
– Low lung or chest wall compliance	• **Chest wall abnormality**
– Auto-PEEP and dynamic hyperinflation	– Flail chest
	– Pain

the respiratory muscles. Early mobility has also been associated with a lower incidence of delirium, which might also result in earlier liberation from mechanical ventilation.

Iatrogenic causes also contribute to a failed SBT. Examples included a partially obstructed endotracheal tube, dead space in the ventilator circuit, or increased airways resistance while breathing aerosolized water from the T-piece.

Gradual Reduction of Support and Automated Weaning

A gradual reduction in synchronized intermittent mandatory ventilation rate has been used for weaning. Similarly, a gradual reduction in the level of pressure support ventilation has been used for weaning. The intent in both cases is to gradually transfer the work-of-breathing from the ventilator to the respiratory muscles of the patient. However, evidence is lacking that gradual reductions of support facilitate liberation more quickly than daily SAT and SBT. Ventilator modes such as SmartCare are available that provide automated weaning. Although these automated modes may be equivalent to clinician-directed weaning, additional data supporting fewer ventilator days are needed before they can be recommended.

Protocols

A successful approach to liberating patients from ventilatory support is the use of protocols implemented by respiratory therapists and nurses. These protocols result in shorter

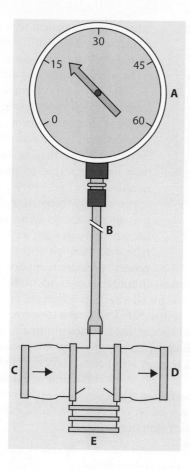

Figure 16-1 Apparatus used to determine PI_{max} for patients with artificial airways. (A) manometer; (B) Connecting tubing; (C) Inspiratory one-way valve with port for thumb occlusion; (D) Expiratory one-way valve with port; (E) 22-mm ID port for attachment to artificial airway. (Determination of maximal inspiratory pressure: a clinical study and literature review. *Respir Care*. 1989; Oct; 34(10):868-878.)

weaning times and shorter lengths of mechanical ventilation than traditional physician-directed weaning. The primary reason for the success of protocols is that they are developed by multidisciplinary teams and are implemented by respiratory therapists and nurses empowered to make clinical decisions. Although protocols can be developed for any approach to weaning, the approach that has been most commonly used is based on SBTs. Elements of a ventilator discontinuation protocol are shown in Figure 16-2.

Extubation

Once the patient has successfully completed an SBT of 30 to 120 minutes, consideration should be given for extubation. Even if the patient has successfully completed an SBT, many clinicians tend to be too conservative, wanting to avoid reintubation. Although reintubation is associated with morbidity and mortality risk, prolonged

Figure 16-2 An approach to ventilator liberation and extubation.

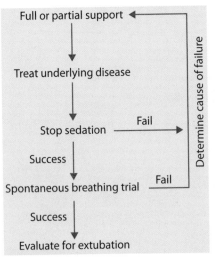

intubation in a patient who can be extubated is also associated with poorer outcomes. A reasonable reintubation rate in general medical or surgical units is about 10% to 20%.

Inability to perform four simple tasks (open eyes, follow with eyes, grasp hand, and stick out tongue), to generate a cough peak flow less than or equal to 60 L/min, and with secretions more than or equal to 2.5 mL/h have been reported to increase the risk of reintubation (Table 16-5). The potential for upper airway obstruction following extubation should always be considered. Deflating the cuff and assessing for air leak around the tube and through the upper airway when positive pressure is applied is sometimes performed to assess this. If no air movement around the tube is identified, this is suggestive of upper airway swelling and potential for airway obstruction after removal of the tube. However, use of the cuff leak test is associated with false-positive and false-negative results. Its use is controversial and should not be used routinely, but rather only in patients with a high probability of upper airway swelling. If upper airway swelling is suspected, a short course of steroid therapy is indicated before extubation, and personnel trained to reintubate should be at the bedside at the time of extubation.

In patients at risk for extubation failure, preventative use of noninvasive ventilation (NIV) is indicated. However, the use of NIV to rescue a failed extubation should be limited to patients with hypercapnic respiratory failure.

Prolonged Mechanical Ventilation and Chronic Critical Illness

The patient with chronic critical illness (CCI) has survived an acute critical illness or injury but has not yet recovered to the point of liberation from life-sustaining

Table 16-5 **Characteristics of Variables for Predicting Extubation Outcome**

Variable	Likelihood ratio	Risk ratio (95% CI)
Cough peak flow ≤ 60 L/min	2.2	4.8 (1.4-16.2)
Secretions ≥ 2.5 mL/h	1.9	3.0 (1.01-8.8)
Unable to perform all four tasks (open eyes, follow with eyes, grasp hand, and stick out tongue)	4.5	4.3 (1.8-10.4)
Any two of the above risks	3.8	6.7 (2.3-19.3)

Data from Salam A, Tilluckdharry L, Amoateng-Adjepong Y, Manthous CA. Neurologic status, cough, secretions and extubation outcomes. *Intensive Care Med.* 2004; Jul; 30(7):1334-1339.

therapies. Such patients are weak, deconditioned, often delirious or comatose, and receiving prolonged mechanical ventilation (PMV). Other forms of organ support such as vasopressors, inotropes, and renal replacement therapy may be required, and the patient may be receiving one of several courses of broad-spectrum antibiotics for ongoing or recurrent infections. A tracheostomy is often in place as well as a feeding tube. The decision about placing a tracheostomy is a point of demarcation often used to identify CCI, as is the need for PMV. A common definition of CCI is PMV more than or equal to 21 consecutive days for more than or equal to 6 h/d. When medically stable, patients who have failed ventilator discontinuation attempts in the ICU should be transferred to long-term acute-care facilities who have demonstrated success and safety in accomplishing ventilator discontinuation. Weaning strategy in the prolonged mechanically ventilated patient should be slow-paced, and should include gradually lengthening SBTs.

Patients with irreversible neuromuscular diseases who require long-term mechanical ventilation are a unique group. Unlike patients with CCI, they have not suffered from acute illnesses or injuries that involve systemic inflammation and multiorgan failure. Therefore their outcomes and resource needs are different than the typical patient with CCI. Important discussions regarding their care usually revolve around safe and effective provision of home mechanical ventilation rather than recovery from multiorgan failure. The relationships between CCI, PMV, and long-term mechanical ventilation are represented schematically in Figure 16-3. Unless there is evidence for clearly irreversible disease (eg, high spinal cord injury, advanced amyotrophic lateral sclerosis), a patient requiring prolonged mechanical ventilatory support for respiratory failure should not be considered permanently ventilator-dependent until 3 months of weaning attempts have failed.

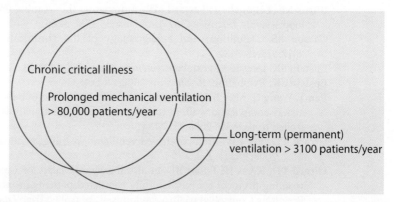

Figure 16-3 Relationship between chronic critical illness (CCI), prolonged mechanical ventilation (PMV), and long-term mechanical ventilation. Most CCI patients require PMV, but not all patients meeting various definitions of PMV would necessarily meet clinical definitions of CCI. Similarly, patients with single-organ dysfunction requiring long-term or home ventilation, such as patients with neuromuscular diseases, are unique and relatively few. Most clinical studies of CCI or PMV exclude those patients. (Reproduced with permission from Carson SS. Definitions and epidemiology of the chronically critically ill. *Respir Care.* 2012; Jun; 57(6):848-858.)

Points to Remember

- The primary prerequisite for ventilator discontinuation is some reversal of the indication for mechanical ventilation.
- Adequate gas exchange should be present, with minimal oxygenation and ventilatory support, before conducting a spontaneous breathing trial (SBT).
- Excessive sedation is a common reason why patients cannot be liberated from mechanical ventilation.
- Weaning parameters are poorly predictive.
- The SBT is the best way to determine if ventilator liberation is possible.
- The poorest weaning outcomes are with the use of synchronized intermittent mandatory ventilation.
- The use of ventilator discontinuation protocols effectively identifies when patients can be liberated from the ventilator.
- Extubation should be considered separately from ventilator liberation.
- A failed SBT is often due to an imbalance between the load on respiratory muscles and the capability of the muscles to meet that load.
- Postextubation noninvasive ventilation can be used to prevent extubation failure or to rescue failed extubation in patients with hypercapnic respiratory failure.

Additional Reading

Blackwood B, Alderdice F, Burns K, et al. Use of weaning protocols for reducing duration of mechanical ventilation in critically ill adult patients: cochrane systematic review and meta-analysis. *BMJ.* 2011;342:c7237.

Branson RD. Modes to facilitate ventilator weaning. *Respir Care.* 2012;57:1635-1648.

Burns KE, Lellouche F, Lessard MR. Automating the weaning process with advanced closed-loop systems. *Intensive Care Med.* 2008;34:1757-1765.

Carson SS. Definitions and epidemiology of the chronically critically ill. *Respir Care.* 2012;57:848-858.

Epstein SK. Decision to extubate. *Intensive Care Med.* 2002;28:535-546.

Epstein SK. Extubation. *Respir Care.* 2002;47(4):483-495.

Fan T, Wang G, Mao B, et al. Prophylactic administration of parenteral steroids for preventing airway complications after extubation in adults: meta-analysis of randomized placebo controlled trials. *BMJ.* 2008;337:a1841.

Girard TD, Ely EW. Protocol-driven ventilator weaning: reviewing the evidence. *Clin Chest Med.* 2008;29:241-252.

Girard TD, Kress JP, Fuchs BD, et al. Efficacy and safety of a paired sedation and ventilator weaning protocol for mechanically ventilated patients in intensive care (Awakening and Breathing Controlled trial): a randomised controlled trial. *Lancet.* 2008;371:126-134.

Haas C, Loik P. Ventilator discontinuation protocols. *Respir Care.* 2012;57:1649-1662.

Hess D, Branson RD. Ventilators and weaning modes. *Respir Care Clin N Am.* 2000;6:407-435.

Hess DR, MacIntyre NR. Ventilator discontinuation: why are we still weaning? *Am J Respir Crit Care Med.* 2011;184:392-394.

Hess DR. The role of noninvasive ventilation in the ventilator discontinuation process. *Respir Care.* 2012;57:1619-1625.

Khamiees M, Raju P, DeGirolamo A, et al. Predictors of extubation and outcome in patients who have successfully completed a spontaneous breathing trial. *Chest.* 2001;120:1262-1270.

King AC. Long-term home mechanical ventilation in the united states. *Respir Care.* 2012;57: 921-932.

King CS, Moores LK, Epstein SK. Should patients be able to follow commands prior to extubation? *Respir Care.* 2010;55:56-65.

MacIntyre NR. Discontinuing mechanical ventilatory support. *Chest.* 2007;132:1049-1056.

MacIntyre NR. Evidence-based ventilator weaning and discontinuation. *Respir Care.* 2004;49:830-836.

MacIntyre NR. Respiratory mechanics in the patient who is weaning from the ventilator. *Respir Care.* 2005;50:275-286.

MacIntyre NR. Evidence based assessments in the ventilator discontinuation process. *Respir Care.* 2012;57:1611-1618.

MacIntyre NR, Cook DJ, Ely EW, et al. Evidence-based guidelines for weaning and discontinuing ventilator support. *Chest.* 2001;120:375S-395S.

Meade MO, Guyatt GH, Cook DJ. Weaning from mechanical ventilation: the evidence from clinical research. *Respir Care.* 2001;46:1408-1415.

Mendex-Tellez P, Needham D. Early physical rehabilitation in the ICU and ventilator liberation. *Respir Care.* 2012;57:1663-1669.

Robertson TE, Mann HJ, Hyzy R, et al. Multicenter implementation of a consensus-developed, evidence-based, spontaneous breathing trial protocol. *Crit Care Med.* 2008;36:2753-2762.

Tanios MA, Epstein SK. Spontaneous breathing trials: should we use automatic tube compensation? *Respir Care.* 2010;55:640-642.

White AC. Long-term mechanical ventilation: management strategies. *Respir Care.* 2012;57: 889-899.

Wittekamp BH, van Mook WN, Tjan DH, et al. Clinical review: post-extubation laryngeal edema and extubation failure in critically ill adult patients. *Crit Care.* 2009;13:233.

Part 2
Ventilator Management

Chapter 17
Acute Respiratory Distress Syndrome

- **Introduction**
- **Overview**
  Clinical Presentation
  Ventilator-Induced Lung Injury
- **Mechanical Ventilation**
  Indications
  Ventilator Settings
  Tidal Volume and Plateau Pressure
  Recruitment Maneuvers
  Other Approaches to PEEP Titration
  Managing Severe Refractory Hypoxemia
  Monitoring
  Liberation
- **Points to Remember**
- **Additional Reading**

Introduction

Acute respiratory distress syndrome (ARDS) is a severe lung injury of diverse etiology. It is frequently related to sepsis and multiorgan failure, and is associated with high mortality. ARDS results in diffuse alveolar damage, pulmonary microvascular thrombosis, aggregation of inflammatory cells, and stagnation of pulmonary blood flow. Because many individuals each year develop ARDS in the United States, it consumes much of the time, energy, and resources in the ICU. It is one of the most changeling causes of ventilatory failure to manage and requires adherence to published guidelines.

Overview

Clinical Presentation

ARDS is characterized by hypoxemia and decreased pulmonary compliance. Bilateral infiltrates are present on the chest radiograph. Pao_2/Fio_2 less than or equal to 200, and no evidence of left heart failure has been the classic definition of ARDS. Recently ARDS has been categorized as severe ($Pao_2/Fio_2 < 100$), moderate (Pao_2/Fio_2 100-200), and mild ($Pao_2/Fio_2 > 200$). This classification is generally accepted but there is controversy over the conditions that should exist during the assessment. Some suggest that the classification should occur immediately on presentation with a positive end-expiratory pressure (PEEP) more than or equal to 5 cm H_2O without a specific Fio_2 requirement. Others have shown that persistent ARDS requires assessment 24 hours after presentation on a PEEP more than or equal to 10 cm H_2O with an Fio_2 more than or equal to 0.5. Regardless of the approach, the term "acute lung injury," defined by a Pao_2/Fio_2 more than 200 but less than or equal to 300, is no longer used to define the least severe form.

Evaluation of ARDS by chest computed tomography (CT) reveals a very heterogeneous disease with areas of consolidation, areas of collapse that are recruitable, and areas of normal lung tissue. Rather than considering ARDS as low compliance lungs, the gas exchanging areas of the lungs should be considered of small volume when compared with normal lungs.

The pathology of ARDS progresses through two phases, although the process may resolve at any point in either phase. The first phase is characterized by an intense inflammatory response resulting in alveolar and endothelial damage, increased vascular permeability, and increased lung water. This phase lasts about 7 to 10 days and then frequently progresses to extensive fibrosis (Phase 2). ARDS has been categorized as pulmonary and extrapulmonary in origin. With pulmonary ARDS, there is direct injury to the lungs as occurs with aspiration, infectious pneumonia, trauma (lung contusion and penetrating chest injury), inhalation injury, near drowning, and fat embolism. With extrapulmonary ARDS, the initial injury is to an organ system distant from the lungs including sepsis syndrome, multiple trauma, burns, shock, hypoperfusion, and acute pancreatitis. Chest wall effects may be more important for extrapulmonary ARDS and the potential for alveolar recruitment might also be greater for extrapulmonary ARDS.

Ventilator-Induced Lung Injury

As a result of the areas of low lung compliance and the heterogeneous nature of this disease, ARDS is one of the most likely pathologies to develop ventilator-induced lung injury. To avoid ventilator-induced lung injury, a plateau pressure (Pplat) less than or equal to 30 cm H_2O, and as low as possible, along with appropriate PEEP that maintains alveolar recruitment is recommended. Pplat is limited to prevent overdistention, whereas an appropriate level of PEEP is maintained to avoid the injury related to cyclical opening and closing of unstable lung units. It is, however, important to remember that the primary cause of ventilator-induced lung injury is an increased alveolar distending pressure, transalveolar pressure (Pplat minus pleural pressure). Pplat may overestimate the transalveolar pressure when the chest wall is stiff. On the other hand, during pressure-controlled patient-triggered ventilation, the transalveolar pressure may exceed the estimated Pplat with significant inspiratory effort.

Mechanical Ventilation

Indications

Patients with ARDS present with hypoxemia and increased work-of-breathing. Respiratory support is indicated to reverse hypoxemia with the application of PEEP, delivery of a high F_{IO_2}, and reduction of the work-of-breathing (Table 17-1). The ability to ventilate may become compromised with CO_2 retention. At this stage, mechanical

Table 17-1 Indications for Mechanical Ventilation in Patients with Acute Respiratory Distress Syndrome

- Increased work-of-breathing
- Oxygenation impairment
- Impending ventilatory failure
- Acute ventilatory failure

ventilation is indicated because of acute ventilatory failure. The use of mask continuous positive airway pressure (CPAP) and noninvasive ventilation is generally not recommended for patients with ARDS. If noninvasive ventilation is attempted for mild ARDS, there should be a very low threshold for intubation.

Ventilator Settings

The first decision when setting up the ventilator is whether support be provided with full or partial ventilatory support. There is evidence supporting the use of neuromuscular paralysis and appropriate sedation, the first 48 hours after intubation in patients with $Pao_2/Fio_2 < 150$. In patients with less severe forms of ARDS, sedation but not paralysis is used to facilitate patient-ventilator interaction.

Initial settings and targets when ventilating a patient with ARDS are shown in Tables 17-2 and 17-3. The initiation to mechanical ventilation is shown in Figure 17-1 and the continued approach to ventilation management is shown in Figure 17-2. Two approaches have been advocated for the ventilation of patients with ARDS. The open lung approach uses pressure-controlled ventilation, maintains a low Pplat while monitoring tidal volume, and uses recruitment maneuvers and high levels of PEEP to maximize alveolar recruitment. The ARDSNet approach focuses on maintaining a low tidal volume while monitoring Pplat and sets PEEP based upon the Fio_2 requirement. One approach emphasizes alveolar recruitment and the other prioritizes avoidance of overdistention. Regardless of the approach, there should be an appropriate balance between overdistention and recruitment, as both are important to avoid ventilator-induced lung injury.

Patient triggering may promote alveolar recruitment in dorsal lung regions, it may facilitate venous return, and it may decrease the requirement for sedation. Some clinicians have advocated ventilator modes that allow spontaneous breathing in patients with ARDS, but further study is needed. In the recovery phase and for mild ARDS, pressure support is useful. For severe ARDS, pharmacologic control of ventilation, including paralysis, may be necessary.

Table 17-2 **Ventilator Settings for Patients with ARDS**

Setting	Recommendation
Mode	A/C (CMV) in most acute stages; pressure support for mild ARDS and during recovery
Rate	20-40/min; avoid auto-PEEP
Volume/pressure control	Pressure or volume
Tidal volume	4-8 mL/kg and plateau pressure ≤ 30 cm H_2O
Inspiratory time	Ensure synchrony in patient-triggered ventilation (0.5-0.8 second), may incorporate a short end-inspiratory pause in passive ventilation
PEEP	10-20 cm H_2O; lowest level to achieve Spo_2/Pao_2 target
Fio_2	As needed to achieve Spo_2/Pao_2 target

Abbreviations: ARDS, acute respiratory distress syndrome; CMV, continuous mandatory ventilation; PEEP, positive end-expiratory pressure.

Table 17-3 Gas Exchange, Pressure, and Tidal Volume Targets

Pao_2:	55-80 mm Hg; Spo_2 88%-95%
$Paco_2$:	40 mm Hg if possible
pH:	7.20-7.40
	Permissive hypercapnia to avoid high Pplat
PEEP:	As necessary to maintain alveolar recruitment (10-20 cm H_2O)
Plateau pressure:	≤ 30 cm H_2O, provided normal chest wall compliance
Tidal volume:	6 mL/kg IBW (4-8 mL/kg IBW)

Abbreviations: IBW, ideal body weight; PEEP, positive end-expiratory pressure.

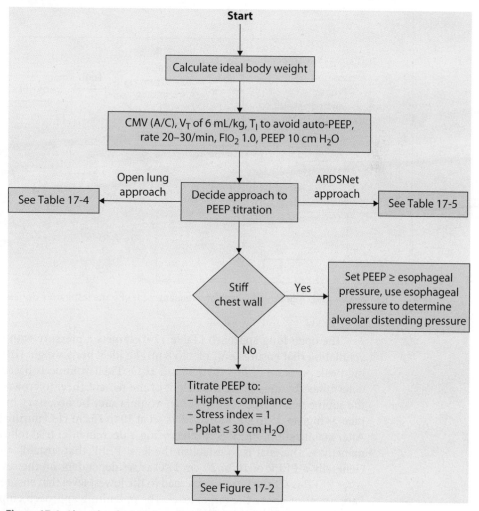

Figure 17-1 Algorithm for initial ventilator management of patients with acute respiratory distress syndrome.

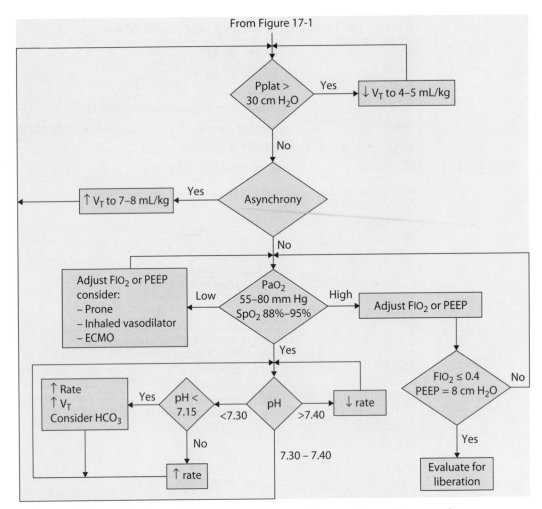

Figure 17-2 Algorithm for ventilator management of acute respiratory distress syndrome.

The open lung approach (Table 17-4) targets a pressure with pressure-controlled ventilation that ensures a V_T of 4 to 8 mL/kg ideal body weight (IBW) while maintaining peak pressure of less than 30 cm H_2O. Tidal volume is based on IBW, which is determined by measuring the height of the patient (heel to crown with the patient in the supine position). Permissive hypercapnia may be necessary in spite of respiratory rates as high as 35 to 40/min. PEEP is set at 10 to 15 cm H_2O during initial stabilization. After stabilization, PEEP is titrated using a decremental trial following a recruitment maneuver. The goal is to establish the least PEEP that sustains alveolar recruitment. Generally a PEEP of 10 to 20 cm H_2O is set dependent on the severity of the ARDS. After PEEP is set the FIO_2 is decreased to the lowest level that ensures that the SpO_2 and PaO_2 are at or above the target level. The open lung approach emphasizes the role of alveolar recruitment.

Table 17-4 Lung Recruitment Maneuver and Decremental PEEP Trial

---

- Ensure hemodynamic stability
- Sedate to apnea
- Recruitment maneuver: Pressure-controlled ventilation, F_{IO_2} 1.0:
  - PEEP 25-35 cm H_2O
  - PIP 40-50 cm H_2O
  - Inspiratory time: 1-3 s
  - Rate: 8-20/min
  - Time: 1-3 min
- Initial recruitment with PEEP 25 cm H_2O, PIP 40 cm H_2O
- Set PEEP at 25 cm H_2O, volume-controlled ventilation with tidal volume 4-6 mL/kg IBW, increase rate, avoid auto-PEEP
  - Measure dynamic compliance after 3-5 min when stable
  - Decrease PEEP by 2 cm H_2O
  - Measure dynamic compliance after 3-5 min when stable
  - Repeat until highest compliance PEEP determined
  - Optimal PEEP is the maximal compliance PEEP + 2 cm H_2O
- Repeat recruitment maneuver and set PEEP at the identified settings, after stabilization adjust tidal volume for Pplat < 30 cm H_2O, then decrease F_{IO_2} until Pao_2 is in target range
- If the recruitment maneuver was tolerated well but the response was poor, repeat the recruitment maneuver with PEEP 30 cm H_2O, PIP 45 cm H_2O after a period of stabilization
- If the recruitment maneuver was tolerated well but the response is still poor, repeat the recruitment maneuver with PEEP 35 cm H_2O, PIP 50 cm H_2O after a period of stabilization
- The maximum recommended recruiting pressure is 50 cm H_2O.

Abbreviations: IBW, ideal body weight; PEEP, positive end-expiratory pressure; PIP, peak inspiratory pressure.

The ARDSNet approach prioritizes avoidance of overdistention. For the acute phase, volume-controlled or pressure-controlled continuous mandatory ventilation (assist/control) is used. The target tidal volume is 6 mL/kg IBW and is maintained between 4 and 8 mL/kg IBW. The target Pplat is less than or equal to 30 cm H_2O, and lower if possible. PEEP is set according to the F_{IO_2}/PEEP combination required to maintain the Pao_2 or Spo_2 within the target range (Table 17- 5). The low PEEP/F_{IO_2} table is used for patients with mild ARDS and the high PEEP/F_{IO_2} table for patients with moderate and severe ARDS. These tables often result in a decremental PEEP titration because high PEEP is required at the onset of intubation and can then be reduced as gas exchange improves. The respiratory rate as high as 35/min is used to maintain pH within the target range. The only factor limiting the setting of rate is the development of auto-PEEP, although auto-PEEP is unusual due to the low compliance and low tidal volume. The primary distinction between the open lung approach and the ARDSNet approach is the focus on lung recruitment maneuvers and decremental PEEP titration with the open lung approach. Both approaches limit V_T and Pplat to avoid overdistention.

Table 17-5 **Combinations of FIO$_2$ and PEEP that have been Used in Patients with the Acute Respiratory Distress Syndrome to Maintain SpO$_2$ at 88% to 95%**

FIO$_2$	0.3	0.4	0.5-0.6	0.7	0.8	0.9	1.0
Low PEEP (mild ARDS)	5	5-8	8-10	10-12	12-14	14-18	20-24
High PEEP (moderate to severe ARDS; greater potential for recruitment)	12-14	14-16	16-18	18-20	20-22	22-24	24

Abbreviations: ARDS, acute respiratory distress syndrome; PEEP, positive end-expiratory pressure.

Tidal Volume and Plateau Pressure

Avoiding overdistention is key to manage the patient with ARDS. Thus, V$_T$ and Pplat are monitored. The overall goal is to maintain the lowest Pplat possible. It the Pplat is more than 30 cm H$_2$O with a tidal volume of 6 mL/kg, there should be a reduction in tidal volume to as low as 4 mL/kg IBW. In the setting of severe acidosis or asynchrony, the V$_T$ can be increased to 8 mL/kg IBW provided that Pplat does not exceed 30 cm H$_2$O. In the setting of asynchrony, the clinician might choose among a higher tidal volume, more sedation, or a mode that promotes synchrony.

Recruitment Maneuvers

The major difference between the ARDSNet approach and the open lung approach is the use of lung recruitment maneuvers and a decremental PEEP trial. The goal of lung recruitment is to maximize the amount of lung volume that can be sustained at a specific PEEP level. The goal of a decremental PEEP trial is to select the minimum PEEP that keeps the lungs open. Once the patient is stabilized after intubation, a lung recruitment maneuver is performed. Stabilization requires hemodynamic stability, because airway pressures 10 to 20 cm H$_2$O above the normal ventilating pressure are applied for a few minutes. Pulse pressure variation should be less than or equal to 13% before attempting a lung recruitment maneuver. The patient should also be sedated to apnea to ensure synchrony during the recruitment maneuver.

Recruitment maneuvers have been performed using a sustained CPAP (eg, 40 cm H$_2$O for 40 seconds) or pressure-controlled ventilation. The pressure-controlled approach seems to be better tolerated than the sustained CPAP maneuver. During these maneuvers the patient is carefully monitored and the maneuvers are stopped if the patient becomes hemodynamically unstable, hypoxemic, or develops a cardiac arrhythmia.

A decremental PEEP trial begins at a level higher than the anticipated PEEP needed and then PEEP is decreased. Identification of the lowest decremental PEEP that sustains the benefit of the recruitment maneuver is determined by monitoring dynamic compliance. This is done on a breath-to-breath basis in volume-controlled ventilation. It only requires 3 to 5 minutes for the compliance to stabilize after the PEEP is decreased. If oxygenation is used, it may take 15 to 30 minutes for stabilization of the Pao$_2$. There is 2 cm H$_2$O PEEP added to the PEEP determined by best compliance because it underestimates PEEP identified by best oxygenation. As PEEP is decreased, compliance initially increases, and then decreases when PEEP is lower than that necessary to maintain recruitment. Once the best PEEP is determined, the recruitment maneuver is repeated since derecruitment occurred during the decremental PEEP trial.

Other Approaches to PEEP Titration

Perhaps the oldest approach to PEEP titration is based on best compliance. The goal is to identify the PEEP level that maximizes recruitment without causing overdistention. It also recognizes that there are some alveoli that cannot be recruited (consolidation) and some require recruiting pressures so high that there is risk of overdistention of open alveoli. Tidal volume is set at 6 mL/kg and PEEP is increased in 2 to 3 H_2O increments, which results in a stepwise alveolar recruitment. After 3 to 5 minutes at each step, Pplat, Spo_2, and blood pressure are assessed. Best PEEP is identified as the level with the best compliance and Pplat less than 30 cm H_2O.

Another approach uses the stress index. For this approach, the ventilator is set on volume-controlled ventilation with a constant inspiratory flow. Upward concavity of the pressure-time waveform represents overdistention and downward concavity of the pressure-time waveform represents tidal recruitment. PEEP and tidal volume are set so that the increase in pressure is linear, suggesting appropriate recruitment without overdistention. This approach also balances the effects of recruitment against those of overdistention.

The chest wall might affect the PEEP requirement, such as with obesity, high intra-abdominal pressure, fluid overload, or chest wall deformity. These effects increase the pleural pressure, causing alveolar collapse and tidal recruitment/derecruitment. In this case, PEEP is increased to match or exceed the esophageal (eg, pleural) pressure, thus counterbalancing the collapsing effect of the chest wall. The result is that Pplat may exceed 30 cm H_2O. In this case, the esophageal pressure is subtracted from the Pplat to determine alveolar distending pressure (Pplat – esophageal pressure). Pplat more than 30 cm H_2O may be safe if the transalveolar pressure is less than 25 cm H_2O. This approach also attempts to balance recruitment and overdistention.

PEEP can also be titrated to the lowest dead space (ie, lowest $Paco_2$ for fixed minute-ventilation), but this is not practical because it requires serial blood gas determinations. PEEP can be titrated using the lower inflection point of the pressure-volume curve, although this approach has fallen out of favor in recent years. PEEP can also be titrated by imaging methods such as CT, but this also is not practical. Regardless of the method used to titrate PEEP, higher levels are appropriate for moderate and severe ARDS, whereas modest levels are appropriate for mild ARDS.

Managing Severe Refractory Hypoxemia

When lung-protective ventilation strategies are applied from the onset of mechanical ventilation, the likelihood of severe refractory hypoxemia is often avoided. Much of the ARDS observed in the past was caused by injurious ventilation strategies. Thus, the first step in managing severe refractory hypoxemia is prevention by lung-protective ventilation to all patients from the onset of mechanical ventilation. In addition, hemodynamic instability and asynchrony affect hypoxemia. Alveolar recruitment and appropriate PEEP improves oxygenation and minimizes lung injury due to tidal recruitment/derecruitment.

Prone position may be beneficial in the setting of refractory hypoxemia. The benefit may be greatest for severe hypoxemia ($Pao_2/Fio_2 < 150$ mm Hg), where being in prone position not only improves oxygenation, but might also afford a survival benefit. If refractory hypoxemia persists despite prone positioning, extracorporeal life support can be considered. Inhaled pulmonary vasodilators may provide short-term improvement in oxygenation, but have not been shown to improve outcome in patients with ARDS. High frequency oscillatory ventilation and airway pressure release ventilation have not been shown to improve outcomes in ARDS.

Monitoring

Hemodynamic monitoring is necessary due to the high PEEP and mean airway pressures sometimes required during ARDS. Pulmonary artery catheters were frequently used in the past to monitor hemodynamic status and to properly titrate fluid therapy and other hemodynamic support. However, pulmonary artery catheters are generally not necessary. Monitoring of arterial blood pressure and central venous pressure is usually adequate to assess fluid status. Daily chest X-rays are used to assess the progression of disease and CT may be helpful. Continuous monitoring of Spo_2 is required, since oxygenation may be difficult to maintain in these patients. Blood gases are indicated when the patient's clinical status changes. Auto-PEEP should be assessed with each ventilator setting change, although it is unusual in patients with ARDS. Reevaluation of Fio_2, PEEP, and Pplat that results in the best gas exchange should occur frequently (Table 17-6).

Liberation

Return to spontaneous breathing following ARDS may be difficult. Patients recovering from ARDS frequently have a high respiratory drive and low lung compliance. Lung function may be compromised for weeks and respiratory muscle weakness may be present. In the recovery phase (ie, when the Fio_2 is 0.40 and the PEEP is 8 cm H_2O with the Pao_2 within the target range), spontaneous breathing trials are initiated. Some patients require tracheostomy. If the patient cannot be extubated, a comfortable level of respiratory support is provided.

Table 17-6 Monitoring During Mechanical Ventilation of Patients with ARDS

- Pulse oximetry, periodic blood gases
- Central venous catheter and continuous blood pressure
- Presence of pneumothorax
- Auto-PEEP
- Tidal volume and plateau pressure

Abbreviations: ARDS, acute respiratory distress syndrome; PEEP, positive end-expiratory pressure.

Points to Remember

- Acute respiratory distress syndrome (ARDS) is a heterogeneous lung disease with areas of consolidation, areas of collapse that are recruitable, and areas of normal tissue.
- The gas exchange area of the lungs in ARDS is small compared with normal (rather than noncompliant).
- ARDS progresses through two phases; the first phase is an intense inflammatory response resulting in alveolar and endothelial damage, increased vascular permeability, and increased lung water and protein; the second phase is characterized by extensive fibrosis.
- With ARDS, Pplat less than or equal to 30 cm H_2O and PEEP to maintain lung recruitment minimizes the risk of ventilator-induced lung injury.
- Mechanical ventilation is indicated in ARDS to reverse shunting and severe hypoxemia, reduce the work-of-breathing, and treat acute respiratory failure.
- Sedation (and sometimes paralysis) should be used to prevent patient-ventilator asynchrony.
- Tidal volumes of 4 to 8 mL/kg ideal body weight are used to maintain a peak alveolar pressure less than or equal to 30 cm H_2O.
- Respiratory rate is limited by the development of auto-positive end-expiratory pressure (auto-PEEP).
- With the open lung approach, lung recruitment maneuvers are performed after the patient is stabilized and PEEP is determined by a decremental PEEP trial, where the least PEEP sustaining the benefit of the lung recruitment maneuver is selected.
- PEEP in early ARDS should be set to maintain alveolar recruitment (10-20 cm H_2O).
- High PEEP is necessary for moderate and severe ARDS, and modest PEEP is necessary for mild ARDS.
- PEEP can also be set based on the tables used in the ARDSNet studies, by incremental PEEP titration to best compliance, and by stress index.
- Esophageal pressure monitoring is used to set PEEP to counterbalance the collapsing effects of the chest wall and to determine end-inspiratory distending pressure.
- Refractory hypoxemia is best avoided by avoiding its development by using lung protective ventilation in all patients.
- Prone positioning, pulmonary vasodilators, and extracorporeal life support (ECLS) may be necessary in patients with refractory hypoxemia.

Additional Reading

ARDS Network. Ventilation with lower tidal volumes as compared with traditional tidal volumes for acute lung injury and the acute respiratory distress syndrome patients. *N Engl J Med.* 2000;342:1301-1308.

Briel M, Meade M, Mercat A, et al. Higher vs lower positive end-expiratory pressure in patients with acute lung injury and acute respiratory distress syndrome: systematic review and meta-analysis. *JAMA.* 2010;303:865-873.

Brower RG, Ware LB, Berthiaume Y, Matthay MA. Treatment of ARDS. *Chest.* 2001;120: 1347-1367.

Chiumello D, Carlesso E, Cadringher P, et al. Lung stress and strain during mechanical ventilation for acute respiratory distress syndrome. *Am J Respir Crit Care Med.* 2008; 178:346-355.

Caironi P. Lung recruitment maneuvers during acute respiratory distress syndrome: open up but not push-up the lung! *Minerva Anesthesiol.* 2011;77:1134-1136.

Collins SR, Blank RS. Approaches to refractory hypoxemia in acute respiratory distress syndrome: current understanding, evidence, and debate. *Respir Care.* 2001;56:1573-1582.

Fan E, Wilcox ME, Brower RG, et al. Recruitment maneuvers for acute lung injury: a systematic review. *Am J Respir Crit Care Med.* 2008;178;1156-1163.

Graf J. Transpulmonary pressure targets for open lung and protective ventilation: one size does not fit all. *Intensive Care Med.* 2012;38:1565-1566.

Guerin C. The preventative role of higher PEEP in treating severely hypoxemic ARDS. *Minerva Anesthesiol.* 2011;77:835-845.

Haas CF. Mechanical ventilation with lung protective strategies: what works? *Crit Care Clin.* 2011;27:469-486.

Hess DR. Approaches to conventional mechanical ventilation of the patient with acute respiratory distress syndrome. *Respir Care.* 2011;56:1555-1572.

Kacmarek RM, Kallet RH. Respiratory controversies in the critical care setting. Should recruitment maneuvers be used in the management of ALI and ARDS? *Respir Care.* 2007; 52:622-635.

Kacmarek RM, Villar J. Lung recruitment maneuvers during acute respiratory distress syndrome: is it useful? *Minerva Anesthesiol.* 2011;77:85-89.

Kallet RH, Corral W, Silverman HJ, Luce JM. Implementation of a low tidal volume protocol for patients with acute lung injury or acute respiratory distress syndrome. *Respir Care.* 2001;46:1024-1037.

Papadakos PJ, Lachmann B. The open lung concept of mechanical ventilation: the role of recruitment and stabilization. *Crit Care Clin.* 2007;23:241-250.

Petrucci N, De Feo C. Lung protective ventilation strategy for the acute respiratory distress syndrome. *Cochrane Database Syst Rev.* 2013;2:CD003844.

Richard JC, Marini JJ. Transpulmonary pressure as a surrogate of plateau pressure for lung protective strategy: not perfect but more physiologic. *Intensive Care Med.* 2012;38:339-341.

Rocco PR, Pelosi P, de Abreu MG. Pros and cons of recruitment maneuvers in acute lung injury and acute respiratory distress syndrome. *Expert Rev Respir Med.* 2010;4:479-489.

Slutsky AS, Ranieri VM. Ventilator-induced lung injury. *N Engl J Med.* 2013;369:2126-2136.

Ware LB, Matthay MA. The acute respiratory distress syndrome. *N Engl J Med.* 2000;342: 1334-1349.

Chapter 18
Obstructive Lung Disease

Objectives

1. Discuss the impact of respiratory muscle dysfunction on the need for mechanical ventilation in patients with chronic pulmonary disease.
2. Discuss the role of auto-positive end-expiratory pressure (auto-PEEP) that develops in patients with obstructive lung disease.
3. List indications for mechanical ventilation in patients with obstructive lung disease.
4. List the initial ventilator settings for obstructive lung disease.
5. Discuss monitoring and ventilator liberation for mechanically ventilated patients with obstructive lung disease.

Introduction

Obstructive pulmonary diseases include chronic obstructive pulmonary disease (COPD), asthma, bronchiectasis, and cystic fibrosis. Patients with this underlying pathology are a significant fraction of those requiring respiratory support. Although this chapter deals primarily with COPD and asthma, the principles related to mechanical ventilation are similar for other obstructive lung diseases.

Overview

With COPD, flow limitation leads to air trapping with increased work-of-breathing and respiratory muscle dysfunction. Asthma is episodic and associated with airways inflammation and bronchospasm. COPD and asthma are chronic diseases that are often managed well in the community. But exacerbations of either can result in respiratory failure necessitating mechanical ventilation.

Respiratory Muscle Dysfunction

Because of the hyperinflation with COPD, the normal dome shape of the diaphragm is flattened and the zone of apposition is decreased. The result is less efficient diaphragmatic function. If the diaphragm is sufficiently flattened, during contraction the lateral rib cage moves inward instead of outward, leading to paradoxical breathing (Table 18-1). Accessory muscles of inspiration (intercostals, scalenes,

Table 18-1 **Characteristics of Normal Breathing Pattern and Paradoxical Breathing**

Normal breathing	*Paradoxical breathing*
• Protrusion of the anterior abdominal wall	• Anterior abdominal wall moves inward
• Expansion of the lateral rib cage	• Lateral rib cage moves inward
• Expansion of the upper chest wall	• Expansion of the upper chest wall

sternomastoid, pectoralis, and parasternal) become the primary muscle groups for breathing. In patients with COPD where chronic respiratory muscle dysfunction has developed, reserve is limited and fatigue can occur with increases in respiratory muscle load.

Auto-Positive End-Expiratory Pressure

Auto-positive end-expiratory pressure (auto-PEEP) is end-expiratory alveolar pressure due to air trapping. Due to the heterogeneity that exists in the lungs, air trapping and auto-PEEP may differ between lung units. As a result, the auto-PEEP level measured is an average value. Long-time constants (Table 18-2) resulting from increased resistance and compliance in COPD necessitate more expiratory time to prevent air trapping and auto-PEEP. Auto-PEEP requires a greater inspiratory pressure to initiate flow into the lungs (difficulty triggering the ventilator) and the hyperinflation resulting from air trapping causes an increased work-of-breathing. The airways resistance with COPD is characterized by flow limitation.

Patients with severe acute asthma also develop air trapping and auto-PEEP. The air trapping occurs due to increased airways resistance with bronchospasm, inflammation, and secretions. Some lung units may be hyperinflated to the point that they compress adjacent lung units. The auto-PEEP and increased resistive load results in large intrathoracic pressure changes during the breathing cycle, resulting in pulsus paradoxus. Hyperinflation causes tidal breathing on a less compliant part of the pressure-volume curve, which decreases compliance and increases the work-of-breathing. The measured auto-PEEP during mechanical ventilation in some patients with asthma may not reflect the magnitude of air trapping because of complete airway obstruction (Figure 18-1). These patients should receive a respiratory pattern to minimize air trapping and breathing effort. Anxiety and a high respiratory drive make this difficult.

Nutrition

It is common that patients presenting with COPD exacerbation are nutritionally depleted, with caloric and protein deficiencies and electrolyte imbalances. This compromises respiratory muscle function and contributes to respiratory failure. Nutritional support is important, but care must be taken to avoid overfeeding, which results in increased carbon dioxide production and, thus, a greater load on the respiratory muscles.

Table 18-2 Pulmonary Time Constant (τ)

- τ = compliance × resistance
- Complete passive exhalation requires 4-5 τ
- Normally τ is about 0.5 s
- With COPD, τ is increased due to high lung compliance and a high airway resistance

---

Abbreviation: COPD, chronic obstructive pulmonary disease.

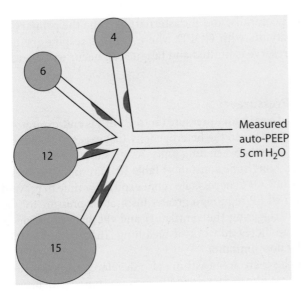

Measured
auto-PEEP
5 cm H_2O

Figure 18-1 Measurement of auto-PEEP in the traditional manner (ie, end-expiratory pause) may be an inaccurate reflection of auto-PEEP if airway closure occurs. In this example, the auto-PEEP measurement will reflect 5 cm H_2O (an average of the lung units with 4 cm H_2O and 6 cm H_2O auto-PEEP). However, some lung units have auto-PEEP levels greater than that measured (12 cm H_2O and 15 cm H_2O).

Mechanical Ventilation

Although often lifesaving, invasive mechanical ventilation should be avoided if possible in patients with COPD. Morbidity (aspiration, barotrauma, nosocomial infection, cardiovascular dysfunction) in chronic pulmonary disease patients is high during invasive mechanical ventilation and some of these patients become ventilator-dependent once intubated. As a result, noninvasive ventilation (NIV) has become standard practice for patients with COPD during an exacerbation. For many of these patients, intubation is avoided with the use of NIV. Moreover, there is a survival benefit afforded to the patient with the use of NIV. With severe acute asthma, NIV can be attempted but success is less likely than with COPD. Use of NIV in severe asthma is an area of controversy, but there is accumulating evidence supporting its use in selected patients with asthma and cystic fibrosis.

Indications

Patients presenting with a COPD exacerbation are hypercapnic, hypoxemic, exhausted, and with respiratory muscle dysfunction (Table 18-3). Mechanical ventilation is indicated to unload the work-of-breathing, rest respiratory muscles, decrease $Paco_2$ to the patient's baseline, and treat hypoxemia.

Table 18-3 Indications for Ventilation in Patients with Chronic Obstructive Pulmonary Disease

- Acute on chronic respiratory failure
- Unloading work-of-breathing
- Resting respiratory muscles

Table 18-4 Indications for Ventilation in Patients with Severe Acute Asthma

- Acute respiratory failure
- Impending respiratory failure
- Severe hypoxemia

A clinical dilemma with asthma is determining when conventional therapy has failed and respiratory support is required. Many patients presenting with acute asthma are young and otherwise healthy, and they can maintain ventilation despite the marked increase in breathing effort. These patients may maintain $Paco_2$ less than or equal to 40 mm Hg until they are completely exhausted. When CO_2 retention occurs, severe hypercapnia and acidosis can rapidly develop. Thus, mechanical ventilation should be provided when $Paco_2$ exceeds 40 mm Hg and sooner if the patient is showing signs of exhaustion (Table 18-4). At this point, the patient is fatiguing and waiting longer before initiating ventilation results in further hypoventilation.

Ventilator Settings for COPD

Mechanical ventilation of the patient with COPD can be challenging. At best, these patients are returned to their baseline characterized by dyspnea, increased work-of-breathing, and abnormal gas exchange. Of primary concern during respiratory assistance of these patients is patient-ventilator synchrony to avoid unnecessary effort and anxiety. Heavy sedation or paralysis is not used beyond the initiation of mechanical ventilation. Ventilator settings that assure patient comfort in addition to adequate gas exchange is important (Table 18-5 and Figure 18-2).

Either pressure-controlled ventilation (PCV) or volume-controlled ventilation (VCV) can be used. An advantage of PCV is that flow varies with the patient's demand. However, in the setting of increased auto-PEEP, tidal volume is reduced with PCV. With VCV, tidal volume does not decrease with increased auto-PEEP, but there is a risk of an increased plateau pressure and overdistention.

Table 18-5 Initial Ventilator Settings for Chronic Obstructive Pulmonary Disease

Setting	Recommendation
Mode	A/C (CMV)
Rate	8-15/min
Volume/pressure control	Pressure or volume
Tidal volume	6-8 mL/kg provided plateau pressure ≤ 30 cm H_2O
Inspiratory time	0.6-1.0 s
PEEP	5 cm H_2O or as necessary to counterbalance auto-PEEP
Fio_2	Usually ≤ 0.50

Abbreviations: CMV, continuous mandatory ventilation; PEEP, positive end-expiratory pressure.

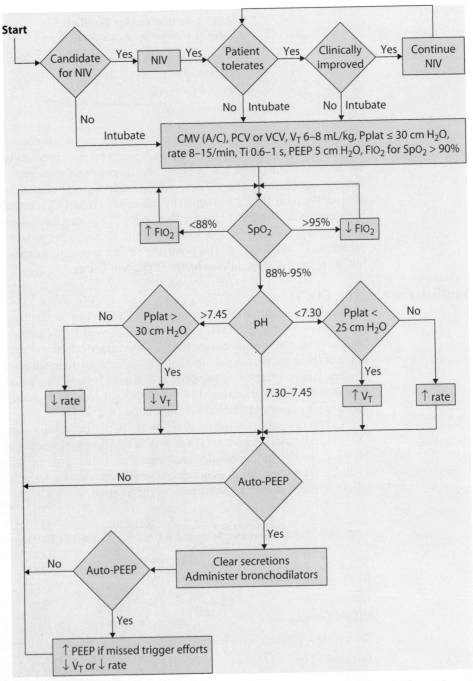

Figure 18-2 Algorithm for the ventilator management of the patient with chronic obstructive pulmonary disease.

Pressure support ventilation (PSV) can be problematic with COPD. Termination of inspiration with PSV is flow-cycled (eg, a fixed fraction of peak flow). Termination of inspiration may be either prolonged or premature, increasing respiratory demand and activating accessory muscles of exhalation to terminate flow if patient and ventilator termination of inspiration is not synchronous. PCV may be preferred over PSV because it allows rate and inspiratory time to be set. In the early phase of respiratory support, a fixed inspiratory time may be better tolerated and is set per patient comfort (0.6-1.0 second).

If VCV is used, flow is set high enough to satisfy inspiratory demand and promote patient comfort. Peak flow should be set to produce an inspiratory time of 0.6 to 1.0 second. When the flow demand of the patient is greatest at the beginning of inspiration, a ramp flow pattern is useful. The lower end-inspiratory flow with the ramp flow pattern may improve gas distribution to long-time constant regions. However, there are some patients who are more comfortable with a constant inspiratory flow pattern. When a shorter inspiratory time (longer expiratory time) is necessary to manage auto-PEEP, a constant inspiratory flow may be necessary. Rate should be set at 8 to 15/min, depending on the degree of hypercapnia and the development of auto-PEEP.

High plateau pressures are usually not a problem in COPD unless auto-PEEP is present. As a result, V_T in the 6 to 8 mL/kg range should be used. Plateau pressure should be kept as low as possible (< 30 cm H_2O) to minimize overdistention.

Auto-PEEP is always a concern when ventilating patients with COPD. Efforts to minimize auto-PEEP and its effects on triggering should be maximized. Therapy to reverse airways resistance (eg, bronchodilators, steroids) and mobilize secretions (eg, bronchoscopy, suctioning) should be used. In addition, minute ventilation should be as low as possible. Auto-PEEP produces a threshold load at the beginning of inspiration, which increases the effort required to trigger the ventilator. A common clinical sign of auto-PEEP is missed triggers. Provided the trigger sensitivity is set properly, the only reason that the patient's rate exceeds the ventilator rate is auto-PEEP. Ensuring that minute ventilation (rate and tidal volume) is not excessive reduces auto-PEEP. However, even if tidal volume is minimized, some patients with COPD are unable to generate sufficient effort to overcome auto-PEEP and trigger the ventilator. In this setting, applied PEEP counterbalances auto-PEEP and improves triggering. PEEP is increased by 1 or 2 cm H_2O increments until patient rate and ventilator rate are equal. The use of 5 cm H_2O PEEP is usually beneficial in patients with COPD, and more than 10 cm H_2O is seldom necessary to counterbalance auto-PEEP. Applying PEEP counterbalances auto-PEEP in the setting of flow limitation with COPD.

The FIO_2 requirement in patients with COPD is rarely more than 0.50. Unloading the work-of-breathing and improving $\dot{V}/\dot{Q}$ matching results in an acceptable PaO_2 with only modest FIO_2 requirement. A PaO_2 of 55 to 80 mm Hg is adequate for these patients.

It is important to avoid overventilation in patients with COPD. $PaCO_2$ should only be decreased to the patient's baseline level. In many patients, this is a $PaCO_2$ of 50 to 60 mm Hg or that required for a near-normal pH (> 7.30). If initial ventilator settings satisfy respiratory drive, these patients usually require minimal sedation. Full respiratory support to rest the respiratory muscles is recommended for the first 24 to 48 hours of ventilation, after which evaluation for liberation should be considered.

Ventilator Settings for Asthma

The major concern when ventilating a patient with severe acute asthma is auto-PEEP. The approach to ventilation should be focused on minimizing auto-PEEP (Table 18-6 and Figure 18-3). This often means that permissive hypercapnia must be allowed, particularly in the early phases of mechanical ventilation. Inhaled bronchodilators and systemic steroids are an important aspect of the management of these patients.

Although either VCV or PCV can be used, VCV is often necessary at the onset of respiratory support. In very severe acute asthma, a high driving pressure is needed to deliver the tidal volume due to the high airways resistance. Although a peak airway pressure of 60 to 70 cm H_2O may be necessary, a plateau pressure less than 30 cm H_2O can still be maintained. The difference between the peak pressure and the plateau pressure is an indication of the degree of airways resistance.

Once the asthma severity improves, the patient can be transitioned to PCV per clinician's bias. With PCV, changes in delivered tidal volume at a fixed pressure are a reflection of changes in resistance and air trapping. As the severity of the asthma improves, delivered V_T with PCV increases. Sedation to minimize asynchrony should be used. Neuromuscular blocking agents may be necessary in some patients, although they should be avoided if possible. Prolonged weakness may occur in some patients following neuromuscular blockade. If adequate sedation is used, full respiratory support can usually be achieved.

To minimize the development of auto-PEEP, a small V_T (4-6 mL/kg) should be used. Delivered tidal volume should be chosen to ensure a plateau pressure less than 30 cm H_2O. Respiratory rate should be set based on the level of air trapping and auto-PEEP. Theoretically, a lower rate minimizes air trapping. However, in some patients with asthma, the rate can be increased to 15 to 20 breaths/min without a marked increase in auto-PEEP. A low tidal volume with a slow rate results in CO_2 retention. Maintaining pH more than or equal to 7.20 is usually sufficient. In young otherwise healthy patients with asthma, an even lower pH may be acceptable. The risk of auto-PEEP, lung injury, and hypotension usually outweighs the risks of acidosis.

Table 18-6 **Initial Ventilator Settings in Patients with Severe Acute Asthma**

Setting	Recommendation
Mode	A/C (CMV)
Rate	8-20/min; allow permissive hypercapnia
Volume/pressure control	Pressure or volume; volume necessary for severe asthma
Tidal volume	4-6 mL/kg and plateau pressure ≤ 30 cm H_2O
Inspiratory time	1-1.5 s; avoid auto-PEEP
PEEP	Use of PEEP is controversial; may attempt to counterbalance auto-PEEP but frequently this does not help
F_{IO_2}	Sufficient to maintain Pao_2 55-80 mm Hg and Spo_2 88%–95%

Abbreviations: CMV, continuous mandatory ventilation; PEEP, positive end-expiratory pressure.

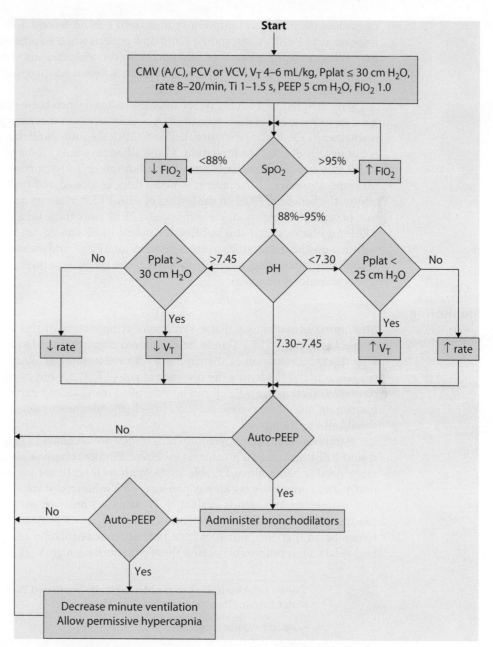

Figure 18-3 Algorithm for mechanical ventilation of the patient with asthma.

Inspiratory time should be short to prolong expiratory time and reduce auto-PEEP. However, better distribution of ventilation can be achieved by lengthening inspiratory time. An initial inspiratory time of 1 second is recommended, with evaluation of the effect on auto-PEEP if inspiratory time is increased to 1.5 second. Provided that the rate is low, the increase in inspiratory time from 1 to 1.5 second does not significantly increase auto-PEEP. A descending ramp flow pattern when volume ventilation is used may enhance distribution of ventilation. However, a shorter inspiratory time can be achieved using a rectangular flow waveform. Peak flow is selected to ensure inspiratory time is appropriate.

An initial FIO_2 of 1 should be set and then reduced when pulse oximetry and blood gas data indicate adequate oxygenation. A controversy with the management of asthma is whether PEEP should be applied. Unlike COPD, the auto-PEEP that occurs in asthma is not usually due to flow limitation. In the absence of flow limitation, the addition of PEEP may not counterbalance auto-PEEP, but rather it may further increase alveolar pressure. Moreover, if the patient is being fully ventilated and making no triggering efforts, the benefit of PEEP in the setting of auto-PEEP might be questioned. Distribution of ventilation may improve with applied PEEP since those lung units without auto-PEEP may be recruited and stabilized. Applied PEEP should not be used in patients with acute asthma if it results in an increase in total PEEP and plateau pressure. If PEEP is applied in this setting, monitoring of gas exchange, plateau pressure, auto-PEEP, and hemodynamics is necessary.

Monitoring

Monitoring of patient-ventilator synchrony is important in this patient population (Table 18-7). Auto-PEEP should be monitored regularly in patients with obstructive lung disease. Evaluation of the expiratory flow waveform or observation for missed triggers is useful to identify the presence of auto-PEEP, but not its magnitude. During passive ventilation, auto-PEEP can be quantified using an end-expiratory hold. Respiratory rate, use of accessory muscles, breath sounds, heart rate, and blood pressure should also be monitored.

Barotrauma and hemodynamic compromise are common in patients with asthma if auto-PEEP and plateau pressure is excessive. Physical examination and chest radiography need to be monitored (Table 18-8). With each ventilator-patient system evaluation, plateau pressure, peak airway pressure, tidal volume, and auto-PEEP levels should be documented and trends evaluated. Continuous pulse oximetry, periodic blood gas measurements, and monitoring of hemodynamics is necessary. It should be remembered that SpO_2 provides little indication of ventilation or acid-base balance. End-tidal CO_2 is not useful because these patients have high V_D/V_T.

Table 18-7 Monitoring of the Mechanically Ventilated Patient with Chronic Obstructive Pulmonary Disease

- Patient-ventilator synchrony
- Auto-PEEP
- Plateau pressure
- Hemodynamics
- Pulse oximetry and arterial blood gases
- Clinical signs of cardiopulmonary distress

Abbreviation: PEEP, positive end-expiratory pressure.

Table 18-8 **Monitoring of the Mechanically Ventilated Patient With Severe Acute Asthma**

- Presence of barotrauma
- Plateau pressure
- Auto-PEEP
- Pulse oximetry and arterial blood gases
- Heart rate and blood pressure

Abbreviation: PEEP, positive end-expiratory pressure.

Liberation

Most important in the process of liberation is to ensure that the acute process that necessitated mechanical ventilation is improving. Second, ensure cardiovascular function is optimized, as many patients with COPD also have cardiovascular disease. Third, optimize electrolyte balance and nutritional status, because nutritional status and some electrolyte imbalances affect respiratory muscle function. Finally, use spontaneous awaking trials and spontaneous breathing trials to identify when liberation is possible.

Most patients with COPD can be fully liberated from mechanical ventilation. Others require long-term support (a difficult subgroup). In those patients who are tracheostomized and require long-term respiratory support, a slow-paced approach may be necessary with spontaneous breathing trials interspersed with periods of respiratory support. Nocturnal ventilation is sometimes required. In some patients with COPD, NIV can be used as a bridge to ventilator independence. NIV can be provided until the patient can breathe independently or requires reintubation.

Liberation of the patient with severe acute asthma is usually more rapid than with COPD. Once the acute phase is adequately treated, ventilator discontinuation should be considered. As the patient's status improves (ie, airflow resistance returning to baseline, auto-PEEP eliminated, and airway pressures and tidal volumes returning to normal, adequate gas exchange), sedation should be decreased or stopped, allowing the patient to resume spontaneous breathing. Once alert and cooperative, a spontaneous breathing trial is performed to assess extubation readiness.

Points to Remember

- Respiratory muscle dysfunction and auto-PEEP are common problems leading to an increase in work-of-breathing in chronic obstructive pulmonary disease (COPD) patients.
- Respiratory muscle dysfunction can lead to acute respiratory failure in patients with COPD.
- Patients with a COPD exacerbation are candidates for noninvasive ventilation (NIV).
- For some patients with COPD, synchrony is better with pressure-controlled ventilation (PCV) than with volume-controlled ventilation (VCV).

- With VCV, peak inspiratory flow should be set to meet inspiratory demand and some patients may be more comfortable with a descending ramp flow pattern.
- With COPD, ventilator rate should be set low with a moderate V_T.
- Counterbalance the effects of auto-positive end-expiratory pressure (auto-PEEP) by applying PEEP in patients with COPD.
- Auto-PEEP is a major problem with severe acute asthma.
- Mechanical ventilation is indicated in acute or impending acute respiratory failure.
- Mechanical ventilation should be considered when $PaCO_2$ rises above 40 mm Hg in patients with severe acute asthma.
- In patients with COPD, target $PaCO_2$ at the patient's baseline level and pH more than 7.30.
- Before attempts at liberation, ensure some reversal of acute pulmonary processes, optimize cardiovascular function, normalize electrolytes, and provide nutritional support.
- In some patients recovering from COPD exacerbation, NIV can be used as a bridge from invasive ventilation to spontaneous breathing.
- Initial ventilation in severe acute asthma frequently requires VCV because of the high driving pressure needed to overcome airways resistance.
- Respiratory rate in severe asthma should be 8 to 20/min and V_T set to keep plateau pressure less than 30 cm H_2O (4-6 mL/kg).
- Permissive hypercapnia may be necessary until the severity of the asthma improves.
- A pH as low as 7.10 may be tolerated in mechanically ventilated patients with severe acute asthma.
- Inspiratory time is set at a level to avoid auto-PEEP in severe asthma.
- Adjust FIO_2 to keep PaO_2 55 to 80 mm Hg.
- With severe asthma, applied PEEP may or may not counterbalance auto-PEEP.
- During mechanical ventilation for patients with severe acute asthma, the use of PEEP is controversial.
- When PEEP is used with severe acute asthma, monitor plateau pressure, auto-PEEP, and hemodynamics.
- Monitor auto-PEEP, plateau pressure, peak airway pressure, tidal volume, and the presence of barotrauma.
- Discontinue respiratory support in severe asthma when tidal volumes, ventilating pressures, and gas exchange have improved.

Additional Reading

Afessa B, Morales I, Cury JD. Clinical course and outcome of patients admitted to an ICU for status asthmaticus. *Chest.* 2001;120:1616-1621.

Afzal M, Tharratt RS. Mechanical ventilation in severe asthma. *Clin Rev Allergy Immunol.* 2001;20:385-397.

Beuther DA. Hypoventilation in asthma and chronic obstructive pulmonary disease. *Semin Respir Crit Care Med.* 2009;30:321-329.

Boldrini R, Fasano L, Nava S. Noninvasive mechanical ventilation. *Curr Opin Crit Care.* 2012;18:48-53.

Brenner B, Corbridge T, Kazzi A. Intubation and mechanical ventilation of the asthmatic patient in respiratory failure. *Proc Am Thorac Soc.* 2009;6:371-379.

Chandramouli S, Molyneaux V, Angus RM, et al. Insights into chronic obstructive pulmonary disease patient attitudes on ventilatory support. *Curr Opin Pulm Med.* 2011;17:98-102.

Fumeaux T, Rothmeier C, Jolliet P. Outcome of mechanical ventilation for acute respiratory failure in patients with pulmonary fibrosis. *Intensive Care Med.* 2001;27:1868-1874.

Koh Y. Ventilatory management of patients with severe asthma. *Int Anesthesiol Clin.* 2001;39:63-73.

Lim WJ, Mohammed Akram R, et al. Noninvasive positive pressure ventilation for treatment of respiratory failure due to severe acute exacerbations of asthma. *Cochrane Database Syst Rev.* 2012;12:CD004360.

MacIntyre N, Huang YC. Acute exacerbations and respiratory failure in chronic obstructive pulmonary disease. *Proc Am Thorac Soc.* 2008;5:530-535.

Mannam P, Siegel MD. Analytic review: management of life-threatening asthma in adults. *J Intensive Care Med.* 2010;25:3-15.

Medoff BD. Invasive and noninvasive ventilation in patients with asthma. *Respir Care.* 2008;53:740-748.

Quon BS, Gan WQ, Sin DD. Contemporary management of acute exacerbations of COPD: a systematic review and metaanalysis. *Chest.* 2008;133(3):756-66.

Rubin BK, Dhand R, Ruppel GL, et al. Respiratory care year in review 2010: part 1. Asthma, COPD, pulmonary function testing, ventilator-associated pneumonia. *Respir Care.* 2011;56:488-502.

Sethi JM. Mechanical ventilation in chronic obstructive pulmonary disease. *Clin Chest Med.* 2000;21:799-818.

Ward NS, Dushay KM. Clinical concise review: mechanical ventilation of patients with chronic obstructive pulmonary disease. *Crit Care Med.* 2008;36:1614-1619.

Chapter 19
Chest Trauma

> **Objectives**
>
> 1. Discuss the clinical presentation of patients with both blunt and penetrating chest trauma.
> 2. Discuss the use of mask continuous positive airway pressure and noninvasive ventilation for patients with chest trauma.
> 3. Discuss the initial ventilator settings for patients with chest trauma.
> 4. Describe the monitoring of mechanically ventilated patients with chest trauma.
> 5. Discuss the weaning of chest trauma patients from ventilatory support.

Introduction

Although the chest wall can absorb significant amounts of trauma without serious injury to the patient, chest trauma is a frequent indication for critical care and mechanical ventilation. Unlike other disease states requiring mechanical ventilation (eg, chronic obstructive pulmonary disease [COPD]), patients suffering chest trauma are typically young and previously healthy and an increasing number are being managed with noninvasive approaches.

Overview

Blunt Chest Trauma

With blunt chest trauma, there are often no exterior signs or symptoms of injury to the chest. Clinical entities associated with blunt chest trauma include fractures, pulmonary contusion, tracheobronchial injury, myocardial and vascular injury, esophageal perforation, and diaphragmatic injury. Fractures can involve the ribs, sternum, vertebrae, clavicles, or scapulae. Of these, rib fractures are the most common. Rib fractures without flailing can be painful, resulting in splinting, atelectasis, and hypoxemia due to ventilation/perfusion mismatching. Isolated rib fractures almost never necessitate mechanical ventilation unless they are associated with other injuries such as pulmonary contusion. Flail chest is a loss of stability of the rib cage caused by multiple rib fractures, which frequently results in significant ventilatory disturbances due to underlying damage to the lung parenchyma, inefficient expansion of the thorax due to paradoxical movement of the chest wall, and pain leading to hypoventilation. Until recently, it was common practice to internally stabilize the rib cage in patients with flail chest by use of positive pressure ventilation and positive end-expiratory pressure (PEEP). Many patients with flail chest are now adequately managed without intubation and mechanical ventilation. This is particularly the case with appropriate pain control and noninvasive ventilation (NIV). It is now generally accepted that mechanical ventilation is only required for patients with flail chest if one of the following is present: shock, closed head injury, need for immediate operation, severe pulmonary dysfunction, or deteriorating respiratory status.

Pulmonary contusion results from high impact blunt chest trauma, which produces leakage of blood and protein from the vascular to the interstitial and alveolar space of the lungs. Clinically, pulmonary contusion is similar in presentation and treatment to acute respiratory distress syndrome (ARDS). If the contusion is localized, high levels of PEEP may produce a paradoxical decrease in arterial oxygenation because blood may be diverted from normal to the injured lung increasing shunt fraction. Mild to moderate forms of pulmonary contusion may not require intubation, and hypoxemia can be adequately treated with oxygen and mask continuous positive airway pressure (CPAP) or NIV.

Tracheobronchial injuries most often occur near the trachea or near the origin of the mainstem bronchi. If they are small and do not result in pneumothorax, these may heal spontaneously. Tracheobronchial injuries that result in large air leaks and pneumothorax require surgical repair. Patients with tracheobronchial injuries may require mechanical ventilation following thoracotomy, particularly if other injuries compromising pulmonary function are present.

Myocardial injuries associated with blunt chest trauma are most often in the form of myocardial contusion. Myocardial contusion can result in arrhythmias, but rarely results in cardiac failure. The need for mechanical ventilation is rare in patients with myocardial contusion who do not have other associated injuries such as rib fractures and pulmonary contusion. Injuries to the thoracic vasculature can result in significant hypotension and the need for emergent thoracotomy. Patients with these injuries typically have multiple chest injuries and require mechanical ventilation.

Diaphragm injury secondary to blunt chest injury is very rare. This injury almost always requires operative repair. Patients with diaphragmatic injury may require postoperative mechanical ventilation and may be difficult to wean due to diaphragmatic weakness.

Penetrating Chest Trauma

Penetrating injuries can affect the lungs, the heart, and/or the vasculature, and almost always require surgical intervention. When associated with tension pneumothorax and/or significant blood loss, penetrating injuries can be immediately life-threatening. A tension pneumothorax can be rapidly corrected by insertion of a chest tube, and mechanical ventilation may not be required. Many penetrating chest injuries require extensive surgical repair, and mechanical ventilation is frequently required postoperatively.

Mechanical Ventilation

Indications

Indications for mechanical ventilation in patients with chest trauma are listed in Table 19-1. None of these indications are absolute, and each is dependent on the corresponding level of respiratory failure. Flail chest with paradoxical chest movement was once considered an absolute indication for positive pressure ventilation. However, many cases of flail chest are now managed effectively without intubation and mechanical ventilation. ARDS is a common complication of chest trauma, and may occur without associated chest contusion. When ARDS occurs in association with chest trauma, its management is similar to that with other causes of ARDS. Pain control is an issue in many patients with chest trauma. If large doses of narcotic pain control are required, respiratory depression may occur and mechanical ventilation may

Table 19-1 Indications for Mechanical Ventilation in Patients With Chest Trauma

- Flail chest with paradoxical chest movement that results in tachypnea, hypoxemia, hypercarbia
- Pulmonary contusion with tachypnea and severe hypoxemia (Pao_2 < 60 mm Hg) breathing 100% O_2
- Rib fractures with chest pain requiring large doses of narcotics for pain control
- Postoperative thoracotomy
- Hemodynamic instability, particularly with marginal respiratory reserve (eg, hypoxemia and tachypnea)
- Severe associated injuries (eg, head trauma)
- Failed noninvasive ventilation

be necessary. Epidural narcotics, patient-controlled analgesia, and intercostal nerve blocks are used to control pain without associated respiratory depression.

Mask CPAP and Noninvasive Ventilation

The use of NIV has become increasingly common in the patient with chest trauma. The early use of NIV in patients with chest trauma facilitates stabilization of the chest, promotes recruitment of collapsed lung regions, and significantly reduces mortality and intubation rate without increasing complications. Some of these patients are managed with 8 to 12 cm H_2O CPAP and Fio_2 adjusted to maintain the Pao_2 more than 60 mm Hg. In some patients, NIV is indicated due to increased work-of-breathing. However, the patient who is requiring increasing levels of CPAP, Fio_2, or ventilatory support should be considered for invasive ventilation. Intubation is usually required if the patient is also hemodynamically unstable.

Ventilator Settings

Recommendations for initial ventilator settings in patients with chest trauma are listed in Table 19-2. Initially, full ventilatory support using volume control or pressure

Table 19-2 Initial Mechanical Ventilation Settings in Patients With Chest Trauma

Setting	Recommendation
Mode	A/C (CMV)
Rate	15-25/min
Volume/pressure control	Pressure or volume
Tidal volume	6-8 mL/kg IBW provided that plateau pressure ≤ 30 cm H_2O; 4-8 mL/kg IBW with ARDS
Inspiratory time	≤ 1 s
PEEP	5 cm H_2O; none with severe air leaks; appropriately titrated if ARDS
Fio_2	1.0

Abbreviations: ARDS, acute respiratory distress syndrome; CMV, continuous mandatory ventilation; IBW, ideal body weight; PEEP, positive end-expiratory pressure.

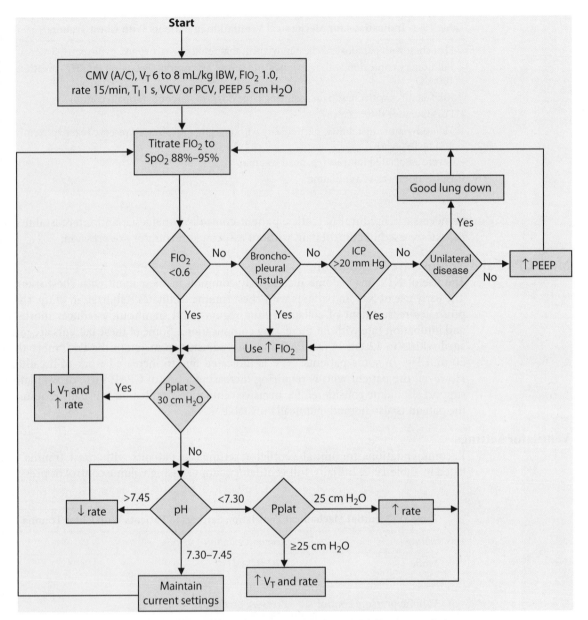

Figure 19-1 An algorithm for mechanical ventilation of the patient with chest trauma.

control is frequently used (Figure 19-1). However, some patients who are well managed for pain and are hemodynamically stable do well on pressure support.

Oxygenation is dependent on F_{IO_2}, PEEP, the extent of pulmonary dysfunction, and hemodynamic stability. The initial F_{IO_2} should be set at 1, and then titrated to the desired level of arterial oxygenation using pulse oximetry. Generally, the initial PEEP level should be set at 5 cm H_2O. If the patient has significant barotrauma (eg, subcutaneous emphysema, pneumothorax, air leaks from chest tubes), then it may be desirable to set the initial PEEP at 0 cm H_2O. If the patient has significant pulmonary shunt, a trial of higher PEEP is appropriate. In patients with chest trauma, however, caution must be exercised when increasing airway pressure because barotrauma is common. As the result of blood loss, hemodynamic instability may result when PEEP is increased, and increasing PEEP may increase intracranial pressure in patients with associated head trauma. If a unilateral pulmonary contusion is present, care must also be exercised when increasing PEEP. With unilateral lung disease, PEEP may result in shunting of blood from higher compliance lung units to low-compliance nonventilated areas, which will result in increasing shunt and hypoxemia. With unilateral pulmonary contusion, lateral positioning with the contused lung up may be more beneficial than increasing PEEP.

With either volume ventilation or pressure ventilation, the plateau pressure should be kept below 30 cm H_2O. In trauma patients with satisfactory lung compliance (eg, postoperative thoracotomy), tidal volumes of 6 to 8 mL/kg of ideal body weight can be used with plateau pressure of less than 30 cm H_2O. Patients with pulmonary contusion and ARDS may require tidal volumes of 4 to 8 mL/kg to keep plateau pressure less than 30 cm H_2O. An initial respiratory rate of 15 to 25/min is often adequate. Respiratory rate is increased if required to establish a desired $Paco_2$. Permissive hypercapnia is generally well tolerated in chest trauma patients, provided that there is no accompanying head trauma with increased intracranial pressure. An inspiratory time less than or equal to 1 second is usually adequate in patients with chest trauma.

Monitoring

Monitoring the mechanically ventilated chest trauma patient is similar in many aspects to that with any mechanically ventilated patient (Table 19-3). Air leak is more likely in patients with chest trauma, and signs of air leak must be assessed frequently. Pneumothorax should be considered following any rapid deterioration of the mechanically ventilated chest trauma patient. Chest trauma patients should be ventilated at the lowest peak alveolar pressure and PEEP level that produces adequate arterial oxygenation. Auto-PEEP must be avoided. Pulmonary embolism is also common in these patients, and should be considered if clinical status rapidly deteriorates. As is the case with many surgical patients, fluid overload frequently occurs and is associated with shunting and

---

Table 19-3 Monitoring of the Mechanically Ventilated Patient With Chest Trauma

- Pneumothorax and extra-alveolar air
- Auto-PEEP, mean airway pressure
- Peak alveolar pressure
- Pulmonary embolism
- Fluid volume status
- Nutritional status

Abbreviation: PEEP, positive end-expiratory pressure.

decreased lung compliance. With prolonged mechanical ventilation, nutritional support is necessary to facilitate healing and weaning from mechanical ventilation.

Liberation

Discontinuation of mechanical ventilation can occur early and quickly in many chest trauma patients, such as those ventilated postoperatively following repair of a penetrating chest injury. Many of these patients have no previous cardiopulmonary disease and recover rapidly if there are no associated problems (eg, head trauma, ARDS). Those who have severe pulmonary contusion and ARDS may have a long mechanical ventilation course that may be complicated with pulmonary infection, empyema, sepsis, and pulmonary embolism. Ventilator liberation may be difficult in some of these patients, particularly if they develop multisystem failure. These patients may require prolonged weaning with periodic spontaneous breathing trials. Weaning may also be difficult in patients with severe chest wall injury or diaphragmatic injury. For patients who are difficult to wean, the goals should be treatment of injuries and preexisting medical conditions, bronchial hygiene (eg, secretion removal), nutritional support, and strengthening and conditioning of respiratory muscles (ie, periods of spontaneous breathing at subfatiguing loads).

> ### Points to Remember
>
> - Chest trauma can be either blunt or penetrating.
> - Indications for mechanical ventilation with chest trauma include flail chest, chest pain requiring large doses of respiratory depressant pain medications, pulmonary contusion, postoperative thoracotomy, hemodynamic instability, or severe associated injuries.
> - Flail chest is not an absolute indication for mechanical ventilation.
> - Mask continuous positive airway pressure and noninvasive ventilation should be considered before the decision to intubate.
> - Chest trauma is commonly associated with severe lung injury.
> - Air leak is a common complication of mechanical ventilation in chest trauma patients.
> - The ventilator course of many chest trauma patients is short and weaning occurs rapidly.
> - In patients with chest trauma who develop acute respiratory distress syndrome, the mechanical ventilation course can be difficult, with prolonged and difficult weaning.

Additional Reading

Chiumello D, Coppola S, Froio S, et al. Noninvasive ventilation in chest trauma: systematic review and meta-analysis. *Intensive Care Med.* 2013;39:1171-1180.

Gentilello LM, Pierson DJ. Trauma critical care. *Am J Respir Crit Care Med.* 2001;163: 604-607.

Harris T, Davenport R, Hurst T, Jones J. Improving outcome in severe trauma: trauma systems and initial management: intubation, ventilation and resuscitation. *Postgrad Med J.* 2012;88:588-594.

Kiraly L, Schreiber M. Management of the crushed chest. *Crit Care Med.* 2010;38(9 Suppl): S469-S477.

Michaels AJ. Management of post traumatic respiratory failure. *Crit Care Clin.* 2004;20:83-99.

Papadakos PJ, Karcz M, Lachmann B. Mechanical ventilation in trauma. *Curr Opin Anaesthesiol.* 2010;23:228-232.

Pettiford BL, Luketich JD, Landreneau RJ. The management of flail chest. *Thorac Surg Clin.* 2007;17:25-33.

Rico FR, Cheng JD, Gestring ML, Piotrowski ES. Mechanical ventilation strategies in massive chest trauma. *Crit Care Clin.* 2007;23:299-315.

Sutyak JP, Wohltmann CD, Larson J. Pulmonary contusions and critical care management in thoracic trauma. *Thorac Surg Clin.* 2007;17:11-23.

Wanek S, Mayberry JC. Blunt thoracic trauma: flail chest, pulmonary contusion, and blast injury. *Crit Care Clin.* 2004;20:71-81.

Wigginton JG, Roppolo L, Pepe PE. Advances in resuscitative trauma care. *Minerva Anestesiol.* 2011;77:993-1002.

Chapter 20
Head Injury

Introduction

Head injury and its associated neurologic dysfunction are common in the United States and other developed countries. The morbidity and mortality associated with this problem are related to acute cerebral edema and other space occupying lesions that increase intracranial pressure (ICP). Head injury is often traumatic in origin. However, similar effects may be seen with surgical (eg, postcraniotomy for tumor resection) and medical (eg, cerebral vascular accident, postresuscitation hypoxia, hepatic failure) problems.

Overview

Physiology

Because the skull is rigid, intracranial volume increases result in an increase in ICP. The relationship between intracranial volume and ICP is described by the cerebral compliance curve (Figure 20-1). Although small increases in intracranial volume are tolerated without an increase in ICP, larger increases in volume result in large increases in ICP. This increase in ICP decreases cerebral blood flow, resulting in cerebral hypoxia. With large increases in ICP, the swelling brain herniates through the tentorium, resulting in compression of the brain stem. Much of the management of head injury relates to efforts to control ICP.

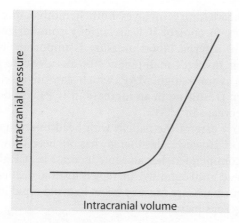

Figure 20-1 Cerebral compliance curve showing the relationship between intracranial pressure and intracranial volume. Normally (low intracranial volume), some cerebral swelling can occur without increasing intracranial pressure. However, a point is reached after which further increases in cerebral swelling result in a large increase in intracranial pressure.

Cerebral perfusion pressure (CPP) is defined as the difference between mean arterial pressure (MAP) and ICP:

$$CPP = MAP - ICP$$

Normally, ICP is less than 10 mm Hg and MAP is about 90 mm Hg, resulting in a normal CPP of more than 80 mm Hg. The target CPP is 50 to 70 mm Hg. CPP less than 50 mm Hg should be avoided. In patients with acute head injury, the ICP is frequently measured. CPP is decreased by either a decrease in MAP or an increase in ICP. Thus, treatments that decrease MAP (eg, positive pressure ventilation, diuresis, vasodilator therapy) decrease CPP, whereas treatments that decrease ICP (hyperventilation, mannitol) increase CPP. A normal physiologic response to an acute increase in ICP is hypertension with bradycardia, which is called the Cushing response.

Mechanical ventilation can increase ICP and decrease CPP because the increased intrathoracic pressure associated with mechanical ventilation. Positive end-expiratory pressure (PEEP) has the potential of decreasing MAP and venous return. A decrease in venous return increases ICP and a decrease in MAP decreases CPP.

Clinical Findings

Increases in ICP can result in abnormal ventilatory patterns such as Cheyne-Stokes breathing, central neurogenic hyperventilation, and apnea with severe injury. Compression of the brainstem (ie, transtentorial herniation) results in dilated nonreactive pupils, posturing (decerebrate and decorticate), and cardiovascular collapse.

Neurogenic Pulmonary Edema

Acute head injury and elevated ICP can result in neurogenic pulmonary edema (NPE). NPE is a noncardiogenic pulmonary edema and is clinically indistinguishable from acute respiratory distress syndrome (ARDS). It results in a decreased functional residual capacity, decreased lung compliance, increased intrapulmonary shunt, and hypoxemia. Treatment of NPE is similar to that of other causes of ARDS, including oxygen therapy and PEEP.

Management

Management of acute head injury involves both hemodynamic and respiratory management. Techniques to control ICP are briefly summarized in Table 20-1. Hemodynamic control of arterial blood pressure is important to maintain CPP. Respiratory management involves maintenance of an adequate $Paco_2$ and Pao_2. Care must be taken to avoid a high MAP, which can adversely affect CPP by decreasing venous return (resulting in an increase in ICP) and decreasing cardiac output (resulting in a decrease in MAP).

In the past, respiratory care of the patient with head injury included the use of iatrogenic hyperventilation. However, this therapy has not been shown to increase survival and is no longer recommended. For an acute increase in ICP, the patient may be temporarily hyperventilated until definitive therapy is instituted, after which the $Paco_2$ is gradually restored to normal. Care must be taken to avoid rapid increases in $Paco_2$, which may produce dangerous increases in ICP.

Table 20-1 **Management of ICP**

Technique	Comments
Hyperventilation	$Paco_2$ of 25-30 mm Hg is useful to acutely lower ICP; $Paco_2$ should be normalized as soon as possible
Mean airway pressure	Mean airway pressure should be kept as low as possible to avoid increases in ICP and decreases in arterial blood pressure
Positioning	30-degree elevation of the head is useful to lower ICP and offset the effect that PEEP may have on intrathoracic pressure and ICP; Trendelenburg's position should be avoided; the head should be kept in a neutral position to facilitate venous outflow from the brain
Dehydration and osmotherapy	Mannitol is useful to treat acute increases in ICP; furosemide and acetazolamide commonly used to promote clearance of fluid from the brain
Sedation and paralysis	ICP increases with agitation, Valsalva maneuvers, coughing, and pain; therapy directed at suppressing these actions often lowers ICP
Corticosteroids	Steroids have been widely used in the past for treatment of cerebral edema, but no benefit has been shown to result from this treatment, and steroids should not be routinely administered for head injury
Barbiturate therapy	High dose barbiturate therapy reduces cerebral oxygen demands and lowers ICP; high dose barbiturate therapy may be a useful treatment in patients with high ICP that does not respond to conventional management
Temperature control	Hyperthermia increases cerebral injury and must be avoided; hypothermia is being increasingly used to lower ICP
Decompressive craniectomy	Removal of part of the skull bone can allow mass expansion without increasing pressure; the role of this therapy is unclear for diffuse edema
Ventriculostomy	Draining a small amount of cerebral spinal fluid can be used to reduce ICP

Abbreviation: ICP, intracranial pressure.

$Paco_2$ has an indirect effect on cerebral vascular tone due to its effect on pH. It is the change in pH that affects the tone of cerebral blood vessels and thus, cerebral blood volume and ICP. A decrease in pH (increased $Paco_2$) causes cerebral vascular dilatation and an increase in ICP. An increase in pH (decreased $Paco_2$) causes a decrease in ICP. During hyperventilation therapy, the brain quickly equilibrates to changes in $Paco_2$ and a new steady state is established within 4 to 6 hours and over time the pH normalizes reducing the benefit of the decreased $Paco_2$. Although iatrogenic hyperventilation is not recommended, permissive hypercapnia may be associated with unacceptable elevations in ICP.

Mechanical Ventilation

As shown in Figure 20-2, increases in $Paco_2$ and decreases in Pao_2 result in increases in ICP. Thus, normal oxygenation and acid-base balance are goals of ventilation in patients with an increased ICP. Increases in alveolar pressure may result in an increase in ICP due to a decrease in venous return and a decrease in cardiac output.

Indications

Indications for mechanical ventilation in patients with head injury are listed in Table 20-2. The most common reason to ventilate these patients is central respiratory depression due to the primary injury. In such patients, lung function may be near normal and mechanical ventilation is straightforward. In patients with traumatic injury, associated injuries to the spine, chest, and abdomen may also require the initiation of mechanical ventilation. Positive pressure ventilation may be necessary due to neurogenic pulmonary edema. Finally, some therapies for acute head injury (eg, barbiturates, sedation, and paralysis) result in central respiratory depression, necessitating mechanical ventilation.

Ventilator Settings

Recommendations for initial ventilator settings for patients with head injury are listed in Table 20-3 and Figure 20-3. Full ventilator support is almost always initially required for these patients, and can be provided by continuous mandatory ventilation (A/C). Because of the depressed neurologic status of these patients and the need to control $Paco_2$, pressure support ventilation as the initial mode in these patients is usually not appropriate. As respiratory status improves and spontaneous breathing becomes acceptable, pressure support ventilation can be used.

Because patients with head injury often have relatively normal lung function, oxygenation is usually not a problem. With these patients, 100% oxygen is initially administered and can be rapidly weaned using pulse oximetry. A Pao_2 more than 80 mm Hg

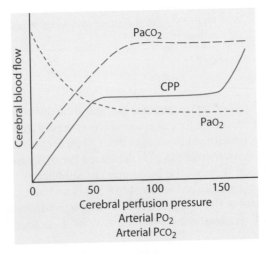

Cerebral blood flow

PaCO₂

CPP

PaO₂

0   50   100   150

Cerebral perfusion pressure
Arterial PO₂
Arterial PCO₂

Figure 20-2 The effects of $Paco_2$, Pao_2, and cerebral perfusion pressure on cerebral blood flow. Note that hypercarbia and hypoxemia increase cerebral blood flow, and thus intracranial pressure. Normally, cerebral blood flow remains relatively constant over a wide range of cerebral perfusion pressures (autoregulation), but this relationship is lost with acute head injury (loss of autoregulation).

Table 20-2 **Indications for Mechanical Ventilation in Patients With Acute Head Injury**

- Depression due to primary neurologic injury
- Associated injuries to the spine, chest, and abdomen
- Neurogenic pulmonary edema
- Treatment with respiratory suppressant medications (barbiturates, sedatives, paralytics)

is often used because this minimizes the potential for periodic episodes of hypoxemia and associated rises in ICP. An initial PEEP level of 5 cm H_2O is usually appropriate and adequate. Although there is concern related to the effects of PEEP on ICP, PEEP usually does not adversely affect ICP at levels less than or equal to 10 cm H_2O. With neurogenic pulmonary edema, the management of oxygenation is similar to that with other causes of ARDS, although care must be taken to avoid the effects of high MAP on ICP. In patients requiring high levels of PEEP, the head of the bed should be raised to minimize the effect of the increased intrathoracic pressure and ICP should be carefully monitored.

The choice of volume-controlled or pressure-controlled ventilation is based on clinician's bias. A tidal volume in the range of 6 to 8 mL/kg ideal body weight can be used provided that plateau pressure is kept below 30 cm H_2O. This is usually not a problem, because these patients typically have a nearly normal lung and chest wall compliance. The ventilatory goal is to maintain the Pco_2 35 to 45 mm Hg and pH 7.35 to 7.45. If the patient has concomitant acute or chronic respiratory disease, a lower tidal volume is selected. A respiratory rate appropriate to achieve normal acid-base balance should be chosen. This can often be achieved at a rate of 15 to 25 breaths/min. An inspiratory time of 1 second is usually adequate.

Table 20-3 **Initial Mechanical Ventilator Settings With Head Injury**

Setting	Recommendation
Mode	CMV (A/C)
Rate	15-25 breaths/min
Volume/pressure control	Volume or pressure
Tidal volume	6-8 mL/kg IBW provided that plateau pressure ≤ 30 cm H_2O
Inspiratory time	1 s
PEEP	5 cm H_2O provided that PEEP does not increase ICP
Fio_2	1.0

Abbreviations: CMV, continuous mandatory ventilation; ICP, intracranial pressure; IBW, ideal body weight; PEEP, positive end-expiratory pressure.

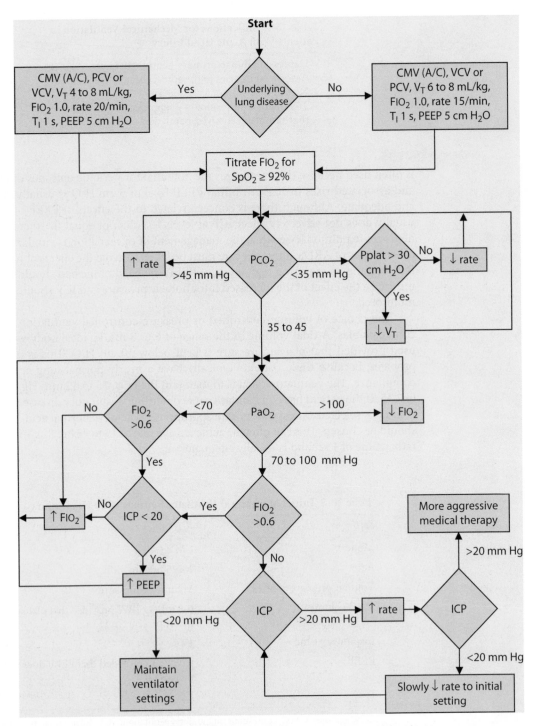

Figure 20-3 An algorithm for mechanical ventilation of the patient with head injury.

Table 20-4 **Monitoring of the Mechanically Ventilated Patient With Head Injury**

- Peak alveolar pressure, mean airway pressure, auto-PEEP
- $Paco_2$ and end-tidal Pco_2
- Intracranial pressure, jugular venous oxygen saturation
- Pulse oximetry
- Heart rate and systemic blood pressure

Abbreviation: PEEP, positive end-expiratory pressure.

Monitoring

Monitoring of mechanically ventilated head-injured patients is similar to that of any mechanically ventilated patient (Table 20-4). If minute ventilation is increased to produce iatrogenic hyperventilation for a short period of time, the presence of auto-PEEP must be evaluated. Capnography may be useful to monitor the level of ventilation in these patients, who often have normal lung function and do not tolerate well an increase in $Paco_2$.

Close observation of ICP should be used when ventilator settings are manipulated. If an ICP monitor is not present, clinical signs of an increased ICP (eg, pupillary response, posturing, changes in level of consciousness) should be evaluated when ventilator changes occur. Although airway clearance is important in these patients, care must be taken to avoid deleterious increases in ICP during suctioning. Nutritional support is necessary to facilitate healing and weaning from mechanical ventilation. Pulmonary embolism can occur in patients with prolonged immobility, and pulmonary infection is also common in these patients.

Jugular venous bulb oxygen saturation ($Sjvo_2$) and brain Po_2 (P_bO_2) from a probe placed into the brain may be used as an index of the adequacy of cerebral oxygenation. The use of these monitors is controversial. If used, $Sjvo_2$ less than 50% or P_bO_2 less than 15 mm Hg are treatment thresholds.

Liberation

Liberation should not be considered until respiratory depressant therapy is no longer required. Ventilator discontinuation can often be initiated before the patient's neurologic function is maximally restored if the ventilatory drive is intact. For some patients, maintenance of a stable airway is required for a longer time than ventilatory support (ie, tracheostomy). However, extubation should not be delayed solely on the basis of depressed neurologic status. Due to central neurologic dysfunction, ventilator liberation, extubation, and decannulation of some of these patients can be prolonged and difficult. Weaning approaches should incorporate spontaneous breathing trials and appropriate rest following a failed trial of spontaneous breathing.

Apnea Test

An apnea test is commonly conducted as part of the diagnosis of brain death. Before conducting the apnea test, the following prerequisites should be met: core temperature more than or equal to 36.5°C, systolic blood pressure more than or equal to 90 mm Hg, euvolemia, normoxemia (or $Pao_2 > 200$ mm Hg breathing 100% oxygen), and eucapnia (or Paco$_2$ > 40 mm Hg in the patient with chronic hypercapnia). The following procedure is used:

- Disconnect the ventilator.
- Administer 6 L/min O$_2$, either by T-piece or by a catheter passed into the trachea.
- Observe the patient closely for signs of respiratory movements. If respiratory movements occur, the apnea test is negative (ie, does not support the clinical diagnosis of brain death), and mechanical ventilation is resumed.
- If respiratory movements do not occur, measure arterial blood gases after 8 minutes and reconnect the ventilator.
- If respiratory movements are absent and Paco$_2$ is more than 60 mm Hg (or 20 mm Hg greater than baseline), the apnea test result is positive and consistent with the clinical diagnosis of brain death.
- If hypotension or desaturation occurs during the apnea test, the ventilator is reconnected and the test is resumed at a later time.
- If no respiratory movements are observed, Paco$_2$ is less than 60 mm Hg, and no adverse effects occur, the test may be repeated with 10 minutes of apnea.

Points to Remember

- The requirement for mechanical ventilation in head-injured patients is usually due to central respiratory depression.
- Cerebral perfusion pressure (CPP) is the difference between mean arterial pressure and intracranial pressure (ICP) and is normally more than 80 mm Hg.
- Positive pressure ventilation can adversely affect CPP.
- Some head-injured patients develop a form of acute respiratory distress syndrome called neurogenic pulmonary edema.
- Normal ICP is less than 10 mm Hg.
- Iatrogenic hyperventilation is used to control acute increases in ICP, but prolonged hyperventilation therapy is not recommended.
- Because many head-injured patients have relatively normal lung function, mechanical ventilation is usually straightforward.
- The effects of mechanical ventilation on ICP must be closely evaluated.
- The neurologic effects of respiratory care procedures such as suctioning must be closely monitored.
- Extubation should not be delayed solely on the basis of depressed neurologic function.
- Weaning some patients may be a prolonged process.
- The apnea test is used to confirm brain death.

Additional Reading

Bein T, Kuhr LP, Bele S, et al. Lung recruitment maneuver in patients with cerebral injury: effects on intracranial pressure and cerebral metabolism. *Intensive Care Med.* 2002;28:554-558.

Bell RS, Ecker RD, Severson MA, et al. The evolution of the treatment of traumatic cerebrovascular injury during wartime. *Neurosurg Focus.* 2010;28:E5.

Berrouschot J, Roossler A, Koster J, Schneider D. Mechanical ventilation in patients with hemispheric ischemic stroke. *Crit Care Med.* 2000;28:2956-2961.

Bratton SL, Chesnut RM, Ghajar J, et al. Guidelines for the management of severe traumatic brain injury. X. Brain oxygen monitoring and thresholds. *J Neurotrauma.* 2007;24(Suppl 1): S65-S70.

Bratton SL, Chestnut RM, Ghajar J, et al. Guidelines for the management of severe traumatic brain injury. XIV. Hyperventilation. *J Neurotrauma.* 2007;249(Suppl 1):S87-S90.

Chintamani, Khanna J, Singh JP, et al. Early tracheostomy in closed head injuries: experience at a tertiary center in a developing country—a prospective study. *BMC Emerg Med.* 2005;5:8.

Coplin WM, Pierson DJ, Cooley KD, et al. Implications of extubation delay in brain-injured patients meeting standard weaning criteria. *Am J Respir Crit Care Med.* 2000;161:1530-1536.

Cormio M, Portella G, Spreafico E, et al. Role of assisted breathing in severe traumatic brain injury. *Minerva Anestesiol.* 2002;68:278-284.

Davis DP, Peay J, Sise MJ, et al. Prehospital airway and ventilation management: a trauma score and injury severity score-based analysis. *J Trauma.* 2010;69:294-301.

Davis DP. Early ventilation in traumatic brain injury. *Resuscitation.* 2008;76:333-340.

Heegaard W, Biros M. Traumatic brain injury. *Emerg Med Clin North Am.* 2007;25:655-678.

Jonathan J, Hou P, Wilcox SR, et al. Acute respiratory distress syndrome after spontaneous intracerebral hemorrhage. *Crit Care Med.* 2013;41:1992-2001.

Martini RP, Deem S, Treggiari MM. Targeting brain tissue oxygenation in traumatic brain injury. *Respir Care.* 2013;58:162-172.

Mascia L, Mastromauro I, Viberti S. High tidal volume as a predictor of acute lung injury in neurotrauma patients. *Minerva Anestesiol.* 2008;74:325-327.

Mascia L, Zavala E, Bosma K, et al. High tidal volume is associated with the development of acute lung injury after severe brain injury: an international observational study. *Crit Care Med.* 2007;35:1815-1820.

Stiefel MF, Udoetuk JD, Spiotta AM, et al. Conventional neurocritical care and cerebral oxygenation after traumatic brain injury. *J Neurosurg.* 2006;105:568-575.

Stocchetti N, Maas AI, Chieregato A, et al. Hyperventilation in head injury: a review. *Chest.* 2005;127:1812-1827.

Suazo JAC, Maas AIR, van den Brink WA, et al. CO_2 reactivity and brain oxygen pressure monitoring in severe head injury. *Crit Care Med.* 2000;28:3268-3274.

Wijdicks EFM. The diagnosis of brain death. *N Engl J Med.* 2001;344:1215-1221.

Chapter 21
Postoperative Mechanical Ventilation

Objectives

1. List indications for mechanical ventilation of postoperative patients.
2. Describe the initial ventilator settings for postoperative patients without prior pulmonary disease, with prior pulmonary disease, and patients with single lung transplantation.
3. Describe monitoring of the ventilated postoperative patient.
4. Discuss weaning of patients requiring postoperative ventilatory support.

Introduction

A frequently encountered category of patients requiring ventilatory support are those in the immediate postoperative period. This is particularly true of patients following thoracic or cardiac surgery, although changes in surgical and anesthesia techniques have decreased the requirement for mechanical ventilation. Generally, these patients do not present complex ventilatory management problems and many are extubated within 24 hours. In addition, many of these patients who present with postoperative hypoxemia or hypercarbia can be successfully managed with mask continuous positive airway pressure (CPAP) or noninvasive ventilation (NIV).

Overview

It has been well established that surgical procedures that include general anesthesia, especially those affecting the thoracic or abdominal cavities, result in impairment of ventilatory function. The reasons for these impairments include the effects of general inhalation anesthetics on hypoxic pulmonary vasoconstriction and a blunting of hypoxemic and hypercapnic ventilatory drive when intravenous narcotics are used. As a result of alteration in the shape and motion of the diaphragm and chest wall, thoracic or cardiac surgery can decrease lung volume by 20% to 30% and upper abdominal surgery can reduce the vital capacity by up to 60%. Many thoracic surgical and cardiac surgical patients have radiographic evidence of atelectasis. In the patient with normal preoperative pulmonary function, this may not present significant postoperative problems. But in patients with preexisting pulmonary disease, some level of postoperative respiratory failure can be expected. Cardiac surgical patients are at risk of diaphragmatic dysfunction due to phrenic nerve injury. In patients with preexisting pulmonary disease, postoperative management can be complex. With the increased use of lung resection surgery, heart and lung transplantation, and complex cardiac surgery performed on older patients, postoperative ventilatory failure is a common reason for ventilatory support.

Mechanical Ventilation

Indications

The primary reason for mechanical ventilation in this group is apnea as a result of unreversed anesthetic agents (Table 21-1). The primary reasons that anesthesia is not

Table 21-1 **Indications for Ventilation in Postoperative Patients**

- Apnea—unreversed anesthetic agents
- Minimize postoperative cardiopulmonary stress
- Preexisting lung disease compromising cardiopulmonary reserve

reversed are iatrogenic hypothermia, the need to reduce cardiopulmonary stress, or the presence of altered pulmonary mechanics. Some cardiac surgeons favor cold cardioplegia to reduce the likelihood of hypoxic injury. These patients receive narcotic anesthesia throughout the procedure and may require 8 to 16 hours for warming and full reversal of anesthesia. Transplant recipients (heart or lung) are ventilated to ensure cardiopulmonary stress is minimized during the initial acclimation period and to minimize any adverse effects of an increased work-of-breathing in the immediate postoperative period. The most difficult group of patients is those with preexisting lung disease whose pulmonary mechanics are adversely affected by surgery, who require ventilatory support because of compromised cardiopulmonary reserve and bronchial hygiene.

Ventilator Settings

Minimal or no prior pulmonary disease It is usually easy to ventilate these patients. Most simply require postanesthesia recovery. Volume or pressure ventilation in the continuous mandatory ventilation (A/C) mode is acceptable (Figure 21-1). Tidal volume may be normal (6-8 mL/kg ideal body weight [IBW]) since lung function is normal. The rate can be set at 12 to 18/min. FIO_2 is titrated to maintain a normal Pao_2 (> 80 mm Hg) and low levels of positive end-expiratory pressure (PEEP) (5 cm H_2O) is applied to maintain functional residual capacity (Table 21-2). In hypothermic patients, minute ventilation is decreased to avoid hypocarbia and alkalosis. As a result, the initial rate may need to be set low and increased as body temperature increases.

Prior pulmonary disease Patients with a history of chronic pulmonary disease are ventilated in the same manner as any patient with chronic pulmonary disease. Air trapping is a concern with chronic obstructive pulmonary disease (COPD). Moderate tidal volume (6-8 mL/kg IBW) and respiratory rate (12-18/min) should be selected. A long expiratory time is needed to avoid auto-PEEP. PEEP is applied to counterbalance auto-PEEP when spontaneous breathing resumes. Plateau pressure (Pplat) less than 25 cm H_2O should be used in patients with COPD. In patients with chronic restrictive pulmonary disease, air trapping is not a problem. Because of reduced lung volumes, however, smaller V_T (4-6 mL/kg predicted body weight) and rapid rates (20-30/min) are set to avoid high Pplat.

Single lung transplant Of all the patients ventilated postoperatively, this group is the most troublesome if one lung has relatively normal pulmonary mechanics (transplanted lung) and the other has mechanics reflecting either obstructive or restrictive disease (native lung). In these patients, the ventilator should be set to ensure the maximum function of the native lung, since this will be the lung presenting the greatest

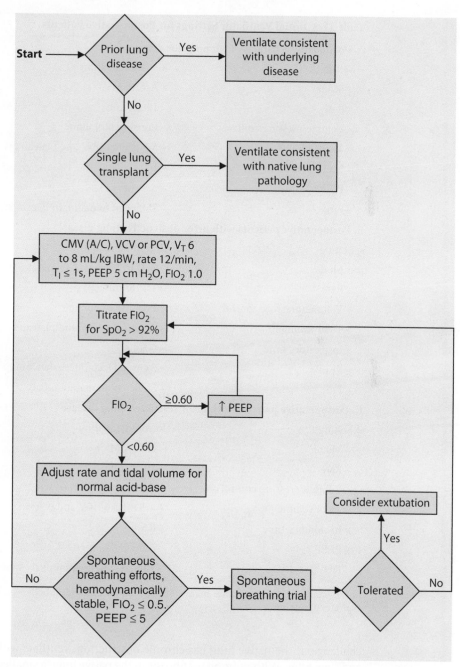

Figure 21-1 An algorithm for mechanical ventilation of the postoperative patient.

Table 21-2 Initial Ventilator Settings for Postoperative Patients

A. Postoperative patients with no prior disease

- Setting
  - Mode
  - Rate
  - Volume/pressure control
  - Tidal volume
  - Inspiratory time
  - PEEP
  - FIO_2

- Recommendation
  - A/C (CMV)
  - 12-18/min
  - Pressure or volume
  - 6-8 mL/kg IBW and plateau pressure $\leq$ 30 cm H_2O
  - 1 s
  - $\leq$ 5 cm H_2O
  - Sufficient to maintain Pao_2 > 80 mm Hg

B. Postoperative patients with prior obstructive lung disease

- Setting
  - Mode
  - Rate
  - Volume/pressure control
  - Tidal volume
  - Inspiratory time
  - PEEP
  - FIO_2

- Recommendation
  - A/C (CMV)
  - 12-18/min
  - Pressure or volume
  - 6-8 mL/kg IBW and plateau pressure $\leq$ 25 cm H_2O
  - 0.5-1 s
  - 5 cm H_2O; counterbalance auto-PEEP
  - Sufficient to maintain Pao_2 > 60 mm Hg

C. Postoperative patients with prior restrictive lung disease

- Setting
  - Mode
  - Rate
  - Volume/pressure control
  - Tidal volume
  - Inspiratory time
  - PEEP
  - FIO_2

- Recommendation
  - A/C (CMV)
  - 20-30/min
  - Pressure or volume
  - 4-6 mL/kg IBW and plateau pressure $\leq$ 30 cm H_2O
  - 0.5-0.8 s
  - 5 cm H_2O
  - Sufficient to maintain Pao_2 > 60 mm Hg

Abbreviations: CMV, continuous mandatory ventilation; IBW, ideal body weight; PEEP, positive end-expiratory pressure.

challenge. If the native lung has chronic obstruction, ventilate with moderate volume and slow rates. With pulmonary fibrosis in the native lung, a smaller V_T and more rapid rate are indicated. In the case of pulmonary fibrosis, there is less concern about air trapping. However, plateau pressure may be high due to reduced compliance.

The greatest ventilatory challenge is the patient with a single lung transplant where the native lung is obstructed and the transplanted lung has become stiff because of fluid, infection, rejection, or acute lung injury. In this setting, it is difficult to dictate ideal ventilator settings because of the differing pathologies in each lung. However, tidal volume should be small. Attention needs to be paid on two variables as adjustments are made. First, concern about plateau pressure because of ventilator-imposed lung injury and damage to the surgical site. Second, air trapping in the obstructed lung resulting in grossly compromised ventilation/perfusion ratios. In this setting, permissive hypercapnia may be necessary with the final ventilator settings being a compromise between conflicting needs.

CPAP and NIV

Many postoperative patients develop respiratory complications postoperatively. Some of these patients can be easily managed with mask CPAP or NIV. Mask CPAP is beneficial in patients who develop respiratory failure following abdominal surgery. In these patients, CPAP can be set at 8 to 12 cm H_2O based on patient tolerance with FIO_2 set to ensure SpO_2 is more than 92%. If patient is hypercarbic, NIV can be applied with PEEP of 5 to 8 cm H_2O, inspiratory pressure set to provide a tidal volume of 4 to 8 mL/kg IBW, respiratory rate for an appropriate $PaCO_2$, and FIO_2 to maintain SpO_2 more than 92%. Cardiac surgical patients and transplant patients may also benefit from mask CPAP or NIV if they develop respiratory failure.

Monitoring

For the majority of postoperative patients, monitoring of gas exchange (pulse oximetry and arterial blood gases), level of consciousness, pulmonary mechanics, and the ability to cough and deep breathe are sufficient to determine if there is a need for continued ventilatory support (Table 21-3). However, in patients with COPD, monitoring of auto-PEEP is also important. These patients are often fluid-positive, which can affect respiratory function. Monitoring fluid balance, including central venous pressure, is often useful. In patients with hemodynamic instability or severe cardiac disease, careful monitoring of pulmonary and systemic hemodynamics is also indicated.

Liberation

Ventilator discontinuation is a simple process for most postoperative patients. When gas exchange is adequate at an FIO_2 of 0.50, the patient is alert and oriented, able to

---

Table 21-3 Monitoring of the Mechanically Ventilated Postoperative Patient

- Pulse oximetry
- Level of consciousness
- Pulmonary mechanics
- Auto-PEEP and plateau pressure
- Fluid balance
- Hemodynamics

Abbreviation: PEEP, positive end-expiratory pressure.

lift the head and take a deep breath, ventilatory support can be discontinued and the patient is extubated. Many clinicians prefer short (30 minutes) spontaneous breathing trials, or a gradual reduction of pressure support to 5 to 10 cm H_2O before discontinuation. However, unless the baseline status is abnormal (ie, COPD), a specific weaning protocol may extend the time ventilation is required. In patients with underlying pulmonary disease or lung transplant patients, more prolonged weaning may be necessary.

Points to Remember

- General anesthesia causes pulmonary vasoconstriction and a blunting of hypoxemic and hypercapnia ventilatory drive.
- Thoracic and cardiac surgery can reduce the functional residual capacity by 20% to 30%, and upper abdominal surgery can reduce the vital capacity by 60%.
- When mechanical ventilation is indicated in postoperative patients, this is likely due to anesthesia that has not been reversed.
- No special ventilatory requirements are needed in postoperative patients without pulmonary disease.
- In patients with obstructive or restrictive lung disease, ventilate according to the primary disease.
- In patients with single lung transplantation, ventilate in a manner most suited for the most diseased lung (usually the native lung).
- Monitoring of postoperative mechanically ventilated patients involves indices of gas exchange, level of consciousness, and pulmonary mechanics.
- In most postoperative patients, the ventilator can be discontinued once F_{IO_2} is reduced and general muscular capability is restored.

Additional Reading

Chiumello D, Chevallard G, Gregoretti C. Non-invasive ventilation in postoperative patients: a systematic review. *Intensive Care Med.* 2011;37:918-929.

Ferreyra GP, Baussano I, Squadrone V, et al. Continuous positive airway pressure for treatment of respiratory complications after abdominal surgery: a systematic review and meta-analysis. *Ann Surg.* 2008;247:617-726.

Glossop AJ, Shephard N, Bryden DC, Mills GH. Non-invasive ventilation for weaning, avoiding reintubation after extubation and in the postoperative period: a meta-analysis. *Br J Anaesth.* 2012;109:305-314.

Granton J. Update of early respiratory failure in the lung transplant recipient. *Curr Opin Crit Care.* 2006;12:19-24.

Pennock JL, Pierce WS, Waldhausen JA. The management of the lungs during cardiopulmonary bypass. *Surg Gynecol Obstet.* 1977;145:917-927.

Tusman G, Böhm SH, Warner DO, Sprung J. Atelectasis and perioperative pulmonary complications in high-risk patients. *Curr Opin Anaesthiol.* 2012;25:1-10.

Chapter 22
Neuromuscular Disease

Objectives

1. Discuss the pathophysiology of ventilatory failure in patients with neuromuscular disease or chest wall deformities.
2. Discuss the indications for invasive and noninvasive ventilation in this patient population.
3. Discuss initial ventilator settings for invasive and noninvasive ventilatory support in this patient population.
4. Discuss monitoring during and weaning from ventilatory support for patients with neuromuscular disease.
5. Discuss the use of the in-exsufflator in patients with neuromuscular disease.

Introduction

Patients with neuromuscular disease or chest wall deformities represent a small percentage of patients receiving ventilatory support. However, they also represent a large percentage of patients requiring long-term ventilatory support. As these patients usually have normal lungs and the reason for ventilatory assistance is an inability to generate sufficient muscular effort to ventilate, providing mechanical ventilation is much easier in this group than with other groups of patients.

Overview

The neurorespirous system includes the central nervous system control centers and feedback mechanisms, spinal cord, motor nerves, and the respiratory muscles that affect chest wall and lung movement. Neuromuscular respiratory failure can be due to dysfunction of the central or the peripheral nervous system (Tables 22-1 and 22-2). The three main components of neuromuscular respiratory failure are inability to ventilate, inability to cough, and aspiration risk. This group of patients can be divided into two general categories—those with a relatively rapid (days to weeks) onset of neuromuscular weakness and those in which neuromuscular weakness is progressive and not reversible.

Rapid Onset

The two primary diseases in this category are myasthenia gravis and Guillain-Barré syndrome. This category also includes patients with prolonged paralysis following the use of neuromuscular blocking agents in the ICU and patients with high spinal cord injury. These patients do not have lung disease, but reversible neuromuscular weakness requiring ventilatory support for varying periods of time prior to return to a stable state where spontaneous breathing is feasible. The exception to this may be the spinal cord-injured patient who may require long-term ventilatory support. Of concern with these patients is their perception that their lungs are being ventilated. As a result, they require large tidal volumes—sometimes exceeding 10 mL/kg, although

Table 22-1 Diseases of the Central Nervous System Associated With Respiratory Dysfunction

Cerebral cortex	Brainstem	Basal ganglia	Spinal cord
Stroke	Infarction ("locked-in syndrome")	Parkinson disease	Trauma
Neoplasm	Neoplasm	Chorea	Infarction or hemorrhage
Cerebral degeneration	Drugs	Dyskinesias	
	Hemorrhage		Dymyelinating disease
Seizures	Progressive bulbar palsy		Disc compression
	Multiple-system atrophy		Syringomyelia
	Poliomyelitis		Tetanus
	Anoxic encephalopathy		Strychnine poisoning
	Encephalitis		Neoplasm
	Multiple sclerosis		Motor neuron disease
	Primary alveolar hypoventilation		Epidural abscess

Reproduced with permission from Benditt JO. The neuromuscular respiratory system: physiology, pathophysiology, and a respiratory care approach to patients. *Respir Care.* 2006; Aug;51(8):829-837.

Table 22-2 Diseases of the Peripheral Nervous System Associated With Respiratory Dysfunction

Motor nerves	Neuromuscular junction	Myopathies
Motor-neuron disease	Drugs	Myotonic dystrophy
Amyotrophic lateral sclerosis	Antibiotics	Muscular dystrophies
Spinal muscular atrophy	Neuromuscular-junction blockers	Polymyositis and dermatomyositis
Guillain-Barré syndrome	Anticholinesterase inhibitors	
Critical-illness neuropathy	Corticosteroids	Thick-filament myopathy
Vasculitides	Lidocaine	Glycogen-storage diseases
Toxins (eg, lithium, arsenic, gold)	Quinidine	Pompe disease
	Lithium	McArdle disease
Metabolic	Antirheumatics	Tarui disease
Diabetes	Toxins	Severe hypokalemia
Porphyria	Botulism	Hypophosphatemia
Uremia	Snake venom	Mitochondrial myopathy
Lymphoma	Scorpion sting	Nemaline body myopathy
Diphtheria	Shellfish poisoning	Acid maltase deficiency
	Crab poisoning	
	Myasthenia gravis	
	Lambert-Eaton myasthenic syndrome	

Reproduced with permission from Benditt JO. The neuromuscular respiratory system: physiology, pathophysiology, and a respiratory care approach to patients. *Respir Care.* 2006; Aug;51(8):829-837.

this is controversial. Because they do not have intrinsic lung disease, plateau pressure (Pplat) is easily kept below 30 cm H_2O.

Gradual Onset

Patients with muscular dystrophy, amyotrophic lateral sclerosis, thoracic deformities (severe scoliosis, kyphosis, or kyphoscoliosis), or postpolio syndrome frequently develop gradual muscular weakness over time, in some cases progressing over years. Many require periodic mechanical ventilation because of acute pulmonary infections and others require chronic ventilatory support because of progressive deterioration in neuromuscular function. For many of these patients, mechanical ventilation is required at some point in their course of disease.

These patients are good candidates for noninvasive ventilation (NIV). At first, these patients may only need nocturnal ventilation. During rapid eye movement (REM) sleep, respiratory control of accessory muscles is lost, resulting in nocturnal hypoventilation when the diaphragm is weak. As the disease progresses, further deterioration in neuromuscular function leads to the need for daytime NIV and invasive ventilatory support may be required.

Mechanical Ventilation

Indications

Ventilatory support in most cases is indicated because of progressive ventilatory muscle weakness leading to ventilatory failure. Oxygenation is not usually an issue. Exceptions are the patients with an acquired neuropathy or myopathy following prolonged mechanical ventilation (polyneuropathy or myopathy of critical illness), pneumonia, atelectasis, or pulmonary edema. Oxygenation may be an issue in these patients because of the primary pathophysiology leading to ventilatory support. However, it is important to remember that most patients with neuromuscular disease develop hypoxemia because they are unable to ventilate. If they are ventilated appropriately, the hypoxemia resolves.

Noninvasive Ventilation

Patients with neuromuscular disease can often be managed with NIV. NIV has been successfully used in both short-term application and long-term applications. NIV is most useful for progressive neuromuscular weakness. NIV in the setting of progressive neuromuscular disease is life-prolonging and improves the quality of life, particularly in patients who do not have bulbar involvement. Usual criteria for NIV in patients with progressive neuromuscular disease are a $Paco_2$ more than 45 mm Hg while awake, or sleep oximetry demonstrates oxygen saturation less than or equal to 88% for more than or equal to 5 minutes, or maximal inspiratory pressure (PI_{max}) is greater than −60 cm H_2O or forced vital capacity (FVC) is less than 50% predicted.

NIV can be provided using either an oronasal or nasal interface. Mouth leak is often problematic, requiring the use of an oronasal mask. In patients using daytime NIV, a mouthpiece can be used sometimes. NIV is most useful in patients where lung function has not been compromised. Typically, an inspiratory positive airway pressure of 8 to 15 cm H_2O is used, although higher settings are needed for some patients.

Unless the patient also has obstructive sleep apnea, an expiratory positive airway pressure of 3 to 4 cm H_2O is sufficient. A backup rate of 10 to 12 breaths/min is needed to manage periodic breathing. Modifications based on air leaks are necessary and large tidal volumes are usually not achievable or necessary. A properly fitting interface is necessary to improve tolerance.

Ventilator Settings

Since these patients have normal lung function, invasive ventilation can be accomplished with low pressures and a low F_{IO_2} (Table 22-3). Volume-controlled ventilation with normal V_T and respiratory rate is usually sufficient. Although high V_T have been recommended by some authorities, that practice is anecdotal and not necessary for most patients. Settings of V_T and respiratory rate that the patient considers comfortable are recommended (Figure 22-1).

In most cases assist/control continuous mandatory ventilation is the mode of choice. If the rate and V_T are set to satisfy the patient's ventilatory demand, many

---

Table 22-3 Initial Ventilator Settings in Patients With Neuromuscular Disease

A. Patients with normal lung volumes

• Setting	• Recommendation
– Mode	– A/C (CMV)
– Rate	– 10 min
– Volume/pressure control	– Volume or pressure
– Tidal volume	– < 10 mL/kg and plateau pressure ≤ 30 cm H_2O
– Inspiratory time	– ≥ 1s
– PEEP	– 5 cm H_2O
– F_{IO_2}	– ≥ 0.21
– Flow waveform	– Rectangular or descending ramp
– Mechanical dead space	– May be necessary to prevent hypocarbia

B. Patients with reduced lung volumes

• Setting	• Recommendation
– Mode	– A/C (CMV)
– Rate	– > 15/min
– Volume/pressure control	– Volume or pressure
– Tidal volume	– ≤ 8 mL/kg and plateau pressure ≤ 30 cm H_2O
– Inspiratory time	– ≤ 1 s (peak flow ≥ 60 L/min with volume ventilation)
– PEEP	– 5 cm H_2O
– F_{IO_2}	– usually ≤ 0.50

Abbreviations: CMV, continuous mandatory ventilation; PEEP, positive end-expiratory pressure.

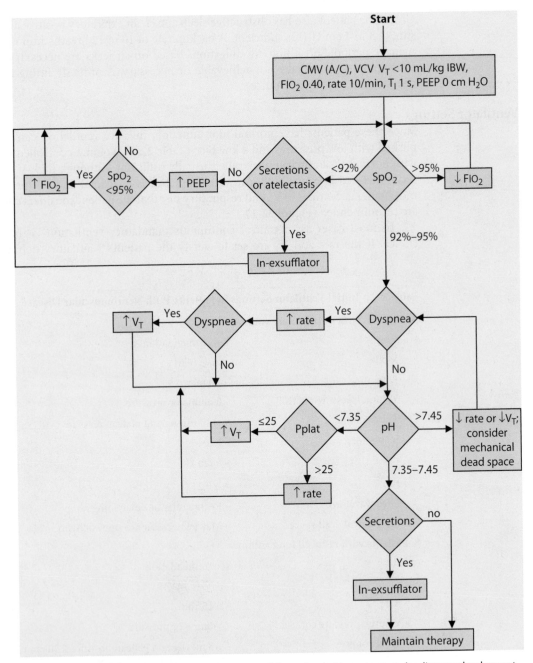

Figure 22-1 An algorithm for mechanical ventilation of the patient with neuromuscular disease who does not have underlying lung disease.

patients allow the ventilator to control ventilation. Inspiratory flow waveforms are set per patient's comfort. A low level of positive end-expiratory pressure (PEEP) is set (eg, 5 cm H_2O) to prevent atelectasis. If large tidal volumes are used, $Paco_2$ can be maintained at a normal level by the addition of 50 to 200 mL of dead space between the ventilator Y-piece and endotracheal tube.

Use of a very high tidal volume, sometimes with the addition of mechanical dead space to avoid excessive respiratory alkalosis, is the practice in some cervical spine injury centers. However, this is controversial and evidence is lacking that this results in better outcomes. Before the decision is made to use large tidal volumes, attempts to use more normal tidal volumes should be made. If a high tidal volume is used in these patients, it should be decreased to 6 to 8 mL/kg if the patient develops acute respiratory failure such as pneumonia.

In patients with reduced lung volumes (ie, thoracic deformities or muscular dystrophies), care must be taken not to overdistend the lungs. Pplat should be maintained as low as possible (< 30 cm H_2O). This requires low tidal volumes (< 8 mL/cm H_2O) with more rapid rates (> 15/min) and shorter inspiratory times (< 1 second). Patients with low lung volumes benefit from the use of PEEP.

Monitoring

Periodic monitoring of blood gases is necessary (Table 22-4). However, frequent blood gases are unnecessary because of the lack of intrinsic lung disease. Spontaneous V_T and respiratory rate, ventilatory pattern, vital capacity (VC), and PI_{max} provide useful information to guide the initiation and termination of ventilatory support. Decisions to initiate ventilatory support due to rapid onset disease are commonly made when VC is less than 10 mL/kg ideal body weight and/or PI_{max} more than −20 cm H_2O. Decisions to begin the process of liberation occur when the above thresholds are reached, and ventilation discontinued when VC is more than 15 mL/kg and PI_{max} is less than −30 cm H_2O with no deterioration after extended periods of spontaneous breathing (> 1 hour).

Liberation

Since these patients are committed to ventilatory support because a primary neuromuscular deficit has resulted in ventilatory muscle weakness and fatigue, liberation can only occur if these indications for ventilation have been reversed. In some patients with severe irreversible disease (eg, high spinal cord injury, end-stage amyotrophic lateral sclerosis), liberation will not be possible and long-term ventilation strategies must be considered. In those patients where the acute process is reversible, appropriate therapy

---

Table 22-4 Monitoring for the Mechanically Ventilated Patient With Neuromuscular Disease or Chest Wall Deformity

- Spontaneous tidal volume and respiratory rate
- Vital capacity and maximal inspiratory pressure
- Periodic arterial blood gases

and time must be allowed for reversal of the neuromuscular deficit. Some patients will require tracheostomy, but this should only be considered if it is consistent with the patient's wishes. The first goal is ventilator independence during waking hours with support at night. Complete ventilator independence is a secondary goal. Because of the nature of these diseases, liberation may take weeks to achieve, and care must be exercised not to fatigue the respiratory muscles during spontaneous breathing trials. Patients should not be pushed to the point that ventilatory pattern changes, VC and PI_{max} deteriorate, or hypercarbia develops.

With many patients in this group, the decision to maintain long-term ventilatory support must be made at some point in their disease process. Specific guidelines for when this should occur are lacking. However, nocturnal NIV should be considered whenever daytime baseline $Paco_2$ is more than 45 mm Hg. When the patient's ventilatory reserve is markedly compromised, even small stressors may facilitate failure. These patients' ability to perform activities of daily living and to handle periodic stress is increased with nocturnal NIV.

In-Exsufflator, Maximum Insufflation Capacity, and Assisted Cough

Patients with neuromuscular diseases and chest wall deformities with ventilatory difficulties are ideal candidates for the in-exsufflator (cough assist). This device simulates a cough by inflating the lungs with pressure, followed by a negative airway pressure to produce a high expiratory flow. This sequence is repeated as necessary to clear secretions. There is considerable anecdotal experience with this therapy in patients with neuromuscular disease. Many of these patients indicate no need for tracheal suctioning when the in-exsufflator is used. Initial application of the in-exsufflator requires low settings to allow acclimation. The inspiratory pressure is then adjusted to 25 to 35 cm H_2O applied for 1 or 2 seconds followed by an expiratory pressure up to −40 cm H_2O for about 1 or 2 seconds. Treatment periods consist of five to six breaths, followed by rest, and repeated until secretions are effectively cleared.

Hyperinflation therapy may be of benefit for patients with neuromuscular disease. This has been described as the maximum insufflation capacity (MIC). It is accomplished by the patient taking a deep breath, holding it, and then stacking consecutively delivered tidal volumes to the maximum volume that can be held with a closed glottis. The air is delivered from a manual or portable volume ventilator. This technique is limited by the ability of the patient to close the glottis (eg, bulbar disease). Some clinicians train the patient in this technique when the vital capacity becomes less than 2 L. MIC can be combined with manually assisted cough to improve secretion clearance. A manually assisted cough consists of an abdominal thrust and/or chest compression (tussive squeeze) after a deep inflation. This can be quantified using a peak flow meter. A peak cough flow of more than 160 L/min is needed to adequately clear airway secretions. The in-exsufflator is usually indicated if the patient with neuromuscular disease cannot generate an unassisted or assisted peak flow more than 160 L/min.

> **Points to Remember**
>
> - Most patients with decreased neuromuscular function do not have intrinsic lung disease.
> - Two subgroups of patients are usually encountered—those with acute onset of weakness that is short-term and reversible, and those with progressive weakness that is nonreversible.
> - Most patients with a gradual onset of weakness are candidates for noninvasive ventilation.
> - Invasive mechanical ventilation is indicated with acute ventilatory failure caused by muscular weakness.
> - In those patients without reduction in lung volumes, larger tidal volumes ($\geq$ 8 mL/kg), long inspiratory times (> 1 second), and moderate rates ($\geq$ 15/min) may be necessary for patient's comfort.
> - Mechanical dead space may be necessary in patients requiring large V_T and $\dot{V}_E$.
> - Use small V_T ($\leq$ 8 mL/kg), rapid rates (> 20/min), and short inspiratory times ($\leq$ 1 second) in patients with reduced lung volumes.
> - Monitor spontaneous ventilatory capabilities: V_T, rate, VC, PI_{max}, and ventilatory pattern.
> - Liberation, when possible, is accomplished by increasing periods of spontaneous breathing trials interspersed with ventilatory support.
> - The mechanical in-exsufflator is useful to mobilize secretions in patients with neuromuscular disease and a weak cough.
> - Patients unable to maintain daytime $Paco_2$ less than 45 mm Hg are candidates for nocturnal chronic ventilatory support.

Additional Reading

Ambrosino N, Carpenè N, Gherardi M. Chronic respiratory care for neuromuscular diseases in adults. *Eur Respir J.* 2009;34:444-451.

Bach JR, Gonçalves MR, Hon A, et al. Changing trends in the management of end-stage neuromuscular respiratory muscle failure: recommendations of an international consensus. *Am J Phys Med Rehabil.* 2013;92:267-277.

Bedlack RS. Amyotrophic lateral sclerosis: current practice and future treatments. *Curr Opin Neurol.* 2010;23:524-529.

Beghi E, Chiò A, Couratier P, et al. The epidemiology and treatment of ALS: focus on the heterogeneity of the disease and critical appraisal of therapeutic trials. *Amyotroph Lateral Scler.* 2011;12:1-10.

Benditt JO, Boitano LJ. Pulmonary issues in patients with chronic neuromuscular disease. *Am J Respir Crit Care Med.* 2013;187:1046-1055.

Benditt JO. Full-time noninvasive ventilation: possible and desirable. *Respir Care.* 2006;51:1005-1015.

Benditt JO. Initiating noninvasive management of respiratory insufficiency in neuromuscular disease. *Pediatrics.* 2009;123;S236-S238.

Benditt JO. The neuromuscular respiratory system: physiology, pathophysiology, and a respiratory care approach to patients. *Respir Care.* 2006;51:829-839.

Bershad EM, Feen ES, Suarez JI. Myasthenia gravis crisis. *South Med J.* 2008;101:63-69.

Birnkrant DJ, Bushby K, Amin RS, et al. The respiratory management of patients with Duchenne muscular dystrophy: a DMD care considerations working group specialty article. *Ped Pulm.* 2010;45:739-748.

Boitano LJ. Equipment options for cough augmentation, ventilation, and noninvasive interfaces in neuromuscular respiratory management. *Pediatrics.* 2009;123(Suppl 4):S226-S230.

Garguilo M, Leroux K, Lejaille M, et al. Patient-controlled positive end-expiratory pressure with neuromuscular disease: effect on speech in patients with tracheostomy and mechanical ventilation support. *Chest.* 2013;143:1243-1251.

Hess DR. The growing role of noninvasive ventilation in patients requiring prolonged mechanical ventilation. *Respir Care.* 2006;51:896-911.

Homnick DN. Mechanical insufflation-exsufflation for airway mucus clearance. *Respir Care.* 2007;52:1296-1307.

Lofaso F, Prigent H, Tiffreau V, et al. Long term mechanical ventilation equipment for neuromuscular patients: meeting the expectations of patients and prescribers. *Respir Care.* 2014;59:97-106.

Lyall RA, Donaldson N, Fleming T, et al. A prospective study of quality of life in ALS patients treated with noninvasive ventilation. *Neurology.* 2001;57:153-156.

Moran FC, Spittle A, Delany C. Effect of home mechanical in-exsufflation on hospitalisation and life-style in neuromuscular disease: a pilot study. *J Paediatr Child Health.* 2013;49:233-237.

Radunovic A, Annane D, Rafiq MK, Mustfa N. Mechanical ventilation for amyotrophic lateral sclerosis/motor neuron disease. *Cochrane Database Syst Rev.* 2013 28;3:CD004427.

Wolfe LF, Joyce NC, McDonald CM, et al. Management of pulmonary complications in neuromuscular disease. *Phys Med Rehabil Clin N Am.* 2012;23:829-853.

Chapter 23
Cardiac Failure

Objectives

1. Describe the effects of positive pressure ventilation on heart-lung interactions.
2. List indications for mechanical ventilation in patients with cardiac failure.
3. Discuss the role of continuous positive airway pressure in patients with cardiac failure.
4. Discuss the monitoring and weaning of patients with cardiac failure.

Introduction

Cardiovascular disease is the leading cause of death in the United States. As a result, many patients present to the emergency department or general patient care units with congestive heart failure or acute myocardial infarction. Many of these patients benefit from the application of positive pressure ventilation. Increasingly the respiratory support is applied noninvasively.

Overview

Heart-Lung Interactions

The normal changes in intrathoracic pressure during spontaneous breathing facilitate venous return and maintains adequate preload to the right heart. In addition, the negative mean intrathoracic pressure reduces left ventricular afterload. Left ventricular dysfunction with myocardial infarction (MI) or severe congestive heart failure results in increased left ventricular preload, pulmonary edema, decreased cardiac output, hypoxemia, and work-of-breathing. Of particular concern is the increase in blood flow required by the diaphragm and accessory muscles as a result of ventricular dysfunction. The respiratory muscles receive as much as 40% of the cardiac output during stress, which can result in a reduction of blood flow to other vital organs.

Effects of Mechanical Ventilation

With positive pressure ventilation, the mean intrathoracic pressure is positive. During inspiration, intrathoracic pressure increases, whereas it decreases with spontaneous breathing. This decreases left ventricular preload and afterload. In the patient with acute left ventricular dysfunction, this may enhance the performance of a compromised myocardium. In the hypovolemic patient, however, these effects may further decrease cardiac output.

The response of the cardiovascular system to positive pressure ventilation is dependent on cardiovascular and pulmonary factors. From a pulmonary perspective, the compliance of the lungs and chest wall affects the transmission of alveolar pressure into the intrathoracic space. The most deleterious effect on hemodynamics occurs with compliant lungs and a stiff chest wall, which results in greater pressure in the intrathoracic space. Cardiovascular volume and tone, pulmonary vascular resistance, and right and left ventricular function determine the effect of intrathoracic pressure on hemodynamics (Table 23-1).

Table 23-1 **Determinants of Cardiovascular Response to Positive Pressure Ventilation**

- **Cardiovascular**
  - Vascular volume
  - Vascular tone
  - Pulmonary vascular resistance
  - Right and left ventricular function
- **Respiratory**
  - Resistance
  - Compliance
  - Homogeneity of resistance and compliance

Positive End-Expiratory Pressure

Since positive end-expiratory pressure (PEEP) elevates intrathoracic pressure, it reduces venous return and decreases preload. In the presence of left ventricular dysfunction with an elevated preload, PEEP generally improves left ventricular function. PEEP may increase pulmonary vascular resistance, thus increasing right ventricular afterload and decreasing left heart filling. PEEP may decrease the compliance of the left ventricle by shifting the intraventricular septum to the left. By increasing the pressure outside the heart, PEEP may improve left ventricular afterload.

Mechanical Ventilation

Indications

Severe heart failure leads to hypoxemia, increased myocardial work, and increased work-of-breathing (Table 23-2). Mechanical ventilation in this setting is indicated to reverse the hypoxemia, reduce the work-of-breathing, and decrease myocardial work. Some patients with severe heart failure develop acute hypercarbia. Therefore the initial treatment includes noninvasive continuous positive airway pressure (CPAP).

Continuous Positive Airway Pressure

The use of mask CPAP in the patient presenting with acute left ventricular failure and pulmonary edema reduces the work-of-breathing and the work of the myocardium. It also increases Pa_{O_2}, decreases Pa_{CO_2}, reduces the need for intubation, and increases

Table 23-2 **Indications for Mechanical Ventilation in Patients With Cardiovascular Failure**

- Increased work of the myocardium
- Increased work–of–breathing
- Hypoxemia

survival. In many patients, CPAP provides sufficient unloading of myocardial and respiratory work while pharmacologic treatment modifies cardiovascular function, avoiding invasive management. Generally, CPAP is most useful in patients who are awake, oriented, and cooperative. If the CPAP mask further agitates the patient, it should be removed and invasive ventilatory support considered. Initial CPAP settings are generally 10 cm H_2O with 100% oxygen.

Noninvasive ventilation (NIV) has also been used to avoid intubation of patients with acute congestive heart failure. For many such patients, the outcomes with CPAP or NIV are equivalent. The specific indication for NIV is hypercarbic ventilatory failure along with the hypoxemic ventilatory failure. However, NIV should be avoided in patients with acute MI, hemodynamic compromise, significant cardiac arrhythmias, and depressed mental status. In these patient presenting with respiratory failure, invasive ventilatory support should be provided rather than NIV.

Ventilator Settings

Since spontaneous breathing potentially diverts blood flow to the respiratory muscles, continuous mandatory ventilation (A/C) should be used (Figure 23-1). Either pressure-control or volume-control ventilation is acceptable. In spite of the pulmonary edema that may be present at the time of initiating ventilatory support, pharmacologic treatment results in rapid resolution. Tidal volumes of 6 to 8 mL/kg ideal body weight are usually adequate with respiratory rates greater than 15/min to achieve eucapnia. Plateau pressure should be less than 30 cm H_2O. Inspiratory time should be short (≤ 1 second). FIO_2 should initially be set at 1 and then titrated per SpO_2 and blood gases. PEEP of 5 to 10 cm H_2O should be applied as support for the failing heart. Care must be exercised with the titration of PEEP because of the complex effects of PEEP on cardiac function. However, most patients with severe left ventricular failure benefit by the application of PEEP (Table 23-3).

Monitoring

Hemodynamics are monitored during pharmacologic therapy and mechanical ventilation (Table 23-4). Pulse oximetry is used to ensure that patients are well oxygenated. Periodic arterial blood gases are needed. Plateau pressure should be monitored. In addition, urine output, and fluid and electrolyte balance should be carefully monitored.

Liberation

Provided no underlying chronic pulmonary disease or secondary pulmonary problems develop and the left heart failure is appropriately managed, weaning can be a relatively easy process. However, in these patients cardiovascular system function is most optimal with increased mean intrathoracic pressure. The elimination of mechanical ventilatory support during a spontaneous breathing trial might result in an increase in left ventricular preload and pulmonary edema. Weaning may progress rapidly to low level pressure support and CPAP, but pulmonary edema may develop when positive pressure ventilation is discontinued. Some patients may develop ischemic changes during weaning. In this case, ventilatory support must be continued until therapy is successful at improving cardiac function (eg, diuresis, afterload reduction).

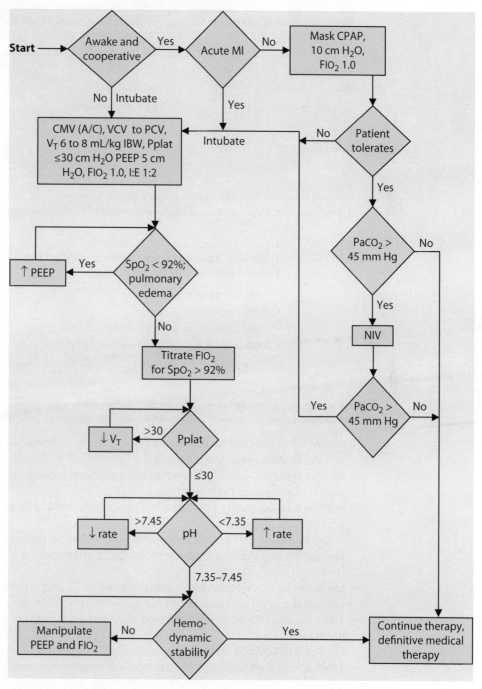

Figure 23-1 An algorithm for mechanical ventilation of the patient with cardiac failure.

Table 23-3 **Initial Ventilator Settings for Acute Congestive Heart Failure**

Setting	Recommendation
Mode	A/C (CMV)
Rate	14-18/min
Volume/pressure control	Pressure or volume
Tidal volume	6-8 mL/kg and plateau pressure $\leq$ 30 cm H_2O
Inspiratory time	$\leq$ 1 s
PEEP	5-10 cm H_2O
F_{IO_2}	1.0

Abbreviations: CMV, continuous mandatory ventilation; PEEP, positive end-expiratory pressure.

Table 23-4 **Monitoring for the Mechanically Ventilated Patient With Cardiovascular Failure**

- Central venous pressure
- Hemodynamics
- Pulse oximetry and periodic arterial blood gases
- Urine output and fluid and electrolyte balance
- β-type natriuretic peptide

Points to Remember

- Severe left ventricular failure results in hypoxemia, increased work-of-breathing, and increased work of the myocardium.
- Positive pressure ventilation reverses the intrathoracic pressure dynamics present during spontaneous breathing.
- Positive end-expiratory pressure (PEEP) decreases preload by increasing mean intrathoracic pressure.
- In the presence of a poorly functioning left ventricle, positive pressure ventilation and PEEP can reduce preload and afterload, improving cardiac function.
- Mask continuous positive airway pressure at 8 to 12 cm H_2O with an F_{IO_2} of 1 may prevent the need for invasive mechanical ventilation.
- 100% oxygen should be administered until blood gas data indicate it can be decreased.
- PEEP of 5 to 10 cm H_2O should be used to reduce preload.
- The decreased intrathoracic pressure during weaning can result in pulmonary edema.
- Proper fluid balance, afterload reduction, and inotropic support is required for the weaning of many patients with severe left heart failure.

Additional Reading

Bellone A, Barbieri A, Bursi F, Vettorello M. Management of acute pulmonary edema in the emergency department. *Curr Heart Fail Rep.* 2006;3:129-135.

Figueroa MS, Peters JI. Congestive heart failure: diagnosis, pathophysiology, therapy, and implications for respiratory care. *Respir Care.* 2006;51:403-412.

Howlett JG. Current treatment options for early management in acute decompensated heart failure. *Can J Cardiol.* 2008;24 Suppl B:9B-14B.

Kapoor JR, Perazella MA. Diagnostic and therapeutic approach to acute decompensated heart failure. *Am J Med.* 2007;120:121-127.

Mekontso Dessap A, Roche-Campo F, Kouatchet A, et al. Natriuretic peptide-driven fluid management during ventilator weaning: a randomized controlled trial. *A J Respir Crit Care Med.* 2012;186:1256-1263.

Methvin AB, Owens AT, Emmi AG, et al. Ventilatory inefficiency reflects right ventricular dysfunction in systolic heart failure. *Chest.* 2011;139:617-625.

Poppas A, Rounds S. Congestive heart failure. *Am J Respir Crit Care Med.* 2002;165:4-48.

Potts JM. Noninvasive positive pressure ventilation: effect on mortality in acute cardiogenic pulmonary edema: a pragmatic meta-analysis. *Pol Arch Med Wewn.* 2009;119:349-53.

Seupaul RA. Evidence-based emergency medicine/systematic review abstract. Should I consider treating patients with acute cardiogenic pulmonary edema with noninvasive positive-pressure ventilation? *Ann Emerg Med.* 2010;55:299-300.

Shirakabe A, Hata N, Yokoyama S, et al. Predicting the success of noninvasive positive pressure ventilation in emergency room for patients with acute heart failure. *J Cardiol.* 2011;57:107-114.

Vital FM, Saconato H, Ladeira MT, et al. Non-invasive positive pressure ventilation (CPAP or bilevel NPPV) for cardiogenic pulmonary edema. *Cochrane Database Syst Rev.* 200816;(3): CD005351.

Yamamoto T, Takeda S, Sato N, et al. Noninvasive ventilation in pulmonary edema complicating acute myocardial infarction. *Circ J.* 2012;76:2586-2591.

Chapter 24
Burns and Inhalation Injury

Objectives

1. Describe the respiratory effects of surface burns and inhalation injury.
2. Discuss issues related to airway injury in patients with inhalation injury.
3. Describe the management of carbon monoxide poisoning.
4. Discuss the indications, initial ventilator settings, monitoring, and ventilator weaning for the patient with surface burns and inhalation injury.
5. Discuss various modes of ventilation that have been proposed to manage patients with burns and inhalation injury.

Introduction

Respiratory complications are common in patients with burn injuries, and respiratory failure is a common cause of mortality in these patients. Pulmonary complications can occur at a number of times along the treatment course of burned patients (Table 24-1). Pulmonary complications are often associated with inhalation injury, but may occur in patients with severe surface burns who do not have inhalation injury. Mechanical ventilation is commonly necessary in these patients who develop respiratory failure.

Overview

Surface Burns

Respiratory failure commonly occurs in patients with major cutaneous burns. Such patients often have associated inhalation injury, and the presence of inhalation injury significantly increases the mortality related with cutaneous burns. However, respiratory failure and the need for mechanical ventilation may occur in the absence of

Table 24-1 **Pulmonary Complications Present at Various Times in Patients With Burns and Smoke Inhalation**

Complications	Time of occurrence
Carbon monoxide poisoning	Within the first hours of exposure
Upper airway obstruction	Within the first 48 h following injury and postextubation
Tracheobronchial obstruction	Within the first 72 h following injury
Pulmonary edema	Hypervolemia due to fluid resuscitation—first 48 h;
	Hypervolemia due to fluid shifts—second to fourth day; sepsis—after the first week
Pneumonia	After the fifth day
Pulmonary embolism	After the first week

Adapted from information in Haponik EF. Smoke inhalation injuries: some priorities for respiratory care professionals. *Respir Care.* 1992;37:609-629.

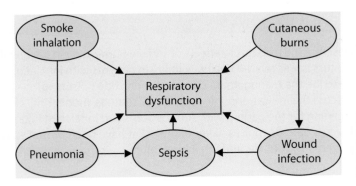

Figure 24-1 Respiratory dysfunction is central to the effects of smoke inhalation and cutaneous burns.

inhalation injury. There are recognized interactions between smoke inhalation and cutaneous burns (Figure 24-1). Pain management is an important aspect of the care of patients with burns, and may be associated with respiratory depression. Appropriate fluid management is difficult in patients with cutaneous burns, and fluid overload with associated hypoxemia and decreased lung compliance may occur. Sepsis can also occur, resulting in respiratory failure due to acute respiratory distress syndrome (ARDS). Burn patients may be hypermetabolic, which increases the ventilation requirement and may result in respiratory failure due to fatigue.

If full thickness circumferential burns of the thorax are present, severe chest wall restriction can occur. This will typically produce respiratory failure, and can make mechanical ventilation difficult. High ventilating pressures may be required, but may not place the patient at risk for overdistention lung injury because the transalveolar pressure may not be high due to the decreased chest wall compliance (Figure 24-2). Severe scarring and eschar formation can also restrict chest wall movement, and can result in difficulty weaning from mechanical ventilation. However, early surgical excision of the burn is commonly practiced, and this has reduced the need for escharotomies to improve chest wall compliance.

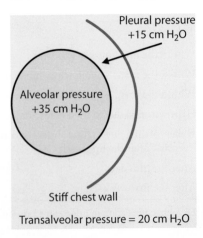

Figure 24-2 Effect of a stiff chest wall on transalveolar pressure. If the chest wall is stiff, there will be a greater increase in pleural pressure. Transalveolar pressure (the difference between the pressure inside and outside the alveolus) will be lower if the pleural pressure is increased. The amount of alveolar distention, and thus the risk of ventilator-induced lung injury, is decreased with a stiff chest wall. This is a setting where esophageal pressure monitoring is useful.

Inhalation Injury

Inhalation injury is associated with increased morbidity and mortality. The effects of inhalation injury can be grouped by those related to thermal injury, parenchymal injury, and systemic toxins. Clinical predictors of inhalation injury are listed in Table 24-2.

Because dry air has a low heat capacity, thermal injury to the lower respiratory tract is rare. However, inhalation of steam and explosive gases such as ether and propane can produce thermal injury to the lower respiratory tract. Thermal injury is almost always confined to the upper airway, which effectively cools hot gas before it reaches the lower respiratory tract. Thermal injury to the upper airway results in laryngeal edema, laryngospasm, swollen vocal cords, and increased mucus production. The diagnosis is made by examination of the upper airway, often using bronchoscopy.

Problems related to thermal injury to the upper airway usually occur within the first 24 to 48 hours. Due to the risk of complete obstruction of the upper airway, the symptomatic patient should be intubated. Many of these patients also require mechanical ventilation due to other severe associated injuries. However, some patients do not require mechanical ventilation, and can breathe adequately once the endotracheal tube bypasses the upper airway obstruction. If respiratory failure does not occur, these patients can often be extubated after several days, provided the upper airway swelling has improved. Bronchoscopic examination of the upper airway may be necessary before extubation, to assess the potential for obstruction if the patient is extubated. Due to the potential of complete upper airway obstruction with extubation, maintenance of a patent airway is paramount and vigilance is necessary to assure the security of the endotracheal tube. Securing the endotracheal tube can be difficult in patients with facial burns, and creative approaches for securing the airway are often necessary to prevent unplanned extubations.

Although thermal injury to the lower respiratory tract is unusual, injury due to the toxic chemical composition of smoke is common. Smoke inhalation can be harmful to both the airways and lower respiratory tract. Smoke inhibits mucociliary transport and induces bronchospasm. Airway obstruction due to retained secretions is particularly problematic in patients with preexisting lung disease, and severe bronchospasm can occur in patients with preexisting asthma.

Table 24-2 Clinical Predictors of Inhalation Injury

- Exposure characteristics: closed space or entrapment, unconscious, inhaled toxin known
- Burns to the face and neck
- Carbonaceous sputum
- Respiratory symptoms: hoarseness, sore throat, cough, dyspnea, chest pain, hemoptysis
- Respiratory signs: pharyngeal inflammation and burns, stridor, tachypnea, cyanosis, abnormal breathing sounds (wheezes, rhonchi, stridor)

Adapted from information in Haponik EF. Smoke inhalation injuries: some priorities for respiratory care professionals. *Respir Care.* 1992;37:609-619.

Table 24-3 **Clinical Effects of Carbon Monoxide Poisoning**

Carboxyhemoglobin level	Physiologic effect
< 1%	No effect
1%-5%	Increase in blood flow to vital organs
5%-10%	Increased visual light threshold, dyspnea on exertion, cutaneous blood vessel dilation
10%-20%	Abnormal vision evoked response, throbbing headache
20%-30%	Fatigue, irritability, poor judgment, diminished vision, diminished manual dexterity, nausea, and vomiting
30%-40%	Severe headache, confusion, syncope on exertion
40%-60%	Convulsions, respiratory failure, coma and death with prolonged exposure
> 60%	Coma; rapid death

ARDS commonly occurs in patients with smoke inhalation. The management of ARDS in this setting is similar to the management of ARDS in other settings, and includes oxygen administration, positive end-expiratory pressure (PEEP), and mechanical ventilation. The management of ARDS resulting from smoke inhalation may be complicated by sepsis, pneumonia, and fluid overload.

Systemic toxins include carbon monoxide (CO), cyanides, and a variety of nitrogen oxides. CO poisoning is the most important and the most common cause of death in fires. The toxicity of CO relates to the very high affinity of hemoglobin for CO, producing carboxyhemoglobin (HbCO). HbCO does not carry oxygen, and inhibits oxygen release from oxyhemoglobin (left-shifted oxyhemoglobin dissociation curve). Clinical effects of HbCO are related to hypoxia (Table 24-3). The diagnosis is made based upon symptoms and measurement of blood HbCO levels. Oxygen saturation and HbCO levels must be measured using CO oximetry. Arterial blood gases frequently demonstrate normal or increased Pao_2, hyperventilation, and metabolic acidosis. The lethal effects of HbCO usually occur early after exposure. In patients who survive CO poisoning, symptoms may persist and occasionally get better and then worse.

The treatment for CO poisoning is oxygen administration. The half-life of HbCO is 4 to 5 hours breathing room air, 45 to 60 minutes breathing 100% oxygen, and 20 to 30 minutes breathing 100% oxygen at three atmospheres (hyperbaric oxygen). Use of 100% oxygen, and hyperbaric oxygen if available, is thus mandatory in the treatment of HbCO. Hyperbaric oxygen is useful even in patients with low HbCO levels who have prolonged neurological symptoms. Airway management and mechanical ventilation may be necessary due to depressed neurological status.

Mechanical Ventilation

Indications

Indications for mechanical ventilation in patients with burn injury and smoke inhalation are listed in Table 24-4. Although many of these patients require mechanical

Table 24-4 Indications for Mechanical Ventilation in Patients With Burn Injury and Smoke Inhalation

- Smoke inhalation or pulmonary burns with respiratory failure (ARDS)
- Severe burns with chest wall restriction
- Respiratory depression due to the pain control
- Respiratory depression due to inhalation of systemic toxins (carbon monoxide)
- Respiratory failure due to secondary infection—pneumonia, sepsis
- Postoperative skin grafting or escharotomy

Abbreviation: ARDS, acute respiratory distress syndrome.

ventilation, airway management and inhalation of 100% oxygen are more important in some patients. For example, 100% oxygen is more important than mechanical ventilation in the spontaneously breathing patient with CO poisoning. Moreover, mechanical ventilation without 100% oxygen in these patients may be lethal. Similarly, spontaneously breathing patients with upper airway obstruction due to smoke inhalation and thermal burns may need an artificial airway, but not necessarily mechanical ventilation.

Ventilator Settings

Recommendations for initial ventilator settings are listed in Table 24-5. An algorithm for initial ventilator management is shown in Figure 24-3. Full ventilatory support is often required initially, and can be provided by continuous mandatory ventilation (A/C). Pressure support is usually not appropriate as an initial ventilatory mode in this patient population. Many of these patients require sedation and paralysis when mechanical ventilation is initiated, and this is particularly true if chest wall compliance is decreased. High frequency percussive ventilation and high frequency oscillatory ventilation have been advocated in some burn centers in the management of these patients. But there is no clear evidence that these approaches are superior to conventional modes

Table 24-5 Initial Mechanical Ventilator Settings With Burns and Smoke Inhalation

Setting	*Recommendation*
Mode	CMV (A/C)
Rate	20-25 breaths/min (lower if auto-PEEP is present)
Volume/pressure control	Either can be used, based on bias of the clinical team
Tidal volume	6-8 mL/kg predicted body weight provided that plateau pressure $\leq$ 30 cm H_2O; 4-8 mL/kg if ARDS is present
Inspiratory time	< 1 s
PEEP	5 cm H_2O; 10-15 cm H_2O if ARDS is present
F_{IO_2}	1.0—particularly with carbon monoxide poisoning

Abbreviations: ARDS, acute respiratory distress syndrome; CMV, continuous mandatory ventilation; PEEP, positive end-expiratory pressure.

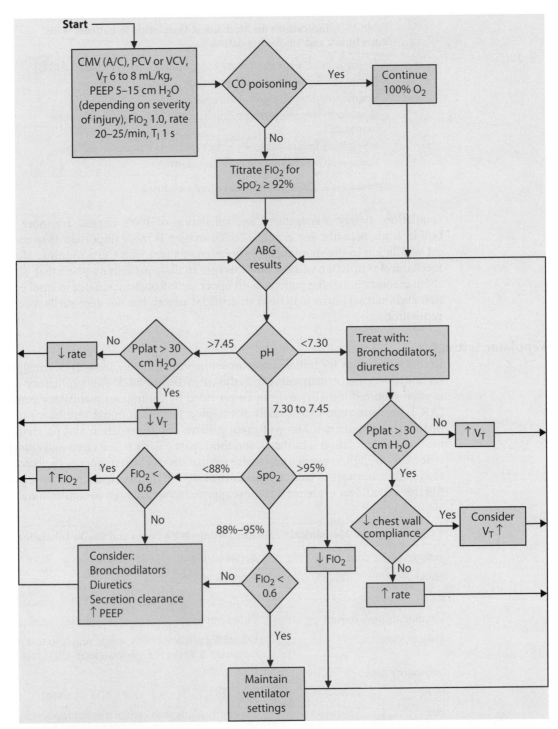

Figure 24-3 An algorithm for initial ventilator settings in the patient with burns and inhalation injury.

of ventilation. There is some evidence that these approaches may be deleterious compared with conventional ventilation.

Oxygenation is dependent on F_{IO_2}, mean airway pressure, and the extent of pulmonary dysfunction. If the patient has CO poisoning, 100% oxygen is required until the measured carboxyhemoglobin level is less than 10%. If CO poisoning is not present, the F_{IO_2} can be titrated to the desired level of arterial oxygenation using pulse oximetry and arterial blood gases. An initial PEEP level of 5 cm H_2O is usually appropriate and may be adequate. In patients with smoke inhalation resulting in ARDS, the management of oxygenation is similar to that with other causes of ARDS.

Either volume-controlled ventilation or pressure-controlled ventilation can be used. The plateau pressure should ideally be kept less than 30 cm H_2O. However, a higher plateau pressure may be necessary in patients with low chest wall compliance. If lung function is relatively normal, tidal volumes of 6 to 8 mL/kg ideal body weight (IBW) can be used. With ARDS, tidal volumes of 4 to 8 mL/kg IBW should be used and the plateau pressure should be kept below 30 cm H_2O if the chest wall is not stiff. With a stiff chest wall, a plateau pressure more than 30 cm H_2O may be safe. An esophageal balloon may be useful; transalveolar pressure should be kept less than 20 cm H_2O. An initial respiratory rate of 20 to 25 breaths/min is usually adequate, and can be increased if required to produce the desired $Paco_2$; higher respiratory rates are often necessary due to the high metabolic rate. Lower rates are necessary if auto-PEEP is present due to high airways resistance. Many patients with burn injury become hypermetabolic, and high minute ventilation may be required to maintain a normal $Paco_2$. In such patients, auto-PEEP is likely, and its presence must be monitored frequently. Permissive hypercapnia is usually well tolerated in these patients, and is usually more desirable than a high respiratory rate with auto-PEEP or a high airway pressure with associated lung injury. Pressure support ventilation or proportional-assistant ventilation can be used during the recovery period.

Monitoring

Monitoring mechanically ventilated burn patients is similar in many aspects to that with any ventilated patient (Table 24-6). Pulse oximetry is unreliable if high HbCO levels are present, and should not be used in this circumstance. Some pulse oximeters measure HbCO noninvasively, but the accuracy of these has been questioned. If minute ventilation is increased, the presence of auto-PEEP must be evaluated. Because chest wall compliance may be decreased with chest wall burns and scar formation, monitoring of esophageal pressure may be useful. Bronchospasm and auto-PEEP can be particularly problematic if the patient has a history of reactive airways disease. Increased production of airway secretions may also occur, requiring suctioning and bronchoscopy. These patients need to be monitored for the development of secondary pulmonary infections. Chest physiotherapy should be avoided in these patients because it increases pain and metabolic rate. Fluid overload is a common problem in these patients, and can result in shunting and decreased lung compliance. Due to the high metabolic rates of these patients, nutritional support is necessary to facilitate healing and weaning from mechanical ventilation. Pulmonary embolism can occur in patients with prolonged immobility, and pulmonary infection is also common in these patients.

Table 24-6 **Monitoring for the Mechanically Ventilated Patient With Burn Injury or Smoke Inhalation**

- Auto-PEEP
- Peak pressure, plateau pressure, and mean airway pressure
- Airway resistance and respiratory system compliance
- Esophageal pressure
- Arterial blood gases
- Pulse oximetry if HbCO < 5%
- Fluid intake and output
- Secondary pulmonary infection
- Cardiac filling pressure (central venous pressure)
- Nutritional status and metabolic rate

Abbreviations: HbCO, carboxyhemoglobin; PEEP, positive end-expiratory pressure.

Liberation

If the extent of injury is not severe, discontinuation of mechanical ventilation for burn patients can occur early and quickly. For some patients, maintenance of a stable airway is a greater issue than ventilatory support. For patients with airway injury, a thorough evaluation of the upper airway (often including bronchoscopy) is required before extubation. If burn injury is severe and associated with ARDS, pulmonary infection, and sepsis, the mechanical ventilation course can be long and difficult. Some of these patients will be difficult to wean, particularly if they develop multisystem failure and malnutrition. These patients require prolonged weaning with periodic spontaneous breathing trials to assess the ability of the patient to breathe without assistance. For patients who are difficult to wean, the goals should be treatment of injuries and underlying preexisting conditions, bronchodilation and bronchial hygiene, nutritional support, and strengthening and conditioning of respiratory muscles.

Points to Remember

- Respiratory complications are common in patients with burn injury and smoke inhalation.
- Thoracic surface burns can result in decreased chest wall compliance.
- Thermal injury can cause severe upper airway injury, but usually does not injure the lower respiratory tract.
- Smoke inhalation can cause bronchospasm and increased production of airway secretions.
- Smoke inhalation can produce acute respiratory distress syndrome.
- Carbon monoxide poisoning is a common cause of mortality in patients with smoke inhalation.
- Breathing 100% oxygen is mandatory to treat carbon monoxide poisoning, and hyperbaric oxygen may be useful.

- Ventilatory requirements of burn patients can be high due to hypermetabolism.
- Decreased chest wall compliance, decreased lung compliance, and increased airway resistance can make ventilation difficult in the patient with burn injury and smoke inhalation.
- In patients with decreased chest wall compliance, an esophageal balloon is helpful to determine a safe distending pressure.
- Once patients begin to breathe spontaneously, pressure support ventilation or proportional-assist ventilation can be applied.
- High frequency percussive ventilation and high frequency oscillatory ventilation have no advantage over conventional ventilation in the management of inhalation injuries.

Additional Reading

Barret JP, Desai MH, Herndon DN. Effects of tracheostomies on infection and airway complications in pediatric burn patients. *Burns.* 2000;26:190-193.

Cancio LC. Airway management and smoke inhalation injury in the burn patient. *Clin Plast Surg.* 2009;36:555-567.

Cartotto R, Ellis S, Smith T. Use of high-frequency oscillatory ventilation in burn patients. *Crit Care Med.* 2005;33(3 Suppl):S175-S178.

Dries DJ. Key questions in ventilator management of the burn-injured patient (first of two parts). *J Burn Care Res.* 2009;30:128-138.

Dries DJ. Key questions in ventilator management of the burn-injured patient (second of two parts). *J Burn Care Res.* 2009;30:211-220.

Ferguson ND, Cook DJ, Guyatt GH, et al. High-frequency oscillation in early acute respiratory distress syndrome. *N Engl J Med.* 2013;368:795-805.

Harrington D. Volumetric diffusive ventilator. *J Burn Care Res.* 2009;30:175-176.

Mlcak RP, Suman OE, Herndon DN. Respiratory management of inhalation injury. *Burns.* 2007;33:2-13.

Mlcak RP. Airway pressure release ventilation. *J Burn Care Res.* 2009;30:176-177.

Peck MD, Koppelman T. Low-tidal-volume ventilation as a strategy to reduce ventilator-associated injury in ALI and ARDS. *J Burn Care Res.* 2009;30:172-175.

Sheridan RL. Airway management and respiratory care of the burn patient. *Int Anesthesiol Clin.* 2000;38:129-145.

Toon MH, Maybauer MO, Greenwood JE, et al. Management of acute smoke inhalation injury. *Crit Care Resusc.* 2010;12(1):53-61.

Young D, Lamb SE, Shah S, et al. High-frequency oscillation for acute respiratory distress syndrome. *N Engl J Med.* 2013;368:806-813.

Chapter 25
Bronchopleural Fistula

Objectives

1. Describe the pathophysiology of bronchopleural fistula.
2. Describe the design and function of underwater seal chest drainage units.
3. List techniques to minimize air leak.
4. Discuss the mechanical ventilation of patients with bronchopleural fistula.

Introduction

Pneumothorax, subcutaneous emphysema, pneumomediastinum, pneumopericardium, and other forms of extra-alveolar air are referred to as barotrauma. A bronchopleural fistula is a persistent leak from the lung into the pleural space, identified by either intermittent (during inspiration) or continuous chest tube air leak. Most barotrauma occurs in patients with trauma, acute respiratory distress syndrome (ARDS), chronic obstructive pulmonary disease (COPD), asthma, and postthoracic surgery. Properly treated extra-alveolar air and bronchopleural fistula are not usually life-threatening problems; however, they do complicate ventilator management.

Overview

Pathophysiology

Extra-alveolar air can develop with trauma, surgical procedures, tumors, and vascular line placement. During mechanical ventilation, extra-alveolar air forms as a result of alveolar rupture to allow gas to enter the adjacent bronchovascular sheath and dissect into the pleural space. Pulmonary disease, high pressure, and overdistention must be present for extra-alveolar gas to develop to a critical level. Extra-alveolar air develops most frequently in COPD and ARDS patients, particularly if complicated by necrotizing pneumonia. Maintaining peak alveolar pressure less than 30 cm H_2O and tidal volume 4 to 8 mL/kg ideal body weight avoids the setting where alveolar rupture is facilitated. Signs and symptoms of a pneumothorax during mechanical ventilation are listed in Table 25-1.

Table 25-1 **Signs and Symptoms of a Pneumothorax During Mechanical Ventilation**

- Increased difficulty ventilating:
  - Volume control: increasing peak airway pressure
  - Pressure control: decreasing tidal volume
- Deteriorating vital signs
  - Initially, increasing pulse and blood pressure
  - Later, cardiovascular collapse and arrest
- Absent or diminished breath sounds on affected side
- Affected side hyperresonant to percussion
- Trachea and mediastinum shifted toward unaffected side

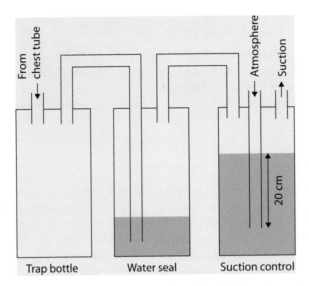

Figure 25-1 (A) Underwater seal chest drainage unit. (B) Two-chamber chest drainage unit. The first chamber (attached to the chest tube) collects pleural drainage and the second chamber serves as the underwater seal. (C) Three-chamber chest drainage unit. The third chamber is used to control the amount of suction applied to the pleural space.

Chest Tubes

Pressure within the pleural space is normally subatmospheric. Once the thorax is entered, gas tends to move into the pleural space. To prevent the extension or development of a pneumothorax, a one-way valve must be attached to the chest tube to prevent air movement into the thorax. This is accomplished by use of an underwater seal (Figure 25-1). The chest tube is placed 2 cm under a column of water and, thus, gas may exit the pleural space when the pressure exceeds 2 cm H_2O. To accommodate fluid drainage, a second container is added to the drainage system. Fluid drains into the collection chamber without affecting the water seal. To facilitate fluid movement and to prevent loculated pockets of air from accumulating in the pleural space, a third chamber is frequently added to control the suction pressure applied to the thoracic space. The pressure applied to the pleural space is low (eg, −20 cm H_2O). In modern commercial systems, each of these chambers is incorporated into a singe device.

Techniques to Minimize Air Leak

Pneumothorax during mechanical ventilation is treated with chest tube drainage and suction. The combination of negative pleural pressure from the chest tube (−20 cm H_2O) and positive pressure from the ventilator establishes a pressure gradient across the lungs and may facilitate the development of a bronchopleural fistula. If a fistula develops, flow through the fistula is determined by the magnitude and duration of the pressure gradient across the lung. Ideally, the approach used to provide mechanical ventilation should minimize ventilating pressure, inspiratory time, and chest tube suction to avoid accumulation of pleural air. Some clinicians recommend independent lung ventilation or high frequency ventilation. Others have proposed manipulation of the chest tube suction system. Two specific approaches to modify chest tube suction are intermittent inspiratory chest tube occlusion and the application of intrapleural pressure equivalent to the level of positive end-expiratory pressure (PEEP). Experience with these maneuvers demonstrates a decrease in the air leak but collapse of lung units is common and neither technique has resulted in improved outcome. In general, a lung protective approach to ventilatory support with emphasis on minimizing airway pressures seems to work very well in the vast majority of patients.

Although air leak from a bronchopleural fistula should be avoided if possible, it is important to recognize that CO_2 elimination occurs through the fistula. The CO_2 concentration leaving the fistula may be similar to that exhaled from the endotracheal tube. In most cases, the fistula does not close until the underlying disease process has resolved. The presence of a bronchopleural fistula is an ominous sign. However, patients usually do not die from a bronchopleural fistula—they die with a bronchopleural fistula.

Mechanical Ventilation

Indications

A bronchopleural fistula or other type of extra-alveolar air is not by itself an indication for mechanical ventilation. Its presence, however, increases the potential for problems with gas exchange. Indications for mechanical ventilation in this setting are apnea, acute ventilatory failure, impending acute ventilatory failure, or oxygenation deficit (Table 25-2).

Ventilator Settings

The goal of ventilator settings is to reduce the pressure gradient across the lung. Thus, the ventilating pressures and PEEP should be minimized (Table 25-3 and Figure 25-2) as much as clinically possible. A ventilatory pattern should be chosen that results in the least gas exiting the fistula, provided gas exchange targets are met. The use of pressure ventilation in this setting controls peak alveolar pressure. However, pressure-controlled ventilation may increase the leak through the fistula because it maintains a higher alveolar pressure throughout the inspiratory phase. The choice of pressure-controlled or volume-controlled ventilation should be determined by the mode that best minimizes air leak through the fistula.

Some of these patients require paralysis to establish the lowest air leak across the fistula and acceptable cardiopulmonary function. Whether spontaneous breathing

Table 25-2 Indications for Mechanical Ventilation

Bronchopleural fistula is not by itself an indication for mechanical ventilation but may be necessary in the following settings:

- Apnea
- Acute ventilatory failure
- Impending acute ventilatory failure
- Oxygenation deficit

Table 25-3 **Mechanical Ventilator Settings for Bronchopleural Fistula**

Setting	Recommendation
Mode	A/C (CMV)
Rate	10-30/min or greater, dependent on underlying disease and air trapping, and the level of air leak
Volume/pressure control	Pressure or volume control; during pressure support adjust the cycle criteria to prevent prolonged inspiration.
Tidal volume	V_T 4-8 mL/kg ideal body weight
Inspiratory time	0.5-0.8 s, depending on air leak
PEEP	As low as possible; depending on oxygenation
FIO_2	High FIO_2 more desirable than high pressure; permissive hypoxemia accepted, Pao_2 > 50 mm Hg

Abbreviations: CMV, continuous mandatory ventilation; PEEP, positive end-expiratory pressure.

should be allowed depends on the severity of the underlying disease process and the hemodynamics and gas exchange during spontaneous breathing. Pressure support ventilation should be used cautiously. With pressure support, inspiration terminates when flow decelerates to a predetermined level. If the leak across the fistula is greater than this level, the ventilator will not appropriately cycle from inspiration to exhalation during pressure support ventilation. Thus, careful setting of cycling criteria is important and these criteria may need to be frequently modified as ventilation continues. Moreover, suction applied to the chest tube may trigger the ventilator.

Permissive hypercapnia and the acceptance of low arterial oxygenation (Pao_2 > 50 mm Hg) are necessary for some of these patients. This is particularly true if the underlying disease state is ARDS, COPD, or trauma. Respiratory rate is set high enough to maximize CO_2 elimination but low enough to minimize fistula leak and air trapping. Depending on the underlying disease state, this may be a rate as low as 10/min or as high as 30/min or more. Tidal volume should also be as low as possible but normally in the 4 to 8 mL/kg ideal body weight range and inspiratory time should be short as possible, normally 0.5 to 0.8 second. All of these maneuvers are designed to minimize the air leak via the fistula. However, because all of these patients present with different levels of leak and pathophysiology, it is important to try various ventilator settings and determine the specific setting that results in the least air leak in the particular patient.

Management of oxygenation is difficult with a bronchopleural fistula, since PEEP used to improve oxygenation increases the leak. As a result, a high FIO_2 is needed. PEEP should be set at the minimal level necessary to maintain open unstable lung units. The goal is to minimize PEEP and mean airway pressure. However, particularly in ARDS and trauma, the oxygenation deficit may be severe and higher levels of PEEP required.

Independent Lung Ventilation

The use of a double lumen endotracheal tube with two ventilators (either synchronized or asynchronous) has been proposed for the management of severe bronchopleural

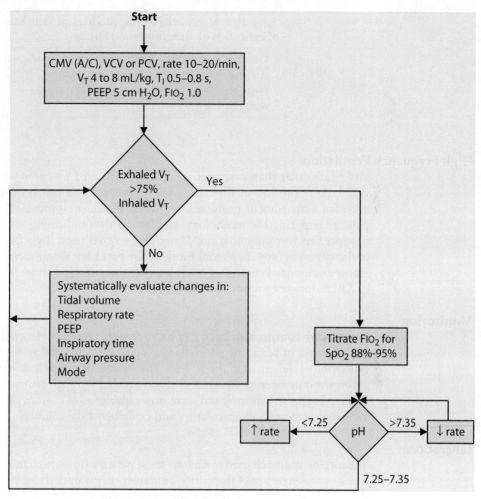

Figure 25-2 An algorithm for mechanical ventilation of the patient with bronchopleural fistula.

fistula. This approach is only recommended when the fistula is the result of disruption of a large airway or where maintenance of an acceptable level of gas exchange is impossible and surgical intervention is planned. This should be considered a short-term solution. Of concern with independent lung ventilation is the potential damage to both the trachea and mainstem bronchi resulting from the use of a double lumen tube, the difficulty of maintaining proper position of the tube, the difficulty with suctioning and secretion clearance, and the technical issues due to the use of two ventilators. Settings on the two ventilators should be based on the pathology of the ventilated lung. Each lung may be ventilated in a similar manner but with lower pressures and volumes to the affected lung or with continuous positive airway pressure alone to the affected lung. The volume of the air leak, as well as hemodynamic and gas exchange stability, are the key variables used to determine the adequacy of ventilator settings.

Table 25-4 **Monitoring During Mechanical Ventilation of Patients With Bronchopleural Fistula**

- Gas exchange: pulse oximetry and arterial blood gases
- Air leak: inspiratory and expiratory V_T
- Hemodynamics: in all patients but especially those with instability

High Frequency Ventilation

Little data other than case reports support improved outcome with high frequency ventilation. The use of high frequency ventilation is not recommended. Lack of accepted management protocols, high cost of the equipment, a limited number of patients requiring the technology, and lack of data indicating improved outcome all support this recommendation. Many centers that used high frequency ventilation in the setting of bronchopleural fistula in the past have abandoned its use. In addition, recent randomized controlled trials indicate that the use of high frequency oscillation in ARDS does not improve mortality.

Monitoring

Key concerns during monitoring of patients with a bronchopleural fistula (Table 25-4) are assurance of adequate gas exchange (pulse oximetry and arterial blood gases) and evaluation of the extent of the air leak. The volume of the air leak is quantified by measuring the difference between inhaled and exhaled V_T. Such estimates of air leak can be made using the monitoring and waveform capabilities of current generation ventilators and many indicate both inspiratory and expiratory tidal volumes.

Liberation

The specific approach used to liberate these patients from mechanical ventilation is not based on the presence of the fistula, but rather on the underlying disease. In general, as the underlying disease improves, the fistula begins to close. The presence of a fistula is not an indication to continue mechanical ventilation. The approach to liberation is not specific to the presence of a bronchopleural fistula.

Points to Remember

- Extra-alveolar air occurs most commonly in patients with trauma, acute respiratory distress syndrome, and chronic obstructive pulmonary disease.
- Disease, high pressure, and overdistention are required for extra-alveolar air to accumulate.
- An underwater seal is necessary to prevent air movement into the pleural space.
- Air leak is minimized by maintaining the lowest possible pressure (peak alveolar, mean airway, and end-expiratory), tidal volume (4-8 mL/kg predicted body weight) and short inspiratory times (0.5-0.8 second).

- The CO_2 concentration in the gas from the fistula may be similar to that exhaled through the ventilator.
- The goal with ventilator settings is to maintain the lowest pressure gradient across the fistula and to achieve minimally acceptable gas exchange targets (permissive hypercapnia, $Pao_2 > 50$ mm Hg).
- Independent lung ventilation is only indicated for large airway leaks, when gas exchange is impossible, and only for short-term use.
- Monitor system pressures, volume of the air leak, gas exchange, and hemodynamics.
- Ventilator liberation is determined by the underlying disease state and not the presence of the fistula per se.

Additional Reading

Ferguson ND, Cook DJ, Guyatt GH, et al. High-frequency oscillation in early acute respiratory distress syndrome. *N Engl J Med*. 2013;368:795-805.

Hasan RA, Al-Neyadi S, Abuhasna S, Black CP. High-frequency oscillatory ventilation in an infant with necrotizing pneumonia and bronchopleural fistula. *Respir Care*. 2011;56: 351-354.

Konstantinov IE, Saxena P. Independent lung ventilation in the postoperative management of large bronchopleural fistula. *Thorac Cardiovasc Surg*. 2010;139:e21-e22.

Malhotra P, Agarwal R, Gupta D, et al. Successful management of ARDS with bronchopleural fistula secondary to miliary tuberculosis using a conventional ventilator. *Monaldi Arch Chest Dis*. 2005;63:163-165.

Shekar K, Foot C, Fraser J, et al. Bronchopleural fistula: an update for intensivists. *J Crit Care*. 2010;25:47-55.

Slinger P, Kilpatrick B. Perioperative lung protection strategies in cardiothoracic anesthesia: are they useful? *Anesthesiol Clin*. 2012;30:607-628.

Young D, Lamb SE, Shah S, et al. High-frequency oscillation for acute respiratory distress syndrome. *N Engl J Med*. 2013 Feb 28;368:806-813.

Chapter 26
Drug Overdose

Introduction

Patients with overdose are a small percentage of those mechanically ventilated. Many of these patients require immediate intubation and mechanical ventilation—often by prehospital personnel. Ventilation of these patients is usually straightforward. However, complications can complicate the course of mechanical ventilation if not managed correctly.

Overview

The patient presenting with a drug overdose is frequently obtunded and unable to effectively maintain spontaneous breathing. However, with some classes of drugs (eg, tricyclic antidepressants) central nervous system hyperactivity may be the initial clinical presentation. If ingested in sufficient quantity, all drugs can result in respiratory depression and necessitate intubation and mechanical ventilation (Table 26-1). In addition, cardiovascular compromise commonly occurs with many types of drug overdoses. Narcotics and sedatives frequently result in hypotension, while tricyclic antidepressants and cocaine can cause life-threatening arrhythmias. The length of ventilatory support may be short or prolonged depending on the drug ingested, the quantity ingested, and the presence of underlying lung disease or complications. Patients may have periods of wakefulness followed by periods of profound respiratory depression. Even when the quantity of ingested drug is insufficient to depress spontaneous breathing, risk of aspiration may still be a primary concern necessitating close observation or intubation for airway protection.

Table 26-1 **Indications for Mechanical Ventilation in Patients With Drug Overdose**

- Apnea
- Acute respiratory failure
- Impending acute respiratory failure

Mechanical Ventilation

Indications

Patients with drug overdose are intubated to facilitate mechanical ventilation and for airway protection. Mechanical ventilation is usually initiated due to apnea or acute ventilatory failure. Oxygenation is often not a concern with these patients unless aspiration has occurred.

Ventilator Settings

These patients are not difficult to ventilate unless aspiration has occurred. They tend to be young and otherwise healthy without underlying lung disease. The ventilatory mode of choice is A/C (continuous mandatory ventilation [CMV]) provided with either pressure or volume ventilation (Table 26-2 and Figure 26-1). Any mode with a backup rate is acceptable. In spite of the fact that the lungs are normal, V_T and airway pressures should always be lung-protective. As a result a V_T of 6 to 8 mL/kg ideal body weight is appropriate with a rate of about 15 to 20/min, dependent on $Paco_2$. If volume-controlled ventilation is selected, an inspiratory time of 1 second is appropriate. With pressure-controlled ventilation, the pressure control level should be set to provide the desired V_T of 6 to 8 mL/kg with an inspiratory time of 1 second. Plateau pressure should be kept less than 30 cm H_2O. Since oxygenation is not a concern unless the patient has aspirated, $Fio_2 \leq 0.40$ is usually adequate to maintain normal Pao_2 (> 80 mm Hg). The use of 5 cm H_2O positive end-expiratory pressure (PEEP) to maintain functional residual capacity is encouraged, provided cardiovascular function is stable and the addition of PEEP does not adversely affect cardiac output. Since many ingested drugs produce peripheral vasodilation, concern regarding airway pressures is warranted.

Monitoring

Regurgitation and aspiration are the primary concerns with overdose patients, and precautions should be taken until the patient is ready for extubation. The cuff on the endotracheal tube should be adequately inflated. Hemodynamic stability is a concern

Table 26-2 Initial Mechanical Ventilator Settings With Drug Overdose

Setting	*Recommendation*
Mode	A/C (CMV)
Rate	15-20/min
Volume/pressure control	Volume or pressure
Tidal volume	6-8 mL/kg ideal body weight
Inspiratory time	1.0 s
PEEP	5 cm H_2O to maintain functional residual capacity
Fio_2	≤ 0.40 is usually adequate
Airway pressures	Lowest necessary to maintain gas exchange

Abbreviations: CMV, continuous mandatory ventilation; PEEP, positive end-expiratory pressure.

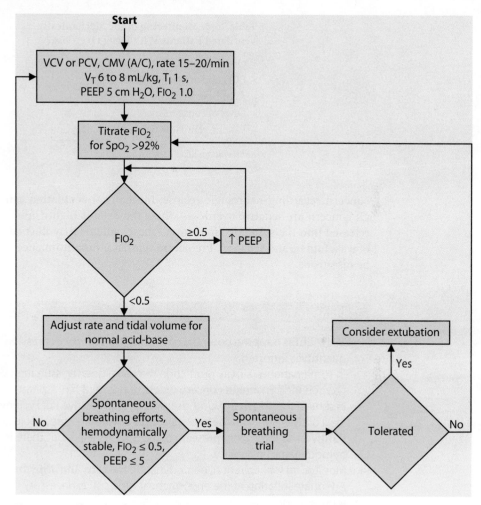

Start

VCV or PCV, CMV (A/C), rate 15–20/min
V_T 6 to 8 mL/kg, T_I 1 s,
PEEP 5 cm H_2O, FIO_2 1.0

Titrate FIO_2
for SpO_2 >92%

FIO_2

≥0.5 → ↑ PEEP

<0.5

Adjust rate and tidal volume for
normal acid-base

Consider extubation

Yes

Spontaneous
breathing efforts,
hemodynamically
stable, FIO_2 ≤ 0.5,
PEEP ≤ 5

No

Yes → Spontaneous
breathing
trial

Tolerated

No

Figure 26-1 Algorithm for mechanical ventilation of the patient with drug overdose.

with many overdose patients since arrhythmias may occur. Monitoring of electro-cardiogram and systemic arterial blood pressure is indicated. Since underlying lung disease is not usually an issue, arterial blood gases are monitored infrequently, but frequent evaluation of acid-base balance may be necessary with some ingested drugs (eg, salicylates). In some cases alkalosis may be indicated to facilitate clearance of the ingested drug. Since mechanical ventilation is indicated for respiratory depression, careful monitoring of the level of consciousness and patient-ventilator synchrony are necessary. Many patients become agitated and combative as their level of neurologic depression decreases (Table 26-3).

Liberation

Discontinuation of ventilatory support is indicated when the drug is sufficiently cleared to allow spontaneous ventilation. Once the patient is awake and there is no

Table 26-3 **Monitoring of the Mechanically Ventilated Patients With Drug Overdose**

- Observation for regurgitation and aspiration
- ECG and arterial pressure
- Acid-base balance
- Level of consciousness
- Patient-ventilator synchrony

Abbreviation: ECG, electrocardiogram.

concern regarding neurologic relapse, mechanical ventilation can be discontinued. Of concern are sedative overdoses where the drug is highly lipid-soluble and slowly released into the systemic circulation. These patients may fluctuate between periods of wakefulness and sedation. Premature ventilator discontinuance in this setting could be disastrous.

Points to Remember

- Many drugs have the potential of causing respiratory depression if sufficient quantity is ingested.
- In some patients, airway protection may be a greater issue than ventilation.
- Oxygenation is rarely a concern unless the patient has aspirated.
- In spite of the absence of lung disease, a lung-protective tidal volume of 6 to 8 mL/kg ideal body weight and the lowest possible airway pressure should always be used.
- Positive end-expiratory pressure of 5 cm H_2O is used, but there is a potential for hemodynamic instability.
- Monitoring for aspiration, hemodynamic stability, and arrhythmias is necessary.
- Adequate inflation of the endotracheal tube cuff is necessary in the case of regurgitation.
- Discontinue ventilatory support when neurologic function has returned to normal.
- Some drugs may cause fluctuation between periods of wakefulness and periods of sedation.

Additional Reading

Devlin JW. The pharmacology of oversedation in mechanically ventilated adults. *Curr Opin Crit Care.* 2008;14:403-407.

Henderson A, Wright M, Pond SM. Experience with 732 acute overdose patients admitted to an intensive care unit over six years. *Med J Aust.* 1993;158:28-30.

Spiller HA, Winter ML, Mann KV, et al. Five-year multicenter retrospective review of cyclobenzaprine toxicity. *J Emerg Med.*1995;13:781-785.

Zuckerman GB, Conway EE Jr. Pulmonary complications following tricyclic antidepressant overdose in an adolescent. *Ann Pharmacother.* 1993;27:572-574.

Chapter 27
Blood Gases

Objectives

1. List causes of hypoxemia and hypoxia.
2. Describe the oxyhemoglobin dissociation curve.
3. Calculate alveolar P_{O_2}.
4. Calculate the various indices of oxygenation.
5. Describe the relationship between $Paco_2$, alveolar ventilation, and carbon dioxide production.
6. Calculate dead space and alveolar ventilation.
7. List causes of respiratory and metabolic acid-base disturbances.
8. Use the anion gap (AG) to differentiate causes of metabolic acidosis.
9. Use the strong ion difference (SID) to differentiate acid-base disturbances.
10. Discuss the controversy related to temperature adjustment of blood gases and pH.
11. Discuss the physiologic variables affecting venous blood gases.
12. Discuss brain tissue oxygen monitoring.

Introduction

Blood gas and pH measurements allow evaluation of oxygenation, ventilation, and acid-base balance. Either arterial or mixed venous blood gases can be assessed. This chapter covers important aspects of blood gas assessment as it relates to the mechanically ventilated patient.

Oxygenation

Partial Pressure of Oxygen

The normal range of Pao_2 is 80 to 100 mm Hg in healthy young persons breathing room air at sea level. Pao_2 decreases with age, altitude, and lung disease. Hypoxemia occurs when the lungs fail to adequately oxygenate arterial blood. Pao_2 is a reflection of lung function and not hypoxia per se. Hypoxia can occur without hypoxemia and vice versa. Causes of hypoxemia and hypoxia are listed in Table 27-1. The best Pao_2 in critically ill mechanically ventilated patients is unknown, but a target Pao_2 of 55 to 80 mm Hg (at sea level) is usually acceptable. Pao_2 must be balanced against the potentially toxic effects of F_{IO_2} and alveolar distending pressure. For mechanically ventilated patients with severe lung disease, permissive hypoxemia may be a desirable alternative to applying potentially injurious ventilator setting to normalize the Pao_2.

Oxygen Saturation

The relationship between Pao_2 and oxygen saturation of hemoglobin (Sao_2) is described by the oxyhemoglobin dissociation curve (Figure 27-1). This is a sigmoid relationship, with hemoglobin having a greater affinity for oxygen at a high P_{O_2} (eg, in the lungs, where the P_{O_2} is high) and a lower affinity for oxygen at a lower P_{O_2} (eg, in the tissues, where P_{O_2} is low). The affinity of hemoglobin for oxygen is also affected by the

Table 27-1 **Clinical Causes of Hypoxemia and Hypoxia**

Hypoxemia

- Decreased inspired oxygen: altitude
- Shunt: atelectasis, pneumonia, pulmonary edema, ARDS
- Diffusion defect: pulmonary fibrosis, emphysema, pulmonary resection
- Hypoventilation: respiratory center depression, neuromuscular disease
- Poor distribution of ventilation: airway secretions, bronchospasm

Hypoxia

- Hypoxemic hypoxia: a lower than normal Pao_2 (hypoxemia)
- Anemic hypoxia: decreased red blood cell count, carboxyhemoglobin, hemoglobinopathy
- Circulatory hypoxia: decreased cardiac output, decreased local perfusion
- Affinity hypoxia: decreased release of oxygen from hemoglobin to the tissues
- Histotoxic hypoxia: cyanide poisoning

environment of the hemoglobin molecule, which can shift the curve to the left or to the right. Shifts of the curve to the right decrease the affinity of hemoglobin for oxygen (promote oxygen unloading), and shifts of the curve to the left increase the affinity of hemoglobin for oxygen (promote oxygen binding). Because of the variable relationship between hemoglobin saturation and Po_2, saturation cannot be precisely predicted from Po_2, and vice versa. To accurately evaluate oxygen saturation, CO-oximetry should be performed. CO-oximetry also allows measurement of total hemoglobin concentration, oxygen saturation, methemoglobin level, and carboxyhemoglobin level.

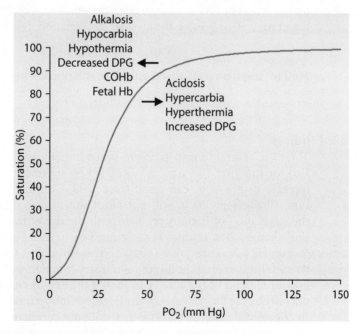

Figure 27-1 Oxyhemoglobin dissociation curve and factors that shift the curve.

Oxygen Content and Oxygen Delivery

Oxygen content (Co_2) is a combination of dissolved oxygen and that combined with hemoglobin (Hb).

$$Co_2 = 1.34 \times [Hb] \times So_2 + 0.003 \times Po_2$$

The amount of oxygen dissolved in plasma is small and related to the Po_2. The importance of Pao_2 is that it determines the Sao_2 and thus the amount of oxygen bound to hemoglobin. Note that a decrease in Pao_2 and Sao_2 may not result in a decrease in Co_2 if there is a concomitant increase in [Hb] (polycythemia).

Oxygen delivery is determined by cardiac output and oxygen content:

$$\text{Oxygen delivery} = \dot{Q}c \times Co_2$$

Note that oxygen delivery to tissues is determined by both $\dot{Q}c$ and Co_2. Thus, hypoxia can result from either a decrease in $\dot{Q}c$ or Co_2. Moreover, a decrease in oxygen delivery may not occur with a decrease in Co_2 if there is a concomitant increase in $\dot{Q}c$.

Alveolar Po_2

Alveolar Po_2 (Pao_2) is a mathematically derived value using the alveolar gas equation:

$$Pao_2 = Fio_2 \times (Pb - Ph_2o) - Paco_2 \times (Fio_2 + (1 - Fio_2)/R)$$

where Fio_2 is the inspired O_2 fraction, Pb is barometric pressure, Ph_2o is water vapor pressure (47 mm Hg at 37°C), and R is the respiratory quotient ($\dot{V}co_2 / \dot{V}o_2$). For calculation of Pao_2, R = 0.8 is commonly used. Note that the effect of R on Pao_2 depends on the Fio_2. For Fio_2 0.60 or greater, the effect of R on Pao_2 becomes negligible. For a high Fio_2 0.60 or greater, the alveolar gas equation thus becomes:

$$Pao_2 = (Pb - Ph_2o) \times Fio_2 - Paco_2$$

For Fio_2 less than 0.60, the alveolar Po_2 is estimated by:

$$Pao_2 = (Pb - Ph_2o) \times Fio_2 - (1.25 \times Paco_2)$$

Pressure-Based Indices

There are several oxygen-pressure-based indices. Each of these relates Pao_2 to either Pao_2 or the Fio_2. $P(a-a)o_2$ is calculated by subtracting the Pao_2 from the Pao_2. An increase in $P(a-a)o_2$ can result from $\dot{V}/\dot{Q}$ disturbances, shunt, or diffusion limitation. Changes in $Paco_2$ will not affect the $P(a-a)o_2$ because $Paco_2$ is included in the calculation of Pao_2. A problem with the use of the $P(a-a)o_2$ is that it changes as Fio_2 changes. The normal $P(a-a)o_2$ is 5 to 10 mm Hg breathing room air, but 30 to 60 mm Hg when breathing 100% O_2. This variability, when the Fio_2 is changed, limits its usefulness as an indicator of pulmonary function with Fio_2 changes and invalidates it as a predictor of the change in Pao_2 if the Fio_2 is changed. The $P(a-a)o_2$ is affected not only by the Fio_2 but also by the degree of intrapulmonary shunt and $\dot{V}/\dot{Q}$ mismatch. In critically ill patients, the $P(a-a)o_2$ does not correlate well with the degree of pulmonary shunt. The $P(a-a)o_2$ is also affected by changes in mixed venous oxygen content.

The Pao_2/Pao_2 is calculated by dividing the Pao_2 by Pao_2. Unlike the $P(A-a)o_2$, the Pao_2/Pao_2 remains relatively stable with Fio_2 changes. A Pao_2/Pao_2 less than 0.75 indicates pulmonary dysfunction due to $\dot{V}/\dot{Q}$ abnormality, shunt, or diffusion abnormality. The Pao_2/Pao_2 is most stable when it is less than 0.55, when the Fio_2 is greater than 0.30, and when the Pao_2 is less than 100 mm Hg. The Pao_2/Pao_2 is more useful than the $P(A-a)o_2$ for comparing the pulmonary function of patients on different Fio_2 and for following a patient's pulmonary function as Fio_2 is changed.

The Pao_2/Fio_2 is easier to calculate than $P(A-a)o_2$ and Pao_2/Pao_2 because it does not require calculation of Pao_2. The Pao_2/Fio_2 is used in the classification of the acute respiratory distress syndrome (ARDS). A Pao_2/Fio_2 of 100 mm Hg or less is consistent with severe ARDS, Pao_2/Fio_2 greater than 100 but less than 200 indicates moderate ARDS, and Pao_2/Fio_2 greater than 200 but less than or equal to 300 indicates mild ARDS, when patients are receiving 5 cm H_2O or greater positive end-expiratory pressure (PEEP).

The oxygenation index (OI) relates Pao_2, Fio_2, and mean airway pressure ($\overline{Paw}$):

$$OI = (Fio_2 \times \overline{Paw} \times 100)/Pao_2$$

Although not commonly used in adults, this index is used to classify respiratory failure in infants and children.

Pulmonary Shunt

Shunting is the portion of the cardiac output that moves from the right side of the heart to the left side of the heart without participating in gas exchange. Shunt is calculated from the oxygen content of pulmonary end-capillary ($Cc'o_2$), arterial (Cao_2) and mixed venous ($C\overline{v}o_2$) blood:

$$\dot{Q}_s/\dot{Q}_T = (Cc'o_2 - Cao_2)/(Cc'o_2 - C\overline{v}o_2)$$

where $\dot{Q}_S$ is shunted cardiac output, $\dot{Q}_T$ is total cardiac output, $Cc'o_2$ is pulmonary end-capillary oxygen content, Cao_2 is arterial oxygen content, and $C\overline{v}o_2$ is mixed venous oxygen content.

The arterial oxygen content (Cao_2) is calculated from arterial blood gas values, and mixed venous oxygen content ($C\overline{v}o_2$) is calculated from pulmonary artery blood gas values. $Cc'o_2$ is calculated based on the assumption that pulmonary end-capillary Po_2 is equal to the alveolar Po_2. When Pao_2 is greater than 150 mm Hg, it is assumed that the end-capillary blood is 100% saturated with oxygen. When a pulmonary artery catheter is not in place to sample mixed venous blood, shunt can be estimated from the equation:

$$\dot{Q}_s/\dot{Q}_t = (Cc'o_2 - Cao_2)/ (3.5 + (Cc'o_2 - Cao_2))$$

The 3.5 vol% can replace $Cao_2 - C\overline{v}o_2$ if there is cardiovascular stability and body temperature is normal. The $Cc'o_2 - Cao_2$ can be replaced by $(Pao_2 - Pao_2) \times 0.003$ in settings where it can be assumed that the Sao_2 is 100%. When the patient has a high Pao_2 (> 150 mm Hg), the modified shunt equation can be used:

$$\dot{Q}_s/\dot{Q}_t = [(Pao_2 - Pao_2) \times 0.003]/[3.5 + (Pao_2 - Pao_2) \times 0.003]$$

Oxygen Delivery and Oxygen Consumption

Oxygen delivery (Do_2) is the volume of oxygen delivered to the tissues each minute and is calculated as:

$$Do_2 = Cao_2 \times \dot{Q}c$$

Normal Do_2 is 1000 mL/min. Of this, the tissues normally extract 250 mL/min ($\dot{V}o_2$), and 750 mL is returned to the lungs. $\dot{V}o_2$ can be calculated using the Fick equation:

$$\dot{V}o_2 = \dot{Q}c \times (Cao_2 - C\bar{v}o_2)$$

Oxygen extraction is the oxygen consumption divided by the oxygen delivery.

Ventilation

Partial Pressure of Carbon dioxide

The adequacy of alveolar ventilation is usually assessed by the arterial partial pressure of carbon dioxide ($Paco_2$) due to the relationship between $Paco_2$, $\dot{V}A$, and $\dot{V}co_2$:

$$Paco_2 = \dot{V}co_2/\dot{V}A$$

Thus, $Paco_2$ is an indication of the body's ability to sustain $\dot{V}_A$ adequate for $\dot{V}co_2$. $\dot{V}co_2$ is determined by metabolic rate and is normally about 200 mL/min. An increase in $\dot{V}co_2$ requires a higher minute ventilation ($\dot{V}_E$). Dead space ventilation also affects the relationship between $\dot{V}_E$ and $Paco_2$; minute ventilation must increase to maintain the same $Paco_2$ in the presence of increased dead space. Clinical causes of hypoventilation (increased $Paco_2$) and hyperventilation (decreased $Paco_2$) are listed in Table 27-2. Although a goal of mechanical ventilation in the past has been to normalize $Paco_2$, an elevated $Paco_2$ (permissive hypercapnia) may be more desirable than the high alveolar distending pressure required to normalize the $Paco_2$.

Dead Space and Alveolar Ventilation

Dead space is that portion of the minute ventilation that does not participate in gas exchange. It consists of anatomic dead space and alveolar dead space. Dead space is calculated using the Bohr equation:

$$V_D/V_T = (Paco_2 - P\bar{E}co_2)/Paco_2$$

Table 27-2 Clinical Causes of Hypoventilation and Hyperventilation

Hypoventilation
- Respiratory center depression: pathologic, iatrogenic
- Disruption of neural pathways affecting respiratory muscles: neuropathy, trauma
- Neuromuscular blockade: disease, paralyzing agents
- Respiratory muscle weakness: fatigue, disease

Hyperventilation
- Respiratory center stimulation: hypoxia, anxiety, central nervous system pathology
- Metabolic acidosis
- Iatrogenic (eg, mechanical ventilation)

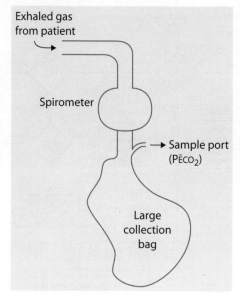

Exhaled gas from patient

Spirometer

Sample port (P̄$_{ECO_2}$)

Large collection bag

Figure 27-2
Collection of exhaled gas for P̄$_{ECO_2}$ determination.

In the Bohr Equation, V_D/V_T is the fraction of the total ventilation that is dead space and P̄$_{ECO_2}$ is the partial pressure of CO_2 in mixed expired gas. Normal V_D/V_T is 0.2 to 0.4. Causes of increased V_D/V_T include pulmonary embolism, positive pressure ventilation, pulmonary hypoperfusion, low tidal volume, and alveolar overdistention. The traditional method to determine P̄$_{ECO_2}$ uses mixed exhaled gas collected for 5 to 15 minutes (Figure 27-2). An arterial blood sample for $Paco_2$ is obtained during this time. However, many current-generation mechanical ventilators have a constant bias flow through the circuit, which complicates the collection of mixed exhaled gas to calculate V_D/V_T. In this case, P̄$_{ECO_2}$ can be calculated from $\dot{V}co_2$ and $\dot{V}_E$ using volumetric capnography.

$$P̄_{ECO_2} = (\dot{V}co_2/\dot{V}_E) \times P_b$$

Because dead space determinations require a leak-free system, they cannot be measured in patients with a bronchopleural fistula.

V_D/V_T correlates with mortality in patients with ARDS; high V_D/V_T is associated with higher mortality. V_D/V_T can also be used to determine the balance between alveolar recruitment and overdistention with titration of PEEP in patients with ARDS. The best level of PEEP is associated with the lowest V_D/V_T, with a PEEP too low and a PEEP too high associated with a higher V_D/V_T.

From the exhaled CO_2 and $\dot{V}_E$, alveolar ventilation ($\dot{V}_A$) can be calculated:

$$\dot{V}_A = \dot{V}_E \times P̄_{ECO_2}/Pb$$

$\dot{V}_A$ can also be calculated from V_D/V_T as:

$$\dot{V}_A = \dot{V}_E - (\dot{V}_E \times V_D/V_T)$$

Acid-Base Balance

Acid-base balance is explained by the Henderson-Hasselbalch equation:

$$pH = 6.1 + log[HCO_3^-]/(0.03 \times Pco_2)$$

Metabolic acid-base disturbances are those that affect the numerator of the Henderson-Hasselbalch equation, and respiratory acid-base disturbances are those things that affect the denominator. The arterial pH is normal (7.40) when the ratio $[HCO_3^-]/(0.03 \times Pco_2)$ is 20:1. The metabolic component of acid-base interpretation is

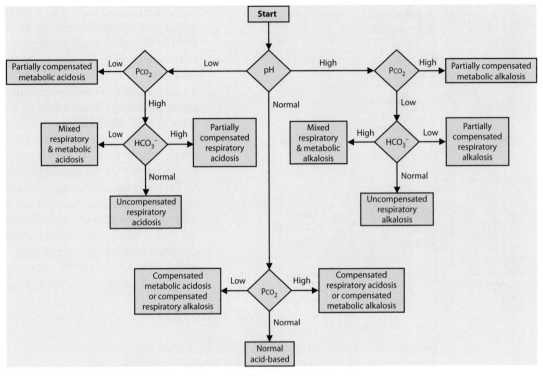

Figure 27-3 Algorithm for acid-base interpretation.

usually given as the $[HCO_3^-]$. The metabolic component can also be expressed as base excess (BE):

$$BE = [HCO_3^-] - 24$$

In other words, $[HCO_3^-]$ less than 24mmol/L corresponds with a negative BE, and $[HCO_3^-]$ greater than 24mmol/L corresponds with a positive BE. An algorithm for classification of acid-base disturbances is shown in Figure 27-3. Clinical causes of metabolic acid-base disturbances are listed in Table 27-3, and the expected degree of compensation for acid-base disturbances is shown in Table 27-4.

Table 27-3 **Clinical Causes of Metabolic Acidosis and Metabolic Alkalosis**

Metabolic acidosis
- Lactic acidosis (eg, hypoxia)
- Ketoacidosis (eg, uncontrolled diabetes)
- Uremic acidosis (eg, renal failure)
- Loss of base from lower gastrointestinal tract (eg, diarrhea)
- Loss of base from kidneys (eg, Diamox, renal tubular acidosis)
- Poisons (eg, methanol, ethylene glycol, aspirin)

Metabolic alkalosis
- Hypokalemia
- Loss of acid from upper gastrointestinal tract (eg, vomiting or gastric suction)
- Bicarbonate administration

Table 27-4 **Expected Compensation for Acid-Base Disturbances**

Respiratory acidosis	*Respiratory alkalosis*
$\Delta HCO_3^- = 0.10 \times \Delta Paco_2$ (acute)	$\Delta HCO_3^- = 0.20 \times \Delta Paco_2$ (acute)
$\Delta HCO_3^- = 0.35 \times \Delta Paco_2$ (chronic)	$\Delta HCO_3^- = 0.5 \times \Delta Paco_2$ (chronic)
Metabolic acidosis	*Metabolic alkalosis*
$Paco_2 = 1.5 \times HCO_3^- + 8$	$Paco_2 = 0.9 \times HCO_3^- + 15$

Note: If the acid-base status exceeds the expected level of compensation, a mixed acid-base disturbance is present.

Anion Gap and Osmol Gap

The anion gap (AG) is useful to differentiate causes of metabolic acidosis. Metabolic acidosis can be associated with a normal AG (hyperchloremic acidosis) or with an increased AG (normochloremic acidosis). The AG is calculated as:

$$AG = [Na^+] - ([Cl^-] + [HCO_3^-])$$

The normal AG is 8 to 12 mmol/L. Causes of metabolic acidosis with an increased AG include lactic acidosis, diabetic ketoacidosis, and azotemic (renal) acidosis. Causes of metabolic acidosis with a normal AG include loss of bicarbonate from the gastrointestinal tract (eg, diarrhea), acetazolamide therapy, or excessive chloride administration (eg, HCl, NH_4Cl). The traditionally defined AG does not take into account the large changes in plasma albumin concentration often seen in critically ill patients. Unless a correction is used, an increased AG may go unrecognized. This has led to the concept of albumin-corrected AG. AG is reduced approximately 2.5 mmol/L for every 1 g/dL fall in albumin:

$$AG \text{ (corrected)} = AG + 2.5 (4.2 - [albumin])$$

The osmol gap is the difference between the measured osmolality of the plasma and that calculated as:

$$Osmol = 2[Na^+] + [glucose]/18 + [BUN]/2.8 + [ethanol]/4.6$$

where osmol is osmolality and BUN is the blood urea nitrogen. If the measured osmolality is more than 10 above that calculated, there may be unmeasured osmotically active particles present, whose metabolites may be organic acids. Metabolic acidosis with an osmol gap is consistent with the presence of the toxins methanol and ethylene glycol.

Strong Ion Difference

The strong ion difference (SID) is a method of evaluating acid-base disturbances based on Stewart's approach to acid-base chemistry. Using Stewart's approach, the only variables that affect pH are the Pco_2, SID, and the concentration of unmeasured strong ions. SID is calculated as:

$$SID = [Na^+ + K^+] - [Cl^-]$$

Table 27-5 Classification of Primary Acid-Base Disturbances Using Stewart's Approach

	Acidosis	*Alkalosis*
Respiratory	↑ P_{CO_2}	↓ P_{CO_2}
Metabolic		
Water excess or deficit	↓ SID, ↓ Na^+	↑ SID, ↑ Na^+
Chloride excess or deficit	↓ Cl^-	↑ Cl^-
Unmeasured strong ion excess	↓ SID, ↑ unmeasured anions	—

Alternatively, SID is calculated as:

$$SID = [HCO_3^-] + 0.28 \times albumin \ (g/L) + inorganic \ phosphate \ (mmol/L)$$

The normal value for SID is 40 mmol/L. Classification of primary acid-base disturbances using SID is shown in Table 27-5. Metabolic acidosis is associated with a decreased SID and metabolic alkalosis is associated with an increased SID.

Mixed Venous Blood Gases

To assess mixed venous blood gases ($P\overline{v}_{O_2}$ and $P\overline{v}_{CO_2}$), blood is obtained from the distal port of the pulmonary artery catheter. Because pulmonary artery catheters are no longer commonly used, blood is drawn from a central venous catheter as a proxy for mixed venous blood. There is a reasonable relationship between central venous blood gases and mixed venous blood gases if the distal tip of the catheter is in the right atrium. Peripheral venous blood gases, however, have little utility for assessment of cardiopulmonary function; they reflect the metabolic conditions of the local tissue and cannot be used to assess respiratory function.

Mixed Venous P_{O_2}

Normal mixed venous P_{O_2} ($P\overline{v}_{O_2}$) is 40 mm Hg and is a global indication of the level of tissue oxygenation. However, normal or supranormal values of $P\overline{v}_{O_2}$ can coexist with severe tissue hypoxia caused primarily by arterial admixture, septicemia, hemorrhagic shock, congestive heart failure, and some febrile states. Further, $P\overline{v}_{O_2}$ reveals little about the oxygenation status of individual tissue beds. Factors affecting $P\overline{v}_{O_2}$ can be illustrated from rearrangement of the Fick equation:

$$C\overline{v}_{O_2} = Ca_{O_2} - \dot{V}_{O_2}/\dot{Q}$$

$C\overline{v}_{O_2}$ (and its components $P\overline{v}_{O_2}$ and $S\overline{v}_{O_2}$) is decreased with decreases in Ca_{O_2} (ie, Pa_{O_2}, S_{O_2}, or Hb), decreases in $\dot{Q}$, or increases in $\dot{V}_{O_2}$. Note that an increase in $\dot{V}_{O_2}$

with a proportional increase in $\dot{Q}$ does not affect $C\bar{v}_{O_2}$ (eg, exercise). Also note that breathing 100% oxygen by persons with normal lung function does not affect $C\bar{v}_{O_2}$ because increasing the Pa_{O_2} affects Ca_{O_2} very little (ie, oxygen is very insoluble in blood and the hemoglobin is nearly 100% saturated when breathing room air). In patients with abnormal lung function, a decrease in $P\bar{v}_{O_2}$ may produce a decrease in Pa_{O_2}.

Mixed Venous and Central Venous Oxygen Saturation

Mixed venous oxygen saturation ($S\bar{v}_{O_2}$) can be determined from a blood sample obtained from the distal port of the pulmonary artery catheter or by an oximeter that monitors $S\bar{v}_{O_2}$ continuously using a system incorporated into the pulmonary artery catheter. The oximeter reflects light from red blood cells near the pulmonary artery catheter, and $S\bar{v}_{O_2}$ is determined as the ratio of transmitted and reflected light. Central venous oxygen (Scv_{O_2}) saturation can be measured when a pulmonary artery catheter is not present. When the central venous catheter tip is 15 cm away from the inlet of the right atrium, Scv_{O_2} overestimates $S\bar{v}_{O_2}$ by 8%, but when the tip of the catheter is in the right atrium, Scv_{O_2} overestimates $S\bar{v}_{O_2}$ by only 1%. $S\bar{v}_{O_2}$ monitoring is used during early goal-directed therapy for sepsis treatment, with a Scv_{O_2} goal 70 % or greater.

Mixed Venous P_{CO_2}

Mixed venous P_{CO_2} ($P\bar{v}_{CO_2}$) is a global indication of tissue P_{CO_2}. Normal $P\bar{v}_{CO_2}$ is 45 mm Hg, which is only slightly greater than Pa_{CO_2}. Under conditions of low perfusion (eg, cardiac arrest), there can be a great disparity between Pa_{CO_2} and $P\bar{v}_{CO_2}$. Under these conditions, a respiratory acidosis can be present at the tissue level and in the venous circulation, concurrent with a respiratory alkalosis in the arterial circulation. Pa_{CO_2} is determined by $\dot{V}_A$, whereas $P\bar{v}_{CO_2}$ is determined by perfusion (Figure 27-4).

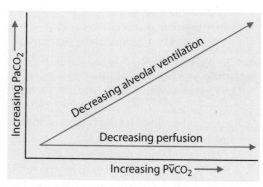

Figure 27-4 Arterial P_{CO_2} is determined by alveolar ventilation, and mixed venous P_{CO_2} is determined by perfusion.

Brain Tissue Po$_2$

There is an increasing interest in monitoring brain tissue oxygenation directly. In traumatic brain injury, brain tissue Po$_2$ (Pbto$_2$) can be monitored directly with a thin, metallic electrode that measures Po$_2$ in a small area of brain tissue. Normal values for Pbto$_2$ are 25 to 30 mm Hg. Higher mortality occurs with increasing duration of Pbto$_2$ less than 15 mm Hg, but it is unknown whether interventions to increase Pbto$_2$, such as increasing Fio$_2$ to increase the Pao$_2$, result in better outcomes.

Temperature Adjustment of Blood Gases and pH

Blood gases and pH are measured at 37°C (normal body temperature). If the patient's temperature is abnormal, the in vivo blood gas and pH values will differ from those measured and reported by the blood gas laboratory. The use of temperature-adjusted values for blood gases and pH is controversial. Although normal values are known for euthermia, normal values during hypothermia and hyperthermia are unknown. The acid-base changes that occur with hypothermia and hyperthermia may be homeostatic. The treatment of acid-base disturbances should be guided by the unadjusted values (ie, those measured at 37°C). Temperature adjustment of blood gases and pH is useful to follow changes in these values with changes in body temperature. Temperature adjusted blood gas values are used during therapeutic hypothermia. Temperature adjusted values should also be used to compare blood gases to exhaled gas values (eg, end-tidal Pco$_2$) and to assess lung function by comparing Pao$_2$ and Pao$_2$. Temperature adjustment allows the clinician to differentiate temperature-related changes from pathophysiologic changes.

Points to Remember

- Arterial blood gas and pH measurements are used to evaluate oxygenation, ventilation, and acid-base balance.
- Pao$_2$ is a reflection of lung function.
- Hemoglobin oxygen saturation is determined by Pao$_2$ and the position of the oxyhemoglobin dissociation curve.
- Pao$_2$ is a function of barometric pressure, Fio$_2$, Paco$_2$, and R.
- P(A-a)o$_2$ is affected not only by pulmonary shunt but also by Fio$_2$ and mixed venous oxygen content.
- $\dot{Q}_s/\dot{Q}_T$ is calculated from Cc'o$_2$, Cao$_2$, and C$\bar{v}$o$_2$.
- Oxygen delivery is the product of arterial oxygen content and cardiac output.
- Paco$_2$ is determined by the relationship between alveolar ventilation and carbon dioxide production.
- V$_D$/V$_T$ is calculated from Paco$_2$ and P$\bar{E}$co$_2$.
- A high V$_D$/V$_T$ is associated with high mortality in patients with ARDS.
- The lowest V$_D$/V$_T$ is associated with best PEEP in patients with ARDS.
- Acid-base balance is explained by the Henderson-Hasselbalch equation.

- Mixed venous oxygenation is a nonspecific indicator of the relationship between oxygen delivery and oxygen consumption.
- Central venous oxygen saturation is monitored as part of early goal-directed therapy for sepsis.
- With conditions such as poor perfusion, there can be a large disparity between arterial P_{CO_2} and mixed venous P_{CO_2}.
- The AG and osmol gap are useful to differentiate causes of metabolic acidosis.
- Blood gases and pH should not be temperature-adjusted to guide treatment of acid-base disturbance.
- Brain tissue P_{aO_2} can be monitored in patients with traumatic brain injury, but it is unclear whether using this monitor to guide practice improves outcomes.
- The SID is a method of evaluating acid-base disturbances in which the only variables that affect pH are the P_{CO_2}, SID, and the concentration of unmeasured strong ions.

Additional Reading

Abdelsalam M, Cheifetz IM. Goal-directed therapy for severely hypoxic patients with acute respiratory distress syndrome: permissive hypoxemia. *Respir Care.* 2010;55:1483-1490.

Androgue HE, Androgue HJ. Acid-base physiology. *Respir Care.* 2001;46:328-341.

Bacher A. Effects of body temperature on blood gases. *Intensive Care Med.* 2005;31:24-27.

Epstein SK, Singh N. Respiratory acidosis. *Respir Care.* 2001;46:366-383.

Fencl V, Jabor A, Kazda A, Figge J. Diagnosis of metabolic acid-base disturbances in critically ill patients. *Am J Respir Crit Care Med.* 2000;162:2246-2251.

Fidkowski C, Helstrom J. Diagnosing metabolic acidosis in the critically ill: bridging the anion gap, Stewart, and base excess methods. *Can J Anaesth.* 2009;56:247-256.

Foster GT, Varziri ND, Sassoon CSH. Respiratory alkalosis. *Respir Care.* 2001;46:384-391.

Guérin C, Nesme P, Leray V, et al. Quantitative analysis of acid-base disorders in patients with chronic respiratory failure in stable or unstable respiratory condition. *Respir Care.* 2010; 55:1453-1463.

Kallet RH. Measuring dead-space in acute lung injury. *Minerva Anestesiol.* 2012;78:1297-1305.

Kellum JA. Clinical review: reunification of acid-base physiology. *Crit Care.* 2005;9:500-507.

Khanna A, Kurtzman NA. Metabolic alkalosis. *Respir Care.* 2001; 46:354-365.

Kraut JA, Madias NE. Approach to patients with acid-base disorders. *Respir Care.* 2001; 46:392-403.

Lim BL, Kelly AM. A meta-analysis on the utility of peripheral venous blood gas analyses in exacerbations of chronic obstructive pulmonary disease in the emergency department. *Eur J Emerg Med.* 2010;17:246-248.

Lucangelo U, Blanch L. Dead space. Measuring dead-space in acute lung injury. *Intensive Care Med.* 2004;30:576-579.

Martini RP, Deem SD, Treggiari MM. Targeting brain tissue oxygenation in traumatic brain injury. *Respir Care.* 2013;58:162-172.

Matousek S, Handy J, Rees SE. Acid-base chemistry of plasma: consolidation of the traditional and modern approaches from a mathematical and clinical perspective. *J Clin Monit Comput.* 2011;25:57-70.

Morris CG, Low J. Metabolic acidosis in the critically ill: Part 1. Classification and pathophysiology. *Anaesthesia.* 2008; 63:294-301.

Morris CG, Low J. Metabolic acidosis in the critically ill: Part 2. Causes and treatment. *Anaesthesia.* 2008;63:396-411.

Ranieri VM, Rubenfeld GD, Thompson BT, et al. Acute respiratory distress syndrome: the Berlin Definition. *JAMA.* 2012;307:2526-2533.

Reinhart K, Kuhn HJ, Hartog C, Bredle DL. Continuous central venous and pulmonary artery oxygen saturation monitoring in the critically ill. *Intensive Care Med.* 2004;30:1572-1578.

Rivers E, Nguyen B, Havstad S, et al. Early goal-directed therapy in the treatment of severe sepsis and septic shock. *N Engl J Med.* 20;345:1368-1377.

Siobal MS, Ong H, Valdes J, Tang J. Calculation of physiologic dead space: comparison of ventilator volumetric capnography to measurements by metabolic analyzer and volumetric CO_2 monitor. *Respir Care.* 2013

Tusman G, Sipmann FS, Bohm SH. Rationale of dead space measurement by volumetric capnography. *Anesth Analg.* 2012;114:866-874.

Story DA. Bench-to-bedside review: a brief history of clinical acid-base. *Crit Care.* 2004; 8:253-258.

Swenson ER. Metabolic acidosis. *Respir Care.* 2001; 46:342-353.

Walley KR. Use of central venous oxygen saturation to guide therapy. *Am J Respir Crit Care Med.* 2011;184:514-520.

Wilkes P. Hypoproteinemia, strong ion difference, and acid-base status in critically ill patients. *J Appl Physiol.* 1998; 84:1740-1748.

Chapter 28
Pulse Oximetry, Capnography, and Transcutaneous Monitoring

Introduction

Noninvasive monitoring of respiratory function is common for mechanically ventilated patients. This is particularly the case with pulse oximetry, which is now available as part of the bedside monitoring system in most critical care units. Although pulse oximetry has become a standard of care during mechanical ventilation, it is important to recognize that there are few, if any, outcome studies to demonstrate the effectiveness of this monitor. Much of the success of pulse oximetry is related to its ease of use, compared to the capnograph and transcutaneous monitors. Capnography is commonly used in the operating room and is popular in some critical care units, while transcutaneous monitoring is used less commonly.

Pulse Oximetry

Principle of Operation

Pulse oximetry passes two wavelengths of light (usually 660 nm and 940 nm) through a pulsating vascular bed and determines oxygen saturation (Spo_2) from the ratio of the amplitudes of the plethysmographic waveforms. New pulse oximetry technology uses eight wavelengths of light to measure Spco (oximetric estimate of carboxyhemoglobin), Sp_{MET} (oximetric estimate of methemoglobin), and Sp_{HB} (oximetric estimate of hemoglobin concentration).

A variety of oximeter probes are available in disposable and nondisposable designs, and they include finger probes, toe probes, ear probes, nasal probes, and foot probes. Most pulse oximeters provide a display of the plethysmographic waveform. Inspection of this waveform allows the user to detect artifacts such as that which occurs with motion and low perfusion. Because pulse oximeters evaluate each arterial pulse, they display heart rate as well as oxygen saturation. The saturation reading should be questioned if the oximeter heart rate differs considerably from the actual heart rate, but good agreement between the pulse oximeter heart rate and the actual heart rate does not guarantee a correct Spo_2 reading.

At saturations greater than 70%, the accuracy of pulse oximetry is about ±4% to 5%. To appreciate the implications of these accuracy limits, one must consider the oxyhemoglobin dissociation curve. If the pulse oximeter displays an SpO_2 of 95%, the true saturation could be as low as 90% or as high as 100%. If the true saturation is 90%, the PaO_2 will be about 60 mm Hg. However, if the true saturation is 100%, the PaO_2 might be very high (≥ 150 mm Hg). Below 70%, the accuracy of pulse oximetry is worse, but the clinical importance of this is questionable. When using SpO_2, one must understand the relationship between SO_2 and PO_2. However, because of the variable and often unknown relationship between SO_2 and PO_2, one should predict PaO_2 from SpO_2 with caution. The relationship between SO_2 and PO_2 also demonstrates the fact that pulse oximetry does not detect hyperoxemia very well.

The pulse oximeter is unique as a monitor in that it requires no user calibration. Manufacturer-derived calibration curves programmed into the software of the device vary from manufacturer to manufacturer and can vary among pulse oximeters of a given manufacturer. For that reason, the same pulse oximeter and probe should be used for each SpO_2 determination on a given patient.

Limitations During Mechanical Ventilation

There are a number of performance limitations of pulse oximetry that should be understood by all clinicians who use these devices. Motion of the probe and high-intensity ambient light can produce inaccurate readings. Motion artifact and low perfusion are common causes of pulse oximetry errors. Manufacturers of pulse oximeters have developed improved software algorithms to calculate SpO_2 in an attempt to eliminate motion artifacts from the pulse signal. Traditional pulse oximeters assume that carboxyhemoglobin and methemoglobin concentrations are low (< 2%). Carboxyhemoglobin and methemoglobin both introduce significant inaccuracy in the SpO_2, and pulse oximetry should not be used when elevated levels of these are present. Vascular dyes also affect the accuracy of pulse oximetry, with methylene blue producing the greatest effect. Because pulse oximeters require a pulsating vascular bed, they are unreliable during cardiac arrest and other low flow states. Nail polish can affect the accuracy of pulse oximetry and it should be removed before pulse oximetry is used. The accuracy and performance of pulse oximetry may also be affected by deeply pigmented skin. The accuracy of pulse oximetry is not affected by hyperbilirubinemia or fetal hemoglobin. Although pulse oximetry is generally considered safe, burns from defective probes and pressure necrosis may occur during monitoring by pulse oximetry.

Continuous pulse oximetry has become a standard of care in critically ill mechanically ventilated patients. For the titration of FIO_2 and positive end-expiratory pressure (PEEP), SpO_2 of 88% to 95% is generally appropriate. Combinations of PEEP and FIO_2 to maintain SpO_2 in this range are used in patients with acute respiratory distress syndrome (ARDS). However, it should be appreciated that pulse oximetry provides little indication of ventilation or acid-base status. Clinically important changes in pH and/or $PaCO_2$ can occur with little change in SpO_2. This is particularly true when the SpO_2 is greater than 95%. Because pulse oximetry also does not evaluate tissue oxygen delivery, a patient can have significant tissue hypoxia in spite of an adequate Spo_2.

Hemodynamics and Pulse Oximetry

Pulsus paradoxus causes variability in the baseline plethysmographic waveform, as can occur in patients with airflow obstruction (Figure 28-1). Respiratory variations in the plethysmographic waveform amplitude during positive pressure ventilation may be useful in predicting fluid responsiveness (Figure 28-2). Plethysmographic indices of fluid responsiveness include respiratory variation in pulse oximetry plethysmographic waveform amplitude (ΔPOP) and the plethysmographic variability index (PVI). ΔPOP and PVI are obtained by continuous analysis of the raw pulse oximeter signal. ΔPOP is calculated as:

$$(POPmax - POPmin)/[(POPmax + POPmin) \times 0.5]$$

where POPmax and POPmin represent the maximal and the minimal amplitudes of the plethysmographic waveform over one respiratory cycle, respectively. PVI is calculated as:

$$[(PImax - PImin)/PImax] \times 100$$

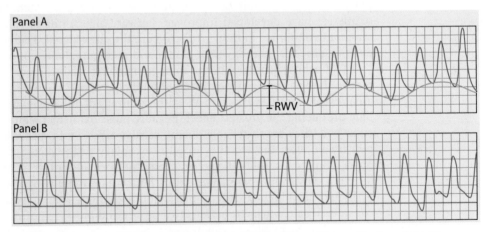

Figure 28-1 Pulse oximeter tracings from a 60-year-old woman with exacerbation of chronic obstructive pulmonary disease who was admitted to the intensive care unit in ventilatory failure.
A. The patient's pulse oximetry tracing at the time of admission reveals respiratory variability in the pulse oximeter plethysmography tracing. Measured pulsus paradoxus at this time was 16 mm Hg.
B. The patient's pulse oximetry tracing after 12 hours of aggressive therapy. Pulsus paradoxus at this time was 8 mm Hg. Note the absence of respiratory waveform variation (RWV) in the baseline of the oximeter tracing after clinical improvement in airflow and resolution of elevated pulsus paradoxus. (Reproduced with permission from Longnecker D, Brown D, Newman M, Zapol W. *Anesthesiology*. 2nd ed. New York, NY: McGraw-Hill; 2012; reproduced from Hartert TV, Wheeler AP, Sheller JR. Use of pulse oximetry to recognize severity of airflow obstruction in obstructive airway disease: correlation with pulsus paradoxus. *Chest*. 1999; Feb;115(2):475-481.)

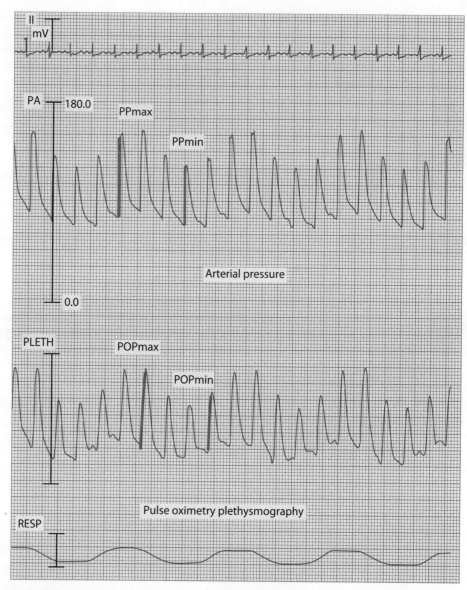

Figure 28-2 Comparison between invasive arterial pressure and pulse oximeter plethysmography recordings. Simultaneous recording of electrocardiographic lead (II), systemic arterial pressure (PA), pulse oximetry plethysmography (PLETH), and respiratory signal (RESP) in one illustrative patient. mV, millivolts; POP, pulse oximetry plethysmographic; PP, pulse pressure. (Reproduced from Cannesson M, Besnard C, Durand PG, et al. Relation between respiratory variations in pulse oximetry plethysmographic waveform amplitude and arterial pulse pressure in ventilated patients. *Crit Care.* 2005; Oct 5;9(5):R562-R568.)

where PImax and PImin are the maximal and the minimal values of the plethysmographic perfusion index (PI) over one respiratory cycle, respectively. PI is the ratio between pulsatile and nonpulsatile infrared light absorption from the pulse oximeter, and it is physiologically equivalent to the amplitude of the plethysmographic waveform.

Capnography

Principle of Operation

Capnography is the measurement of CO_2 at the airway, and display of a waveform is called the capnogram. CO_2 can be measured using mass spectrometry, Raman spectroscopy, or infrared absorption. Most capnographs use infrared absorption at 4.26 μm. The measurement chamber is placed at the airway with a mainstream capnograph or gas is aspirated through fine-bore tubing to the measurement chamber inside the capnograph with the sidestream device. There are advantages and disadvantages of each design and neither is clearly superior.

There are potential technical problems related to the use of capnography. These include the need for periodic calibration and interference from gases such as N_2O. Water is particularly a problem because it occludes sample lines in the sidestream capnograph and condenses on the cell of mainstream devices. Manufacturers use a number of features to overcome these problems, including water traps, purging of the sample line, use of a water permeable sample line, heating of the mainstream cell, and automated calibration.

Normal Capnogram

The normal capnogram is illustrated in Figure 28-3. During inspiration, P_{CO_2} is zero. At the beginning of exhalation, P_{CO_2} remains zero as gas from anatomic dead space leaves the airway (phase I). The P_{CO_2} then sharply rises as alveolar gas mixes with dead space gas (phase II). During most of exhalation, the curve levels and forms a

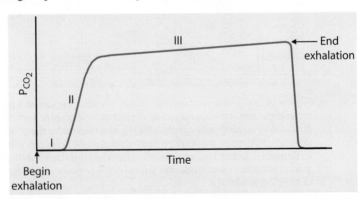

Figure 28-3 Time-based capnogram. I, anatomic dead space; II, transition from anatomic dead space to alveolar plateau; III, alveolar plateau. (Reproduced with permission from Longnecker D, Brown D, Newman M, Zapol W. *Anesthesiology.* 2nd ed. New York, NY: McGraw-Hill; 2012.)

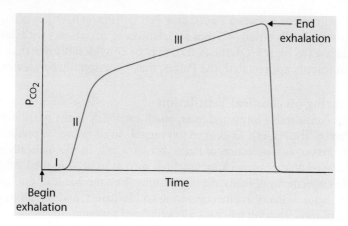

Figure 28-4 Capnogram with obstructive lung disease. (Reproduced with permission from Longnecker D, Brown D, Newman M, Zapol W. *Anesthesiology.* 2nd ed. New York, NY: McGraw-Hill; 2012.)

plateau (phase III). This represents gas from alveoli and is called the alveolar plateau. The P_{CO_2} at the end of the alveolar plateau is called end-tidal P_{CO_2} ($P_{ET}CO_2$). The slope of phase III of the capnogram is increased in patients with obstructive lung disease (Figure 28-4).

End-Tidal P_{CO_2}

The $P_{ET}CO_2$ presumably represents alveolar P_{CO_2} (P_ACO_2). P_ACO_2 is determined by the ventilation-perfusion ratio ($\dot{V}/\dot{Q}$) (Figure 28-5). With a normal $\dot{V}/\dot{Q}$, the P_ACO_2 approximates the arterial P_{CO_2} (P_aCO_2). If the $\dot{V}/\dot{Q}$ decreases, P_ACO_2 rises toward mixed venous P_{CO_2} ($P_{\bar{v}}CO_2$). With a high $\dot{V}/\dot{Q}$ (ie, dead space), P_ACO_2 will approach the inspired P_{CO_2}. $P_{ET}CO_2$ can be as low as the inspired P_{CO_2} (zero) or as high as the $P_{\bar{v}}CO_2$. An increase or decrease in $P_{ET}CO_2$ can be the result of changes in CO_2 production (ie, metabolism), CO_2 delivery to the lungs (ie, circulation), or alveolar ventilation. However, because of homeostasis, compensatory changes may occur so that $P_{ET}CO_2$ does not change. In practice, $P_{ET}CO_2$ is a nonspecific indicator of cardiopulmonary homeostasis and usually does not indicate a specific problem or abnormality.

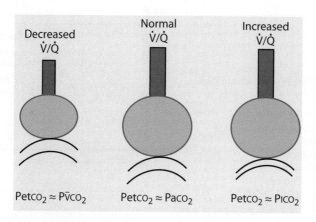

Figure 28-5 Relationship between $P_{ET}CO_2$ and $\dot{V}/\dot{Q}$. (Reproduced with permission from Longnecker D, Brown D, Newman M, Zapol W. *Anesthesiology.* 2nd ed. New York, NY: McGraw-Hill; 2012.)

The gradient between $Paco_2$ and $Petco_2$ [P(a-et)CO$_2$] is often calculated. This gradient is usually small (< 5 mm Hg). However, in patients with dead space–producing disease (ie, high $\dot{V}/\dot{Q}$), the $Petco_2$ may be considerably less than $Paco_2$. Although not commonly appreciated, the $Petco_2$ may occasionally be greater than the $Paco_2$.

Use and Limitations During Mechanical Ventilation

There is considerable intra- and interpatient variability in the relationship between $Paco_2$ and $Petco_2$. The P(a-et)CO$_2$ is often too variable to allow precise prediction of $Paco_2$ from $Petco_2$. $Petco_2$ as a reflection of $Paco_2$ is useful only in mechanically ventilated patients who have relatively normal lung function, such as in head-injured patients. $Petco_2$ is not useful as a predictor of $Paco_2$ during weaning from mechanical ventilation. Use of $Petco_2$ as a predictor of $Paco_2$ is often deceiving and incorrect, and should be used with caution for this purpose in adult mechanically ventilated patients.

A useful application of capnography is the detection of esophageal intubation. Because there is normally very little CO_2 in the stomach, intubation of the esophagus and ventilation of the stomach results in a near-zero $Petco_2$. A potential problem with the use of capnography to confirm endotracheal intubation occurs during cardiac arrest, with false-negative results because of very low $Petco_2$ values related to decreased pulmonary blood flow. Relatively inexpensive disposable devices that produce a color change in the presence of exhaled CO_2 are available to detect esophageal intubation.

$Petco_2$ may also be useful for assessing the adequacy of cardiopulmonary resuscitation (CPR). The onset of cardiac arrest results in a decrease of $Petco_2$ to zero. With the initiation of CPR, $Petco_2$ immediately increases with return of spontaneous circulation. Capnography during CPR is recommended in the guidelines of the American Heart Association. A low $Petco_2$ should prompt assessment of the quality of CPR. A persistent $Petco_2$ less than 10 mm Hg during CPR suggests a poor outcome.

Volumetric Capnometry

Although the traditional capnogram is time based, it can be volume based if expiratory flow is measured. The volume-based capnogram (Figure 28-6) is displayed with Pco_2

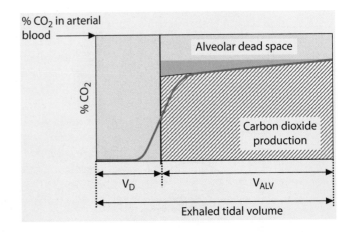

Figure 28-6 The volumetric capnogram. (Reproduced with permission from Longnecker D, Brown D, Newman M, Zapol W. *Anesthesiology*. 2nd ed. New York, NY: McGraw-Hill; 2012.)

on the vertical axis and volume on the horizontal axis. Airway dead space volume (ie, anatomic dead space), alveolar dead space volume, and the volume of exhaled CO_2 (ie, $\dot{V}CO_2$) can be determined from the volume-based capnogram. Note that the determination of alveolar dead space requires knowledge of the $PaCO_2$ in addition to the exhaled capnogram.

Transcutaneous PO_2 and PCO_2

Transcutaneous PO_2 ($PtCO_2$) uses an electrode attached to the skin. To measure a $PtCO_2$ approximating PaO_2, the electrode must be heated to approximately 44°C. The increase in PO_2 caused by heating balances the decrease in PO_2 caused by skin oxygen consumption and the diffusion of oxygen across the skin. In adults, the $PtCO_2$ is frequently less than PaO_2. $PtCO_2$ is also affected by perfusion, and it may reflect oxygen delivery to the skin under the electrode. $PtCO_2$ monitoring is almost never used because there are concerns about its accuracy, it is labor intensive, and because use of pulse oximetry is widespread.

For transcutaneous PCO_2 ($PtCCO_2$), reasonably good correlation with $PaCO_2$ can be obtained at a temperature of 37°C. Because $PtCCO_2$ is consistently greater than $PaCO_2$, manufacturers incorporate a correction factor so that the $PtCCO_2$ displayed approximates the $PaCO_2$. The closeness with which $PtCCO_2$ approximates $PaCO_2$ is the result of a complex set of physiologic events and thus it is incorrect to think of $PtCCO_2$ as $PaCO_2$. Decreased perfusion causes the $PtCCO_2$ to increase. A miniaturized single sensor combining the measurement of SpO_2 and $PtCCO_2$ is commercially available. This device is attached to the earlobe. Because there are concerns about accuracy of transcutaneous monitoring and because it is labor intensive, it has not received widespread acceptance in mechanically ventilated adults.

Points to Remember

- Pulse oximetry uses the principles of oximetry and plethysmography to measure SpO_2.
- Accuracy of pulse oximetry is ± 4% to 5%, the implications of which are determined by the oxyhemoglobin dissociation curve.
- Limitations of pulse oximetry include motion artifact, interference from carboxyhemoglobin and methemoglobin, interference from vascular dyes and nail polish, and inability to detect hyperoxemia.
- A reasonable target SpO_2 is 88% to 95% in mechanically ventilated patients.
- Capnography is the measurement of CO_2 at the airway.
- $PetCO_2$ depends on the $\dot{V}/\dot{Q}$ ratio.
- $PetCO_2$ is often an imprecise indicator of $PaCO_2$.
- $PetCO_2$ may be useful to detect esophageal intubation and to evaluate the quality of CPR.
- Owing to technical and physiologic limitations, transcutaneous monitoring is seldom used.

Additional Reading

Barker SJ, Badal JJ. The measurement of dyshemoglobins and total hemoglobin by pulse oximetry. *Curr Opin Anaesthesiol.* 2008;21:805-810.

Barker SJ, Curry J, Redford D, Morgan S. Measurement of carboxyhemoglobin and methemoglobin by pulse oximetry: a human volunteer study. *Anesthesiology.* 2006;105:892-897.

Bendjelid K, Schütz N, Stotz M, et al. Transcutaneous P_{CO_2} monitoring in critically ill adults: clinical evaluation of a new sensor. *Crit Care Med.* 2005;33:2203-2206.

Blanch L, Romero PV, Lucangelo U. Volumetric capnography in the mechanically ventilated patient. *Minerva Anestesiol.* 2006;72:577-585.

Bolliger D, Steiner LA, Kasper J, et al. The accuracy of non-invasive carbon dioxide monitoring: a clinical evaluation of two transcutaneous systems. *Anaesthesia.* 2007;62:394-399.

Broch O, Bein B, Gruenewald M, et al. Accuracy of the pleth variability index to predict fluid responsiveness depends on the perfusion index. *Acta Anaesthesiol Scand.* 2011;55:686-693.

Cannesson M, Delannoy B, Morand A, et al. Does the Pleth variability index indicate the respiratory-induced variation in the plethysmogram and arterial pressure waveforms? *Anesth Analg.* 2008;106:1189-1194.

Eberhard P. The design, use, and results of transcutaneous carbon dioxide analysis: current and future directions. *Anesth Analg.* 2007;105(6 Suppl):S48-S52.

Feiner JR, Bickler PE, Mannheimer PD. Accuracy of methemoglobin detection by pulse CO-oximetry during hypoxia. *Anesth Analg.* 2010;111:143-148.

Feiner JR, Severinghaus JW, Bickler PE. Dark skin decreases the accuracy of pulse oximeters at low oxygen saturation: the effects of oximeter probe type and gender. *Anesth Analg.* 2007;105(Suppl):S18-S23.

Marik PE, Cavallazzi R, Vasu T, Hirani A. Dynamic changes in arterial waveform derived variables and fluid responsiveness in mechanically ventilated patients: a systematic review of the literature. *Crit Care Med.* 2009;37:2642-2647.

McMorrow RC, Mythen MG. Pulse oximetry. *Curr Opin Crit Care* 2006;12:269-271.

Sandroni C, Cavallaro F, Marano C, et al. Accuracy of plethysmographic indices as predictors of fluid responsiveness in mechanically ventilated adults: a systematic review and meta-analysis. *Intensive Care Med.* 2012;38:1429-1437.

Seguin P, Le Rouzo A, Tanguy M, et al. Evidence for the need of bedside accuracy of pulse oximetry in an intensive care unit. *Crit Care Med.* 2000;28:703-706.

Shamir MY, Avramovich A, Smaka T. The current status of continuous noninvasive measurement of total, carboxy, and methemoglobin concentration. *Anesth Analg.* 2012;114:972-978.

Sinha P, Soni N. Comparison of volumetric capnography and mixed expired gas methods to calculate physiological dead space in mechanically ventilated ICU patients. *Intensive Care Med.* 2012;38:1712-1717.

Urbano J, Cruzado V, López-Herce J, et al. Accuracy of three transcutaneous carbon dioxide monitors in critically ill children. *Pediatr Pulmonol.* 2010;45:481-486.

Van de Louw A, Cracco C, Cerf C, et al. Accuracy of pulse oximetry in the intensive care unit. *Intensive Care Med.* 2001;27:1606-1613.

Verhovsek M, Henderson MP, Cox G, et al. Unexpectedly low pulse oximetry measurements associated with variant hemoglobins: a systematic review. *Am J Hematol.* 2010;85:882-885.

Walley KR. Use of central venous oxygen saturation to guide therapy. *Am J Respir Crit Care Med.* 2011;184:514-520.

Weaver LK, Churchill SK, Deru K, Cooney D. False positive rate of carbon monoxide saturation by pulse oximetry of emergency department patients. *Respir Care.* 2013;58(2):232-240.

Yin JY, Ho KM. Use of plethysmographic variability index derived from the Massimo pulse oximeter to predict fluid or preload responsiveness: a systematic review and meta-analysis. *Anaesthesia.* 2012;67:777-783.

Chapter 29
Hemodynamic Monitoring

Objectives

1. Discuss important heart-lung interactions during mechanical ventilation.
2. List indications for hemodynamic monitoring.
3. Describe the use of direct and derived hemodynamic measurements.
4. Describe the effect of positive pressure ventilation on hemodynamic measurements.
5. Describe how pulse pressure variation (PPV) can inform the response to fluid administration.

Introduction

Invasive hemodynamic monitoring is commonly used with critically ill, mechanically ventilated patients. Because of the interactions between mechanical ventilation and hemodynamics, it is important that clinicians providing ventilatory support understand the basics of hemodynamic monitoring.

Heart-Lung Interactions

The heart and lungs share a common space in the thorax and, thus, are linked anatomically. With each breath, the lungs and thorax change both in volume and in pressure. These fluctuations affect cardiac function through changes in heart rate, preload, afterload, venous return, and contractility of the heart. Changes in intrapleural pressure can affect preload and afterload; positive pressure ventilation can decrease preload and afterload. Pulmonary vascular resistance (PVR) is dependent on lung volume; positive end-expiratory pressure (PEEP) may restore lung volume to the normal functional residual capacity (FRC) and decrease PVR. If applied in excess, however, PEEP can increase lung volume above FRC and increase the PVR. The descent of the diaphragm with respiration compresses the abdominal compartment and increases abdominal pressure, which increases the abdominal vascular pressures and increases the driving pressure for venous return. During positive pressure ventilation, the increase in abdominal pressure may partially compensate for the increase in right atrial pressure induced by the positive pressure. The application of PEEP can have complicated effects on the venous return depending on the change in abdominal pressure and the filling pressure of the ventricle. Ventricular interdependence occurs such that changes in the performance of one ventricle affects the other. The rise in right ventricular volume that accompanies an acute increase in the PVR will act to decrease LV compliance via effects on the ventricular septum.

Hemodynamic Monitoring

Indications and complications for arterial and pulmonary artery catheters are listed in Table 29-1 and normal hemodynamic values are listed in Table 29-2.

Table 29-1 Indications and Contraindications for Arterial and Venous Cannulation

Arterial cannulation
- Indications: continuous blood pressure monitoring, frequent blood gases
- Complications: hemorrhage, infection, ischemia (embolus, thrombus, spasm)

Central venous catheter
- Indications: fluid administration, nutritional support, CVP measurements, central venous blood gases
- Complications: pneumothorax, embolus and thrombus formation, infection

Pulmonary artery cannulation
- Indications: PCWP measurements, cardiac output measurements, mixed venous blood gases
- Complications: pneumothorax, arrhythmias, embolus and thrombus formation, infection, cardiovascular injury

---

Direct Measurements

Common sites for indwelling arterial catheters are the radial, brachial, axillary, and femoral arteries. Because of the presence of collateral circulation, the radial artery usually is the vessel of choice. Direct measurement of arterial blood pressure allows continuous display of systolic pressure, diastolic pressure, and mean arterial pressure.

Table 29-2 Normal Values for Direct Measured and Derived Hemodynamic Values

Direct measurements	
Central venous pressure	< 6 mm Hg
Pulmonary capillary wedge pressure	4-12 mm Hg
Pulmonary artery pressure	
systolic	20-30 mm Hg
diastolic	6-15 mm Hg
mean	10-20 mm Hg
Systemic arterial blood pressure	
systolic/diastolic	120/80 mm Hg
mean	80-100 mm Hg
Cardiac output	4-8 L/min
Heart rate	60-100 beats/min

Derived measurements	
Cardiac index	2.5-4 L/min/m^2
Stroke volume	60-130 mL
Pulmonary vascular resistance	110-250 dynes $\times$ s$\cdot$cm^{-5}
Systemic vascular resistance	900-1400 dynes $\times$ s$\cdot$cm^{-5}
Right ventricular stroke work index	8-10 g$\cdot$m/m^2/beat
Left ventricular stroke work index	50-60 g$\cdot$m/m^2/beat

Central venous pressure (CVP) is measured from a catheter located in the superior vena cava or right atrium. CVP reflects right atrial pressure, which reflects right ventricular end-diastolic pressure and the performance of the right ventricle. In patients with normal cardiac reserve and PVR, CVP reflects preload.

A pulmonary artery catheter is used to evaluate intravascular pressure and cardiac output. However, the use of the pulmonary artery catheter has decreased significantly in recent years after publication of studies that questioned whether its use resulted in improved patient outcomes. The pulmonary artery catheter is a special balloon tipped flow-directed catheter used for pulmonary artery pressure (PAP) and pulmonary capillary wedge pressure (PCWP) monitoring. The standard catheter consists of a proximal port (at the level of the right atrium to infuse fluids, measure CVP, and inject cold solution for cardiac output), distal port (in the pulmonary artery), a balloon (which is inflated for PCWP measurements), and a thermistor (to measure temperature and calculate cardiac output). Pulmonary artery catheters can also be used to monitor mixed venous oxygen saturation, right ventricular ejection fraction, and to provide temporary cardiac pacing. An elevated PAP may indicate left-to-right shunt, left ventricular failure, mitral stenosis, or pulmonary hypertension. When the balloon is inflated, the catheter floats forward to a small branch of the pulmonary artery. Blood flow past the balloon is thus obstructed, and PCWP is measured (Figure 29-1). PCWP (also called pulmonary artery wedge pressure or pulmonary artery occlusion pressure) is a reflection of left atrial pressure. An elevated PCWP may indicate left ventricular failure, mitral stenosis, or cardiac insufficiency.

Thermodilution cardiac output is measured by injecting a cold solution into the central circulation (right atrium). The downstream temperature change in the pulmonary artery allows cardiac output to be calculated. A thermistor located near the tip of the pulmonary artery catheter measures the blood temperature in the pulmonary artery. The temperature of the patient, the temperature of the injection solution, and the change in blood temperature are the variables used to compute cardiac output. A continuous thermodilution cardiac output technique emits a safe amount of heat into the blood without using a fluid injectate, and cardiac output is computed by analysis of temperature changes in the pulmonary artery using signal processing techniques. Pulse contour waveform analysis techniques allow minimally invasive continuous cardiac output monitoring without the need for a pulmonary artery catheter.

Derived Measurements

Cardiac output is often normalized to patient size by dividing cardiac output ($\dot{Q}c$) by body surface area (BSA):

$$CI = \dot{Q}c/BSA$$

where CI is cardiac index. The volume of blood ejected from the ventricle with each contraction, stroke volume (SV), can be calculated by dividing cardiac output by heart rate (f_c):

$$SV = \dot{Q}c/f_c$$

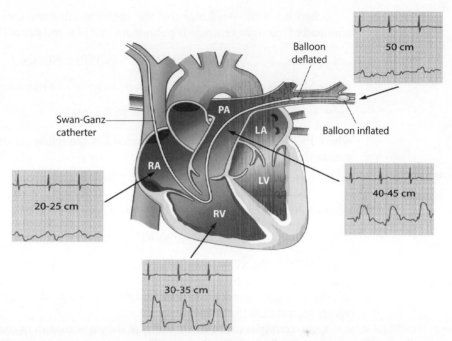

Figure 29-1 Pressure waveforms recorded by the pulmonary artery catheter. As the catheter is advanced from the venous cannulation site, the first waveform recorded will be the central venous pressure trace. Passage of the catheter from the right atrium (RA) into the right ventricle (RV) is accompanied by a marked increase in systolic pressure. As the catheter tip enters the pulmonary artery (PA), a dicrotic notch may appear in the systolic wave and the diastolic pressure will increase in magnitude and will be downsloping in contrast to the upsloping diastolic pressure in the right ventricle (RV). With further advancement of the catheter, the balloon will occlude blood flow and the tip will record the pulmonary artery occlusion pressure, characterized by disappearance of the systolic pressure wave and reappearance of venous *a*, *c*, and *v* waves. Numbers show the approximate depth when inserting the PAC from the right internal jugular vein. (Modified with permission from Mark JB. *Atlas of Cardiovascular Monitoring.* New York, NY: Churchill Livingstone; 1998:Fig. 3.1.)

Figure 29-2 The relationship between measured and derived hemodynamic parameters and cardiac output.

Stroke volume   Heart rate

Cardiac output

Preload	Afterload	Contractility
CVP	PVR	RVSWI
PCWP	SVR	LVSWI

SV can also be normalized to patient size:

$$SVI = CI/f_c$$

where SVI is stroke volume indexed.

Hemodynamic monitoring allows preload, afterload, and contractility to be assessed. This provides the clinician with the information necessary to assess cardiac output (Figure 29-2). Preload is determined by myocardial stretch at end diastole (end-diastolic tension). An increase in blood volume and an increase in venous tone will increase preload. A decrease in blood volume (eg, diuretic administration) will decrease preload. The CVP is an indicator of right ventricular preload, and PCWP is an indicator of left ventricular preload. Excessive preload is associated with cardiac failure and insufficient preload is associated with hypovolemia or sepsis.

Afterload is the resistance that the ventricle must overcome to eject blood. The afterload of the right ventricle is pulmonary vascular resistance (PVR):

$$PVR = [(MPAP - PCWP) \times 80] / \dot{Q}c$$

where MPAP is the mean PAP. PVR can be indexed to patient size:

$$PVRI = PVR \times BSA$$

where PVRI is the PVR index. The afterload of the left ventricle is systemic vascular resistance (SVR):

$$SVR = [(MAP - CVP) \times 80] / \dot{Q}c$$

where MAP is mean systemic arterial pressure. SVR can also be indexed to patient size:

$$SVRI = SVR \times BSA$$

where SVRI is the SVR index. Afterload is determined primarily by vascular tone; an increase in vascular tone increases afterload and a decrease in vascular tone decreases afterload. Thus, vasodilating agents decrease afterload, whereas vasoconstricting agents increase afterload.

Contractility is the intrinsic ability of the myocardium to contract, independent of preload and afterload. The contractility of the right ventricle is determined by the right ventricular stroke work index (RVSWI):

$$RVSWI = SVI \times (MPAP - CVP) \times 0.0136$$

The contractility of the left ventricle is determined by the left ventricular stroke work index (LVSWI):

$$LVSWI = SVI \times (MAP - PCWP) \times 0.0136$$

Contractility is manipulated by use of inotropic and beta-blocking agents. Inotropic agents increase contractility, and β-blocking agents decrease contractility.

Airway Pressure and Hemodynamics

Effect of Pressure Changes During Respiratory Cycle

Although intravascular pressures are measured, it is actually transmural pressure (the difference between intraluminal pressure and pleural pressure) that is important. Thus, changes in intrapleural pressure affect transmural pressure measurements. During spontaneous breathing, pleural pressure decreases during inspiration and increases during expiration. Pleural pressure increases during inspiration and decreases during exhalation during positive pressure ventilation. At end exhalation, pleural pressure is the same for spontaneous breathing and positive pressure breathing (Figure 29-3). For that reason, intrathoracic pressure measurements should always be recorded at end exhalation.

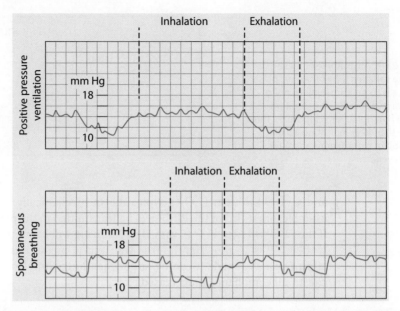

Figure 29-3 Pulmonary artery pressure waveform with spontaneous breathing (top) and positive pressure breathing (bottom). Note that end-expiratory pressure is equal for both waveforms.

Because CVP is affected by pleural pressure, changes in CVP during the respiratory cycle can be used to evaluate patient effort during spontaneous or assisted ventilation. A large decrease in CVP during inhalation suggests that the patient has a high inspiratory load and may have a high work of breathing. A large increase in CVP during a passive positive pressure breath means that lung compliance is high relative to chest wall compliance, and thus much of the airway pressure is transmitted to the pleural space.

Effect of PEEP on Hemodynamic Measurements

Positive pressure ventilation can also affect measurements of PCWP. This may occur due to catheter tip position and due to the effect of PEEP on pleural pressure. If the catheter tip is positioned in zone 1 of the lungs (ventilation without perfusion), PCWP reflects alveolar pressure rather than left atrial pressure. This rarely occurs because catheter floatation will usually direct the catheter tip into zone 3 (perfusion in excess of ventilation), but it may occur if PAP is low and PEEP is high.

The degree to which PEEP (and all airway pressure) is transmitted to the pleural space is determined by the compliance of the lung and chest wall:

$$\Delta Ppl/\Delta P_{aw} = C_L/(C_L + C_W)$$

where ΔPpl is the change in pleural pressure, ΔP_{aw} is the change in airway pressure, C_L is lung compliance, and C_W is chest wall compliance. Because chest wall compliance and lung compliance are normally equal, only half of the PEEP pressure will be transmitted to the pleural space. When lung compliance is reduced, as often occurs with acute respiratory failure, less than half of the PEEP pressure will be transmitted to the pleural space and affect CVP measurements. For example, assume that C_W is 100 mL/cm H_2O

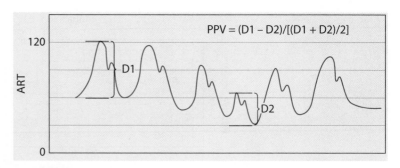

Figure 29-4 An example of pulse pressure variation (PPV). Maximal pulse pressure is 60 mm Hg; minimal pulse pressure is 36 mm Hg. The resulting PPV (24 mm Hg/48 mm Hg) is 50%. This is more than 12%, indicating a high likelihood of hypovolemia and fluid responsiveness.

and C_L is 50 mL/cm H_2O (a typical C_L in mechanically ventilated patients). In this example, one-third of the PEEP will be transmitted to the pleural space and affect CVP. If the PEEP is 12 cm H_2O (9 mm Hg), 3 mm Hg will be transmitted to the pleural space. If the CVP is 15 mm Hg, the true transmural pressure is 12 mm Hg. Although this effect is usually small, it can be large when lung compliance is relatively normal and chest wall compliance is decreased.

Pulse Pressure Variation

Positive pressure ventilation causes lung volume to phasically vary by increasing pressure during the inspiratory phase, causing proportional increases in intrathoracic pressure as the lungs expand against the chest wall and diaphragm. This results in changes in right atrial pressure. Increasing right atrial pressure transiently decreases venous return to the right ventricle, and intrathoracic blood volume decreases. After several heartbeats, the decreased flow reaches the left ventricle and its output also transiently decreases. In nonvolume responsive states, intrathoracic blood volume changes very little during ventilation. Arterial pulse pressure variation (PPV) during ventilation identifies patients as being volume responsive. Positive pressure ventilation-induced PPV may identify volume responders if PPV is greater than 12% (Figure 29-4). A important limitation of PPV to assess volume responsiveness is that it is less accurate when tidal volume is less than 8 mL/kg; thus it is less accurate during lung-protective ventilation.

Fluid Management in ARDS

The Fluid and Catheter Treatment (FACT) trial conducted by the ARDS Network evaluated the role of conservative fluid management in patients with ARDS. In this study, 1000 patients were randomized to two different protocols, a liberal versus a conservative fluid management, based on CVP or PCWP. Although there was no significant 60-day mortality difference between the groups, patients in the conservative strategy group with a lower CVP had significantly more days alive and free of mechanical ventilation, and discharged from the ICU. These important results did not occur at the expense of increased organ failures in these patients at 7 and 28 days. In a fluid conservative approach, fluid intake is restricted and urinary output is increased in an attempt to decrease lung edema. Evidence does not support improved outcomes with the use of albumin or other colloids compared to those resuscitated with normal saline.

Points to Remember

- A number of heart-lung interactions are important during mechanical ventilation.
- Direct hemodynamic measurements include arterial blood pressure, CVP, PAP, PCWP, and cardiac output.
- Derived hemodynamic measurements include SV, PVR, SVR, right ventricular stroke work, and left ventricular stroke work.
- Hemodynamic measurements are used to evaluate preload, afterload, and contractility.
- Because of vascular pressure fluctuations that occur during breathing, vascular pressures should always be recorded at end exhalation.
- The effect of PEEP on vascular pressure measurements is determined by lung compliance and chest wall compliance.
- PPV reflects fluid responsiveness.

Additional Reading

Morgan P, Al-Subaie N, Rhodes A. Minimally invasive cardiac output monitoring. *Curr Opin Crit Care.* 2008;14:322-326.

Neamu RF, Martin GS. Fluid management in acute respiratory distress syndrome. *Curr Opin Crit Care.* 2013;19:24-30.

Pinsky MR. Heart-lung interactions during mechanical ventilation. *Curr Opin Crit Care.* 2012;18:256-260.

Schmidt GA. Cardiopulmonary interactions in acute lung injury. *Curr Opin Crit Care.* 2013;19:51-56.

Truijen J, van Lieshout JJ, Wesselink WA, Westerhof BE. Noninvasive continuous hemodynamic monitoring. *J Clin Monit Comput.* 2012;26:267-278.

Wheeler AP, Bernard GR, Thompson BT, et al. Pulmonary-artery versus central venous catheter to guide treatment of acute lung injury. *N Engl J Med.* 2006;354:2213-2224.

Wiedemann HP, Wheeler AP, Bernard GR, et al. Comparison of two fluid-management strategies in acute lung injury. *N Engl J Med.* 2006;354:2564-2575.

Chapter 30
Basic Pulmonary Mechanics During Mechanical Ventilation

Introduction

Pulmonary mechanics are frequently measured on mechanically ventilated patients. Some such as PIP and Pplat are recorded as part of patient-ventilator system checks. Others can be easily made at the bedside with no equipment but that available on the ventilator (eg, airway pressure, flow, and volume).

Assessment of Mechanics During Mechanical Ventilation

Airway Pressure

A typical airway pressure waveform during volume-controlled ventilation (VCV) is shown in Figure 30-1. With VCV, pressure increases as volume is delivered. If a constant flow pattern is chosen, there should be a constant increase in pressure during inspiration. With a descending ramp flow pattern, the inspiratory pressure waveform will be more rectangular. PIP varies with resistance, flow, tidal volume, respiratory system compliance, and PEEP.

An end-inspiratory pause of sufficient duration (0.5-2 seconds) allows equilibration between proximal airway pressure and alveolar pressure (Palv). This measurement should be made on a single breath and removed immediately to prevent the development of auto-PEEP. During the end-inspiratory pause, there is no flow and a pressure plateau develops as proximal airway pressure equilibrates with Palv (Figure 30-2).

The pressure during the inspiratory pause is the Pplat and represents peak Palv. Because it reflects Palv, Pplat should usually be kept at less than 30 cm H_2O and always should be kept as low as possible.

The difference between PIP and Pplat is due to the resistive properties of the system (eg, pulmonary airways, artificial airway), and the difference between Pplat and total PEEP is due to respiratory system compliance. The measurement of Pplat is valid only if the patient is passively ventilated—active breathing invalidates the measurement. The measurement is also not valid if leaks are present.

During pressure-controlled ventilation (PCV), PIP and peak Palv may be equal due to the flow waveform with this mode of ventilation (Figure 30-3). With PCV, flow decreases during inspiration and is often followed by a period of zero flow at end inspiration. During this period of no flow, proximal airway pressure should be equal to Palv. If flow does not reach zero before the end of inspiration during PCV, an end-inspiratory pause maneuver

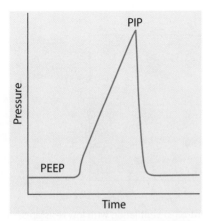

Figure 30-1 A typical airway pressure waveform during volume ventilation.

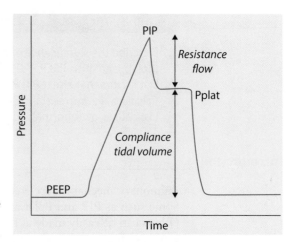

Figure 30-2 Plateau pressure is determined using an end-inspiratory pause.

is needed to determine Pplat. With all other factors held constant (eg, tidal volume, compliance, PEEP), Palv is identical for volume- and pressure-control ventilation. Because lung injury is related to peak Palv (ie, Pplat), the importance of the decrease in PIP that occurs when changing from volume to pressure ventilation is questionable.

Auto-PEEP

An end-expiratory pause is used to determine auto-PEEP (Figure 30-4). This method is valid only if the patient is not spontaneously breathing and there are no system leaks (eg, circuit leak or bronchopleural fistula). For patients who are triggering the ventilator, an esophageal balloon catheter is needed to measure auto-PEEP. During the end-expiratory pause, there is equilibration between end-expiratory pressure and proximal airway pressure. Auto-PEEP is the difference between set PEEP and total PEEP measured with this maneuver. All current-generation ventilators have the capability of measuring auto-PEEP using an end-exhalation pause maneuver.

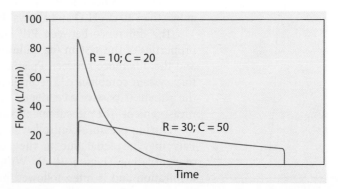

Figure 30-3 Typical airway flow waveforms for pressure-controlled ventilation with low resistance and low compliance (eg, acute respiratory distress syndrome [ARDS]), and with high resistance and high compliance (eg, chronic obstructive pulmonary disease [COPD]).

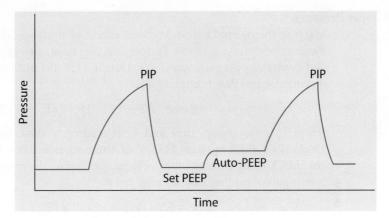

Figure 30-4 Auto-PEEP is determined using an end-expiratory pause.

Auto-PEEP is determined by the tidal volume, respiratory system compliance, airways resistance, and expiratory time:

$$\text{Auto-PEEP} = V_T / [C \times (e^{K_E/T_E} - 1)]$$

where $K_E = 1/(R_E \times C)$, e is the base of the natural logarithm, T_E is expiratory time, R_E is expiratory airways resistance, and C is respiratory system compliance. Because set PEEP may counterbalance auto-PEEP, the presence of auto-PEEP is most appropriately measured with no PEEP set on the ventilator. Auto-PEEP causes dynamic hyperinflation, hemodynamic instability, ventilation-perfusion mismatch, and difficulty triggering the ventilator.

Measurements of auto-PEEP and Pplat reflect average alveolar pressures. Because of the inhomogeneity of the lungs with disease, some lung units have an auto-PEEP (or Pplat) higher or lower than that measured. This is of particular concern with measures of auto-PEEP due to airway closure during exhalation (Figure 30-5).

Figure 30-5 The effect of airway closure on measurement of auto-PEEP. Although the auto-PEEP is high in some lung units, the level measured is only that in lung units where the airway remains open at end exhalation.

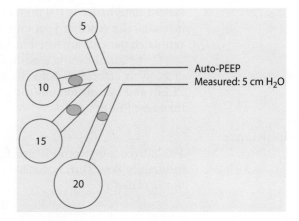

Mean Airway Pressure

Many of the desired and deleterious effects of mechanical ventilation are related by mean airway pressure ($\overline{P}aw$). Factors affecting mean airway pressure are PIP, PEEP, I:E, and inspiratory pressure waveform. During PCV, the inspiratory pressure waveform is rectangular and $\overline{P}aw$ is estimated as:

$$\overline{P}aw = (PIP - PEEP) \times (T_I/T_T) + PEEP$$

where T_I is inspiratory time and T_T is total cycle time. For example, with a PIP of 25 cm H_2O, PEEP of 10 cm H_2O, T_I of 1 second, rate 20/min ($T_I/T_T = 0.33$), $\overline{P}aw$ is 15 cm H_2O. During constant-flow volume ventilation, the inspiratory pressure waveform is triangular, and $\overline{P}aw$ can be estimated as:

$$\overline{P}aw = 0.5 \times (PIP - PEEP) \times (T_I/T_T) + PEEP$$

For example, with a PIP of 25 cm H_2O, PEEP 5 cm H_2O, T_I 1.0 seconds, rate 30/min ($T_I/T_T = 0.5$), $\overline{P}aw$ is 15 cm H_2O. Many current-generation microprocessor ventilators display $\overline{P}aw$ from integration of the airway pressure waveform. Because expiratory resistance is usually greater than inspiratory resistance, Paw is not equivalent to Palv. The difference between mean alveolar pressure ($\overline{P}aw$) and $\overline{P}aw$ is estimated by the following relationship:

$$\overline{P}alv - \overline{P}aw = \dot{V}_E/60 \times (R_E - R_I)$$

Compliance

The difference between Pplat and total PEEP is determined by the compliance of the lungs and chest wall. Thus, compliance can be calculated as:

$$C = V_T/(Pplat - PEEP)$$

The V_T used in this equation is the actual tidal volume delivered to the patient, and it should be corrected for the effects of volume compressed in the ventilator circuit. PEEP should include any auto-PEEP that is present. Pplat should be determined from an end-inspiratory breath-hold that is long enough to produce equilibration between proximal airway pressure and alveolar pressure. Normal respiratory system compliance is 100 mL/cm H_2O and should be greater than 50 mL/cm H_2O in mechanically ventilated patients. Causes of a decrease in compliance in mechanically ventilated patients are listed in Table 30-1.

Compliance can be used to determine the best PEEP setting. The optimal level of PEEP is associated with the highest compliance. Low lung volume (insufficient PEEP) and overdistention (too much PEEP) are associated with a lower compliance than best PEEP.

Resistance

The difference between PIP and Pplat is determined by inspiratory resistance and end-inspiratory flow. During constant-flow volume ventilation, inspiratory resistance can be calculated as:

$$R_I = (PIP - Pplat)/\dot{V}_I$$

Table 30-1 Causes of decreased compliance and increased resistance in mechanically ventilated patients

Compliance	Resistance
Lung effects:	Bronchospasm
Congestive heart failure	Secretions
ARDS	Small endotracheal tube
Consolidation	Mucosal edema
Low lung volume	Low lung volume
Overdistention	
Fibrosis	
Mainstem intubation	
Lung resection	
Pleural effects:	
Pneumothorax	
Pleural effusion	
Chest wall effects:	
Abdominal distention	
Morbid obesity	
Chest wall deformity	

where $\dot{V}_I$ is the inspiratory flow. Expiratory resistance can be estimated from the time constant (τ) of the lung: $R_E = \tau/C$ (Figure 30-6). Expiratory resistance can also be estimated as $R_E = (Pplat - PEEP)/\dot{V}_E$, where $\dot{V}_E$ is peak expiratory flow. Causes of increased resistance during mechanical ventilation are listed in Table 30-1. Inspiratory resistance is less than expiratory resistance due to the increased diameter of airways during inspiration. Normal airways resistance is 1 to 2 cm H_2O/L/s and should be less than 10 cm H_2O/L/s in intubated mechanically ventilated patients.

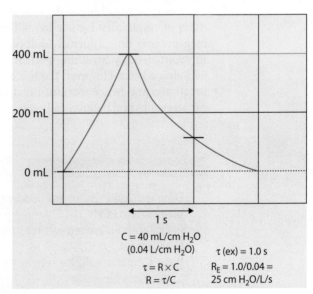

Figure 30-6 Use of the tidal volume waveform to measure time constant (τ) and calculate expiratory airways resistance.

$$C = 40 \text{ mL/cm } H_2O$$
$$(0.04 \text{ L/cm } H_2O)$$
$$\tau = R \times C$$
$$R = \tau/C$$
$$\tau \text{ (ex)} = 1.0 \text{ s}$$
$$R_E = 1.0/0.04 = 25 \text{ cm } H_2O\text{/L/s}$$

Least Squares Fitting Method

This method allows dynamic estimation of respiratory mechanics without the need for measurement of Pplat through use of the equation of motion:

$$Pvent + Pmus = V/C + \dot{V}R + PEEP + auto\text{-}PEEP$$

If the respiratory muscles are relaxed (Pmus = 0), and if many measures of Pvent (airway pressure), volume, and flow are made during inspiration, it is possible to calculate resistance, compliance, and auto-PEEP using an iterative least squares fitting method. This is the method used by ventilators that display resistance and compliance on every breath without flow interruption. Because it assumes that the respiratory muscles are relaxed, this method becomes less accurate during spontaneous breathing modes. If resistance, compliance, and auto-PEEP are known, it is possible to calculate Pmus.

Work-of-Breathing

Inspiratory work-of-breathing performed by the ventilator can be estimated during constant-flow passive inflation of the lungs by the following calculation:

$$W = (PIP - 0.5 \times Pplat)/100 \times V_T$$

For example, if PIP = 30 cm H_2O, Pplat = 25 cm H_2O, and tidal volume = 0.4 L, then W = 0.07 kg·m, or 0.18 kg·m/L. The units for work-of-breathing are kilogram-meter (kg·m) or joules (J); 0.1 kg·m = 1.0 J. Work-of-breathing is often normalized to the tidal volume (work/L). Normal work-of-breathing is ≈ 0.5 J/L. Work-of-breathing will increase with an increase in resistance, a decrease in compliance, or an increase in tidal volume. Although work-of-breathing is not commonly calculated, it is reasonable to expect that ventilator libetration will be difficult with a high work-of-breathing.

Power of breathing is the rate at which work is done, and may be a better assessment of respiratory muscle loads than work of breathing per breath because it is a measure over time, (normal adult power of breathing is 4-8 J/min). Work-of-breathing in spontaneously breathing patients has traditionally required use of an esophageal balloon catheter. However, the use of an artificial neural network may allow power of breathing, and hence work-of-breathing is calculated noninvasively without the need for an esophageal balloon catheter.

Points to Remember

- During VCV, PIP is determined by tidal volume, inspiratory flow, resistance, compliance, and PEEP.
- Peak Palv is estimated by measuring airway pressure during an end-inspiratory breath-hold.
- Pplat should usually be kept at less than 30 cm H_2O and should always be kept as low as possible.

- Auto-PEEP is estimated by measuring airway pressure during an end-expiratory breath-hold.
- Mean airway pressure is calculated from PIP, PEEP, and T_I/T_T.
- Compliance is calculated from V_T, Pplat, and PEEP.
- Inspiratory resistance is calculated from PIP, Pplat, and inspiratory flow.
- Work-of-breathing is increased with increases in resistance, compliance, and V_T.

Additional Reading

Banner MJ, Euliano NR, Brennan V, et al. Power of breathing determined noninvasively with use of an artificial neural network in patients with respiratory failure. *Crit Care Med.* 2006;34:1052-1059.

Bekos V, Marini JJ. Monitoring the mechanically ventilated patient. *Crit Care Clin.* 2007;23:575-611.

Blanch L, Bernabé F, Lucangelo U. Measurement of air trapping, intrinsic positive end-expiratory pressure, and dynamic hyperinflation in mechanically ventilated patients. *Respir Care.* 2005;50:110-124.

Blankman P, Gommers D. Lung monitoring at the bedside in mechanically ventilated patients. *Curr Opin Crit Care.* 2012;18:261-266.

Henderson WR, Sheel AW. Pulmonary mechanics during mechanical ventilation. *Respir Physiol Neurobiol.* 2012;180:162-172.

Lucangelo U, Bernabè F, Blanch L. Lung mechanics at the bedside: make it simple. *Curr Opin Crit Care.* 2007;13:64-72.

Lucangelo U, Bernabé F, Blanch L. Respiratory mechanics derived from signals in the ventilator circuit. *Respir Care.* 2005;50:55-67.

Stenqvist O. Practical assessment of respiratory mechanics. *Br J Anaesth.* 2003;91:92-105.

Zanella A, Bellani G, Pesenti A. Airway pressure and flow monitoring. *Curr Opin Crit Care.* 2010;16:255-260.

Chapter 31
Advanced Pulmonary Mechanics During Mechanical Ventilation

1. Draw normal pressure, flow, and volume waveforms for pressure- and volume-controlled ventilation.
2. Describe the effects of abnormal respiratory system mechanics on pressure, flow, and volume waveforms during pressure- and volume-controlled ventilation.
3. Discuss the use of flow- and pressure-volume curves during mechanical ventilation.
4. Describe the use of the stress index during mechanical ventilation.
5. Describe the use of esophageal pressure to measure pleural pressure during mechanical ventilation.
6. Discuss the use of intra-abdominal pressure measurements during mechanical ventilation.
7. Explain how lung volume can be measured during mechanical ventilation.

Introduction

It is useful to assess respiratory mechanics in many mechanically ventilated patients using the pressure and volume displays on the ventilator. Additional information can be gained by observing the graphic waveforms of pressure, volume, and flow. In this chapter, mechanics based on the waveform displays of the ventilator, pressure-volume curves, esophageal pressure, intra-abdominal pressure, and measurement of end-expiratory lung volume (EELV) are discussed.

Scalars

Pressure

Some ventilators measure pressure directly at the proximal airway. Others approximate inspiratory pressure by measuring pressure in the expiratory circuit during inspiration and approximate expiratory pressure by measuring pressure in the inspiratory circuit during exhalation.

With patient-triggered breaths, airway pressure drops below baseline to trigger the ventilator. Active patient effort may continue after the initiation of a patient-triggered breath, which produces scooping out of the airway tracing (Figure 31-1). This suggests that the inspiratory flow of the ventilator should be increased if volume-controlled ventilation is used. Alternatively, pressure-controlled or pressure-support ventilation might be used and the rise time can be adjusted to better meet the patient's flow demand. The depth and duration of the negative pressure deflection prior to a patient-triggered breath indicates the response of the ventilator and the magnitude of the patient effort.

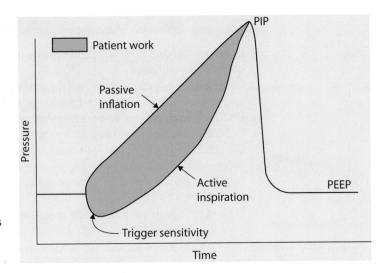

Figure 31-1 Active inspiration during positive pressure ventilation produces scooping of the airway pressure waveform.

A typical airway pressure waveform is shown in Figure 31-2. During exhalation, the pressure should be the set positive end-expiratory pressure (PEEP) level. During inhalation, the airway pressure waveform is determined by the flow set on the ventilator and the patient's respiratory demand. With constant-flow volume-controlled ventilation, airway pressure should increase linearly during the inspiratory phase. With pressure-controlled and pressure-support ventilation, airway pressure during inhalation approximates a square wave. The shape of the pressure waveform is also affected by the rise in time setting on the ventilator.

Flow

Although some ventilators measure flow directly at the proximal endotracheal tube, most measure it in the ventilator using inspiratory and expiratory pneumotachometers.

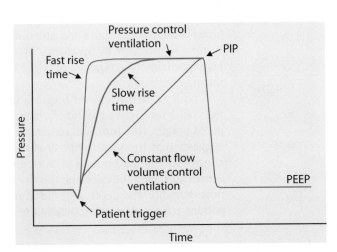

Figure 31-2 Airway pressure waveforms during mechanical ventilation.

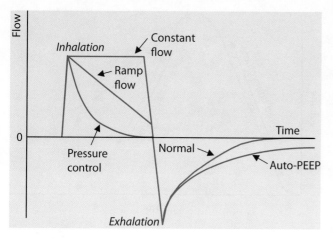

Figure 31-3
Airway flow waveforms during mechanical ventilation.

Flow measured directly at the airway is not affected by factors such as circuit leaks and the compressible volume of the ventilator circuit.

A typical airway flow waveform is illustrated in Figure 31-3. With volume-controlled ventilation, the inspiratory flow waveform is determined by the flow setting on the ventilator. With pressure-controlled ventilation, inspiratory flow decreases according to the patient's respiratory mechanics. If an end-inspiratory pause is set with volume-controlled ventilation, or a long inspiratory time is used with pressure-controlled ventilation, a period of zero flow occurs at the end of the inspiratory phase.

The shape of the expiratory flow waveform is determined by respiratory mechanics, active exhalation, and inspiratory efforts that do not trigger the ventilator. Exhalation is normally passive. With normal resistance and compliance, expiratory flow quickly reaches a peak and then decreases throughout exhalation. Flow at end exhalation indicates that auto-PEEP is present but does not indicate the amount of auto-PEEP. Although useful, the end-expiratory flow is thus an insensitive and imprecise indicator of auto-PEEP. If the patient makes an ineffective inspiratory effort, such as occurs in the setting of auto-PEEP, an upward notching is seen in the expiratory flow waveform with each ineffective effort (Figure 31-4).

Volume

Most monitoring systems used with mechanical ventilators do not measure volume directly. Flow is integrated to produce volume ($\int \dot{V}dt$). The volume waveform depends on the flow pattern set on the ventilator. With a constant inspiratory flow, volume delivery is constant during inspiration. With pressure-controlled ventilation, most of the volume is delivered early in the inspiratory period. A leak distal to the point of volume measurement (eg, leak around the endotracheal tube, bronchopleural fistula) produces a difference between the inspiratory and expiratory tidal volume (Figure 31-5).

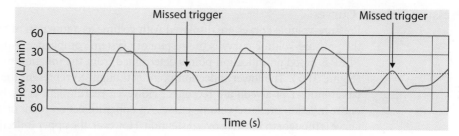

Figure 31-4 Flow waveform of a patient with auto-PEEP and missed trigger efforts. Note the effect of a missed trigger effort on the expiratory flow pattern.

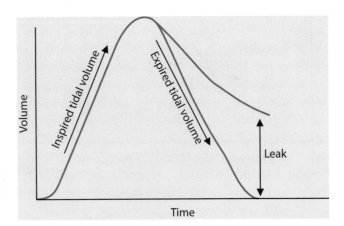

Figure 31-5 Airway volume waveforms during mechanical ventilation. Illustrated is how the volume waveform can be used to assess leak.

Loops

Pressure, flow, and volume can be displayed not only as time scalars but also as flow-volume and pressure-volume loops. This information is similar to that obtained in the pulmonary function laboratory with two exceptions. Loops during mechanical ventilation are obtained during tidal volume breathing, whereas loops in the pulmonary function laboratory are obtained with a vital capacity maneuver. Also, loops during mechanical ventilation are passive, whereas loops produced in the pulmonary function laboratory are with forced inhalation and exhalation.

Flow-Volume Loops

Flow-volume loops are displayed with flow as a function of volume. Some systems display expiratory flow in the positive position, whereas other systems display expiratory flow in the negative position. During inspiration, the shape of the flow-volume loop is determined by the flow setting on the ventilator with volume-controlled ventilation. During exhalation, the shape of the flow-volume loop is determined by respiratory mechanics. The expiratory flow-volume loop has a characteristic concavity with obstructive lung disease (Figure 31-6). With reversible airflow obstruction, the expiratory flow-volume loop may change shape following bronchodilator administration, indicating an improvement in expiratory flow.

Pressure-Volume Curves

Pressure-volume curves are displayed with volume as a function of pressure. The slope of the pressure-volume curve is the respiratory system compliance. An approach for setting PEEP is based on inflection points determined from the inflation pressure-volume curve (Figure 31-7). The lower inflection point is thought to represent the pressure at which a large number of alveoli are recruited. However, recruitment is likely to occur along the entire inflation pressure-volume curve. An upper inflection point on the pressure-volume curve is thought to indicate overdistention. However, the upper inflection point might represent the end of recruitment rather than the point of overdistention.

The most common methods used to measure pressure-volume curves are the use of a super syringe (Figure 31-8), inflation with a constant slow flow (< 10 L/min), and the

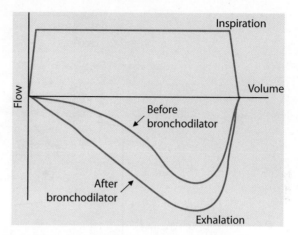

Figure 31-6 Flow-volume loops and the effect of bronchodilator therapy.

measurement of plateau pressures (Pplat) at various inflation volumes. Correct interpretation of the pressure-volume curve during non-constant-flow ventilation (eg, pressure-controlled ventilation), and with higher inspiratory flows, is problematic (Figure 31-9).

In spite of enthusiasm for the use of pressure-volume curves to set the ventilator in patients with acute respiratory distress syndrome (ARDS), a number of issues preclude routine use. Measurement of the pressure-volume curve requires sedation, and often paralysis, to correctly make the measurement. It is often difficult to identify the inflection points and may require mathematical curve fitting to precisely identify the inflection points.

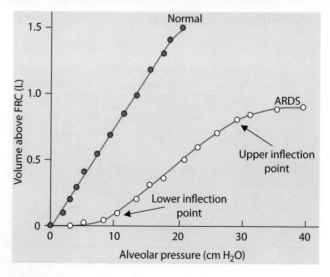

Figure 31-7 Inflation pressure-volume curves during passive mechanical ventilation. The pressure-volume curve for ARDS illustrates a lower inflection point and upper inflection point. (Adapted from: Bigatello LM, Hurford WE, Pesenti A. Ventilatory management of severe acute respiratory failure for Y2K. Anesthesiology. 1999; Dec; 91(6):1567-1570.)

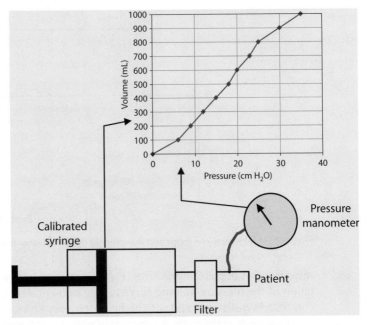

Figure 31-8 Equipment used to measure a pressure-volume curve using a super syringe.

Esophageal pressure measurement is needed to separate lung from chest wall effects. Although the inflation limb of the pressure-volume curve is most commonly measured, the deflation limb may be more useful than the inflation limb. Finally, and perhaps most importantly, the pressure-volume curve treats the lungs as a single compartment, but the

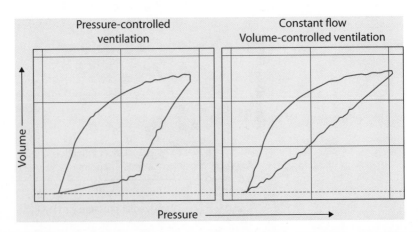

Figure 31-9 Dynamic pressure volume curves as displayed on the ventilator. The only difference between the two curves is a change from pressure-controlled to volume-controlled ventilation. This demonstrates that dynamic pressure-volume curves cannot be used to detect inflection points.

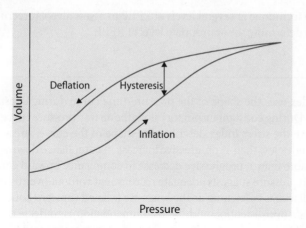

Figure 31-10 Inflation and deflation pressure-volume curves illustrating hysteresis.

lungs of patients with ARDS are heterogeneous. This likely explains why recruitment has been shown to occur along the entire inflation pressure-volume curve.

One approach to setting PEEP is to perform a recruitment maneuver (such as continuous positive airway pressure of 40 cm H_2O for 40 seconds or the use of pressure control ventilation at a PEEP of 20-25 cm H_2O with a driving pressure of 15-20 cm H_2O for 1-3 minutes) followed by a decremental PEEP titration (starting at a high level of PEEP and decreasing the PEEP stepwise while observing for signs of de-recruitment). The intent with this approach is to shift ventilation from the inflation limb to the deflation limp of the pressure-volume curve. As can be seen in Figure 31-10, this results in a greater lung volume for the same applied PEEP. While this is theoretically attractive, whether or not it affects important patient outcomes is unclear.

PEEP-induced lung recruitment can be assessed by performing pressure-volume curves and measuring EELV corresponding to different PEEP levels. Lung recruitment at a given airway pressure is defined as the difference in lung volume between pressure-volume curves starting at different EELVs corresponding to different levels of PEEP (Figure 31-11). Several current-generation ventilators are able to measure pressure-volume curves using a

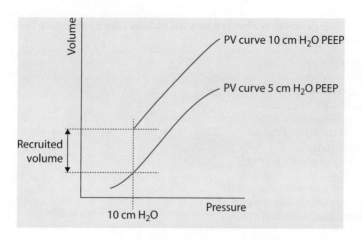

Figure 31-11 Pressure-volume curve technique to determine recruited lung volume with two levels of PEEP.

slow inflation technique at several levels of PEEP to assess alveolar recruitment and inflection points to determine the appropriate level of PEEP.

Stress Index

The stress index uses the shape of the pressure-time curve during constant-flow tidal volume delivery. During constant inspiratory flow, the airway pressure curve is fitted to a power equation where the stress index describes the shape of the curve; stress index = 1, straight curve; stress index less than 1, progressive increase in compliance downward concavity; and stress index more than 1, progressive decrease in compliance upward concavity. Thus, a linear increase in pressure suggests adequate recruitment without overdistention (stress index = 1). If compliance is worsening as the lungs are inflated (upward concavity, stress index > 1), this suggests overdistention and the recommendation is to decrease PEEP or decrease tidal volume. If the compliance is improving as the lungs are inflated (downward concavity, stress index < 1), this suggests tidal recruitment and potential for additional recruitment with PEEP, and thus a recommendation to increase PEEP (Figure 31-12). The stress index is one of several approaches for selection of PEEP in patients with ARDS (Table 31-1). However, just like the pressure-volume curve, it treats the lungs as a single compartment, but the lungs of patients with ARDS are heterogeneous.

Esophageal Pressure

Esophageal pressure is a surrogate for intrapleural pressure. In critically ill patients in a supine position, the absolute value for esophageal pressure often overestimates the true intrapleural pressure due to the weight of the mediastinal viscera. However, a properly placed esophageal balloon will accurately reflect changes in pleural pressure regardless of patient position. The esophageal balloon is placed in the lower third of the esophagus and about 0.5 to 1 mL of air is added to the balloon.

In the spontaneously breathing subject, proper placement can be evaluated using the Baydur maneuver, in which airway and esophageal pressures are evaluated during airway

Table 31-1 Procedures That can be Used to Select the Appropriate Level of PEEP in a Patient With ARDS.

Gas exchange
   Oxygenation (PEEP/F_{IO_2} tables)
   Dead space
Respiratory mechanics
   Compliance
   Pressure-volume curve
   Stress index
   Transpulmonary pressure
Imaging
   Chest computed tomography
   Electrical impedance tomography
   Ultrasound

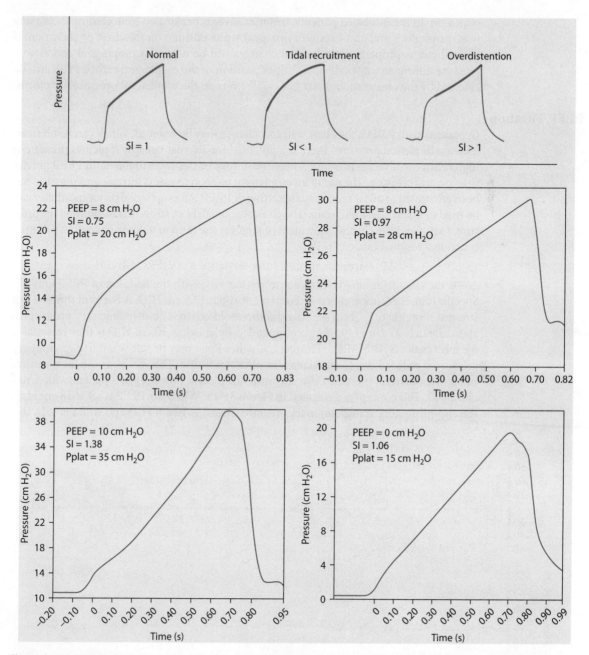

Figure 31-12 TOP. Normal stress index (SI), a stress index illustrating tidal recruitment, and another stress index illustrating overdistention. MIDDLE. Stress index in a patient early in the course of acute respiratory distress syndrome (ARDS). In this case the stress index improved as PEEP was increased. (Reproduced with permission from Hess DR. Approaches to conventional mechanical ventilation of the patient with acute respiratory distress syndrome. *Respir Care*. 2011; Oct;56(10):1555–1572.) BOTTOM. Stress index (SI) in a patient late in the course of ARDS. In this case the stress index improved as PEEP was decreased. (Reproduced with permission from Hess DR. Approaches to conventional mechanical ventilation of the patient with acute respiratory distress syndrome. *Respir Care*. 2011; Oct;56(10):1555–1572)

occlusion. In the intubated patients, this maneuver is performed by occluding the airway (end-inspiratory and end-expiratory pauses) while pushing on the chest or abdomen. If the catheter is properly placed, equal changes will be noted for esophageal and airway pressure during airway occlusion. Proper position of the esophageal catheter can also be assessed by the observation of cardiac oscillations on the esophageal pressure waveform.

PEEP Titration

In patients with ARDS, the chest wall compliance may be reduced, which can result in an increase in pleural pressure. There is a potential for alveolar collapse if pleural pressure is high relative to alveolar pressure. Therefore, it may be desirable to maintain PEEP greater than pleural pressure. The use of an esophageal balloon to assess intrapleural pressure has been advocated to allow more precise setting of PEEP. An esophageal balloon catheter can be used to assess stress and stain. The clinical equivalent of stress is transpulmonary pressure. (ΔP_L), and the clinical equivalent of strain is the ratio of volume change (ΔV) to the functional residual capacity (FRC):

$$\Delta P_L \text{ (stress)} = \text{specific lung elastance} \times \Delta V/FRC \text{ (strain)}$$

ΔV is the change in lung volume above resting FRC with the addition of PEEP and V_T. Specific lung elastance is relatively constant at about 13.5 cm H_2O. A harmful threshold of strain is more than 2. Thus, the harmful threshold of stress (transpulmonary pressure) is approximately 27 cm H_2O. The recommended Pplat below 30 cm H_2O is thus reasonable for most patients with ARDS. However, a higher Pplat may be safe when transpulmonary pressure is reduced due to an increase in pleural pressure. This makes a case for measurement of esophageal pressure (as a surrogate for pleural pressure) in a patient with a stiff chest wall. This concept is illustrated in Figure 31-13. When the PEEP is set at 18 cm H_2O, the end-inspiratory transpulmonary pressure (stress) is 12 cm H_2O and strain is 1. In this

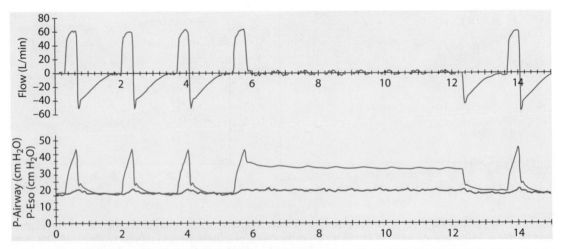

Figure 31-13 An example of a patient with severe ARDS, in whom the PEEP is titrated to 18 cm H_2O so that the PEEP matches the esophageal pressure. The plateau pressure is 32 cm H_2O. The esophageal pressure during the plateau pressure measurement is 20 cm H_2O. Thus, end-inspiratory transalveolar pressure (stress) is 12 cm H_2O in this case.

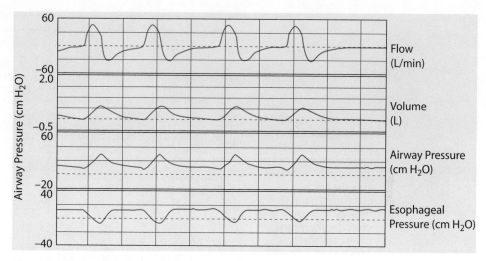

Figure 31-14 The change in esophageal pressure (bottom tracing) may be used to assess patient effort with each inspiration during pressure support ventilation.

case, stress at 12 cm H_2O and strain at 1 are both in the safe range, despite that the Pplat is greater than 30 cm H_2O.

Patient Versus Ventilator Work-of-Breathing

Patients often exert work during mechanical ventilation, particularly during patient-triggered modes. The work performed by the patient may be high and difficult to assess by usual means such as contraction of accessory muscles and asynchronous breathing. Measuring esophageal pressure, proximal airway pressure, and flow makes it possible to estimate the amount of inspiratory work done by the ventilator and the amount done by the patient. The sum of ventilator work and patient work is the total inspiratory work-of-breathing. Some bedside monitoring systems calculate and display these measurements on a breath-by-breath basis. Normal inspiratory work-of-breathing is 0.5 J/L (0.05 kg-m/L). High inspiratory work (> 1.5 J/L or > 15 J/L/min) results in fatigue and failure to wean from mechanical ventilation. Patient effort can also be assessed by the esophageal pressure decrease during inspiration (Figure 31-14).

Auto-PEEP With Spontaneous Breathing

During passive ventilation, auto-PEEP can be assessed by use of an end-expiratory hold. During active breathing, an esophageal balloon is needed to assess auto-PEEP. With a patient-triggered breath, inspiratory flow will not occur at the proximal airway until the pleural pressure change equals the auto-PEEP level. Auto-PEEP can thus be quantified by observing the pleural pressure change required to produce flow at the proximal airway (Figure 31-15). Because auto-PEEP may be a fatiguing load for the spontaneously breathing patient, methods should be used to decrease the amount of auto-PEEP (eg, application of external PEEP, administration of bronchodilators).

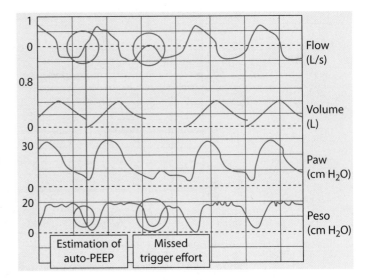

Figure 31-15 Airway pressure, flow, and volume graphics with esophageal pressure in a patient with auto-PEEP. Note the decrease in esophageal pressure required to trigger the ventilator, the missed trigger, and that flow does not return to zero at end exhalation.

Transmission of Pressure to the Pleural Space

Esophageal pressure measurements can also be used to estimate the amount of airway pressure transmitted to the pleural space during passive positive pressure ventilation. The pleural pressure produced during passive inflation depends on tidal volume and chest wall compliance (Figure 31-16). If the lungs are passively inflated, chest wall compliance can be calculated as the tidal volume delivered divided by the change in

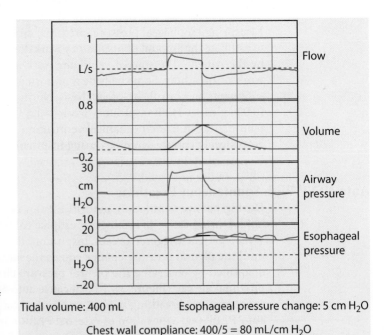

Figure 31-16 Use of esophageal pressure to calculate chest wall compliance.

Tidal volume: 400 mL   Esophageal pressure change: 5 cm H_2O

Chest wall compliance: 400/5 = 80 mL/cm H_2O

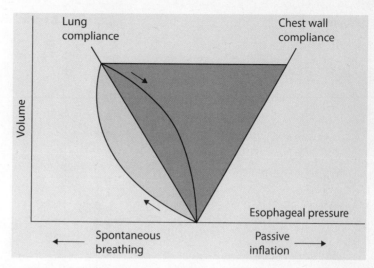

Figure 31-17 The Campbell diagram. The slope of the pressure-volume curve during spontaneous breathing represents lung compliance. The chest wall compliance line is the slope of the esophageal pressure-volume curve generated during passive positive pressure ventilation. The area between the lung compliance line and the chest wall compliance line represents elastic work-of-breathing (shaded area). The area between the lung compliance line and the inspiratory pressure-volume curve represents the resistive work-of-breathing (shaded area). The total spontaneous inspiratory work-of-breathing is the sum of the resistive work and the elastic work.

esophageal pressure. In the absence of an esophageal balloon, respiratory variation of the central venous pressure can be used to estimate changes in pleural pressure. The Campbell diagram can be used to calculate the work-of-breathing due to chest wall compliance, lung compliance, and airways resistance (Figure 31-17).

Intra-abdominal Pressure

Gastric Pressure

One approach to measurement of intra-abdominal pressure is to place a balloon catheter into the stomach. The pressure in the balloon represents gastric pressure and is a reflection of intra-abdominal pressure. During spontaneous breathing, pressures can be measured simultaneously in the esophagus and the stomach. The difference between the pressure in the stomach and the esophagus is called transdiaphragmatic pressure (Pdi). Pdi is a reflection of the strength of the diaphragm. Accordingly, Pdi is used to assess diaphragm weakness. A decrease in gastric pressure during inhalation occurs with diaphragm paralysis (Figure 31-18).

Bladder Pressure

Another method for measurement of intra-abdominal pressure is to measure bladder pressure in a patient with a Foley catheter. This is most commonly performed to assess the presence of abdominal compartment syndrome. In the mechanically ventilated patient, measurement of bladder pressure may be useful to assess the effect of abdominal pressure on chest wall compliance.

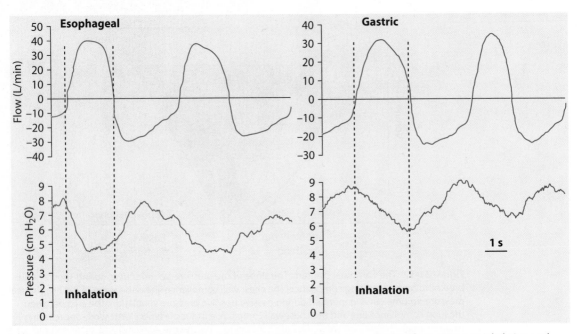

Figure 31-18 Esophageal (left) and gastric (right) pressures. Positive flow represents inhalation, and negative flow represents exhalation. Both esophageal and gastric pressures decrease during inhalation, consistent with diaphragmatic paralysis. (From Lecamwasam HS, Hess D, Brown R, et al. Diaphragmatic paralysis after endovascular stent grafting of a thoracoabdominal aortic aneurysm. *Anesthesiology.* 2005; Mar; 103(3):690-692.)

Lung Volume

EELV can be measured during mechanical ventilation using a nitrogen washout technique during a step change in F_{IO_2}. EELV is made with two measurements in a series of 20 breaths. The step change in F_{IO_2} to determine EELV is usually 0.1. Accuracy is best at F_{IO_2} of 0.4 to 0.65. Prior to the F_{IO_2} step change, the patient should be stable and the F_{IO_2} should be constant for at least 5 minutes. It might seem reasonable to measure EELV to evaluate the effect of PEEP titration, and thus, lung strain. However, PEEP-induced changes in EELV not only reflect recruitment or de-recruitment, but also the change can result from inflation or deflation of already open lung units.

Points to Remember

- Much qualitative information can be obtained by observing the airway pressure waveform.
- Failure of the expiratory flow to decrease to zero indicates the presence of auto-PEEP

- With a large leak from the lungs (around airway cuff or through a bronchopleural fistula), expiratory volume will be less than inspiratory volume.
- Flow-volume loops can be used to assess response to bronchodilators.
- The Pressure-volume curve can be used to assess appropriate PEEP setting and overdistention.
- Stress index can be used to assess tidal recruitment and overdistention.
- Esophageal pressure is used as a suffogate for pleural pressure.
- Esophageal pressure can be used to assess PEEP setting, patient work-of-breathing, auto-PEEP during spontaneous breathing, and chest wall compliance.
- Measurement of intra-abdominal pressure may be useful to assess transdiaphragmatic pressure and the effect of intra-abdominal pressure on chest wall compliance.

Additional Reading

Albaiceta GM, Blanch L, Lucangelo U. Static pressure-volume curves of the respiratory system: were they just a passing fad? *Curr Opin Crit Care*. 2008;14:80-86.

Benditt, JO. Esophageal and gastric pressure measurements. *Respir Care*. 2005;50:68-77.

Blanch L, López-Aguilar J, Villagrá A. Bedside evaluation of pressure-volume curves in patients with acute respiratory distress syndrome. *Curr Opin Crit Care*. 2007;13:332-337.

Branson RD, Johannigman JA. Innovations in mechanical ventilation. *Respir Care*. 2009;54: 933-947.

Dellamonica J, Lerolle N, Sargentini C, et al. PEEP-induced changes in lung volume in acute respiratory distress syndrome: two methods to estimate alveolar recruitment. *Intensive Care Med*. 2011;37:1595-1604.

Grasso S, Stripoli T, De Michele M, et al. ARDS net ventilatory protocol and alveolar hyperinflation: role of positive end-expiratory pressure. *Am J Respir Crit Care Med*. 2007;176:761-767.

Harris RS. Pressure-volume curves of the respiratory system. *Respir Care*. 2005;50:78-99.

Harris RS, Hess DR, Venegas JG. An objective analysis of the pressure-volume curve in the acute respiratory distress syndrome. *Am J Respir Crit Care Med*. 2000;161:432-439.

Hess DR. Approaches to conventional mechanical ventilation of the patient with acute respiratory distress syndrome. *Respir Care*. 2011;56:1555-1572.

Hess DR, Bigatello LM. The chest wall in acute lung injury/acute respiratory distress syndrome. *Curr Open Crit Care*. 2008;14:94-102.

Hickling KG. Best compliance during a decremental, but not incremental, positive end-expiratory pressure trial is related to open-lung positive end-expiratory pressure: a mathematical model of acute respiratory distress syndrome lungs. *Am J Respir Crit Care Med*. 2001;163:69-78.

Lecamwasam HS, Hess D, Brown R, Kwolek CJ, Bigatello LM. Diaphragmatic paralysis after endovascular stent grafting of a thoracoabdominal aortic aneurysm. *Anesthesiology*. 2005;102:690-692.

Loring SH, O'Donnell CR, Behazin N, et al. Esophageal pressures in acute lung injury: do they represent artifact or useful information about transpulmonary pressure, chest wall mechanics, and lung stress? *J Appl Physiol*. 2010;108:515-522.

Lu Q, Constantin JM, Nieszkowska A, et al. Measurement of alveolar derecruitment in patients with acute lung injury: computerized tomography versus pressure-volume curve. *Crit Care*. 2006;10:R95.

Lucangelo U, Bernabé F, Blanch L. Respiratory mechanics derived from signals in the ventilator circuit. *Respir Care.* 2005;50:55-67.

Olegard C, Sondergaard S, Houltz E, et al. Estimation of functional residual capacity at the bedside using standard monitoring equipment: a modified nitrogen washout/washin technique requiring a small change of the inspired oxygen fraction. *Anesth Analg.* 2005;101: 206-212.

Rouby JJ, Arbelot C, Brisson H, Lu Q, Bouhemad B. Measurement of alveolar recruitment at the bedside: the beginning of a new era in respiratory monitoring? *Respir Care.* 2013;58: 539-542.

Stenqvist O. Practical assessment of respiratory mechanics. *Br J Anesthesiol.* 2003;91:92-105.

Talmor D, Sarge T, Malhotra A, et al. Mechanical ventilation guided by esophageal pressure in acute lung injury. *New Engl J Med.* 2008;359:2095-2104.

Terragni PP, Filippini C, Slutsky AS, et al. Accuracy of plateau pressure and stress index to identify injurious ventilation in patients with acute respiratory distress syndrome. *Anesthesiology.* 2013;119:880-889.

Chapter 32
Nutritional Assessment

Introduction

Nutritional assessment and nutritional support are important considerations during mechanical ventilation (Figure 32-1). Assessment of nutritional status and determination of nutritional requirements for mechanically ventilated patients requires the teamwork of physicians, dietitians, respiratory therapists, and nurses. Too few calories cause respiratory muscle catabolism and muscle weakness. Too many calories—particularly carbohydrate calories—increase metabolic rate and can result in respiratory muscle fatigue or hypercapnia due to increased CO_2 production ($\dot{V}CO_2$).

Oxygen Consumption, Carbon Dioxide Production, and Energy Expenditure

The relationship between metabolism, oxygen consumption ($\dot{V}O_2$), and $\dot{V}CO_2$ is dependent on the substrate metabolized. $\dot{V}CO_2$ divided by $\dot{V}O_2$ is the respiratory quotient (R). R is 1 for carbohydrate metabolism, 0.7 for fat metabolism, 0.8 for protein metabolism, 8.7 for lipogenesis, and 0.25 for ketogenesis. Whole-body R is normally 0.7 to 1. With balanced metabolism, R is 0.8, carbohydrate metabolism raises it toward 1, and fat metabolism lowers it toward 0.7. With lipogenesis, the overall R may be greater than 1, but it seldom exceeds 1.2. With ketogenesis, the overall R may be less than 0.7 but is seldom less than 0.65.

The principal function of the cardiopulmonary system is to provide the O_2 needed for energy production and to clear the CO_2 produced. An increase in metabolic rate increases $\dot{V}O_2$ and $\dot{V}CO_2$, increases ventilation requirement, and forms the relationship between breathing ($\dot{V}O_2$ and $\dot{V}CO_2$) and nutrition expenditure (energy as Kcal). Excessive caloric intake, particularly with carbohydrates, results in increased $\dot{V}CO_2$.

Effects of Starvation

If mechanically ventilated patients receive inadequate nutritional support, they may suffer the effects of starvation. The initial response to starvation is an increase in glycogen and fat metabolism. Glycogenolysis provides glucose, which is necessary for

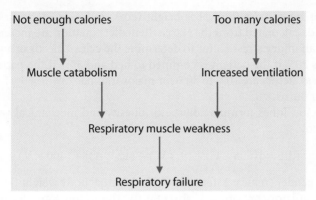

Figure 32-1 The relationship between nutrition and respiration. Either too few or too many calories can result in respiratory failure.

cerebral metabolism. Glycogen stores are depleted after 4 to 5 days of fasting. Lipolysis of adipose tissue triglycerides produces ketones, which can also be metabolized by brain cells. Gluconeogenesis also occurs, primarily due to the breakdown of muscle and visceral proteins. By the third day of fasting, ketogenesis and gluconeogenesis are at maximal rates. There is also a decrease in metabolic rate with starvation that slows the rate at which nutritional stores are depleted. There are numerous effects of starvation on respiratory function (Table 32-1), the most serious of which is loss of respiratory muscle mass due to catabolism.

Nutritional Assessment

From height and weight, the basal energy expenditure (BEE) can be estimated using the Harris-Benedict equation:

$$BEE = 66 + 13.7 \times W + 5 \times H - 6.8 \times A \text{ (males)}$$
$$BEE = 655 + 9.66 \times W + 1.8 \times H - 4.7 \times A \text{ (females)}$$

Table 32-1 Effects of Starvation on Respiratory Function

- Respiratory muscle function: catabolism of muscle protein results in weakening of respiratory muscles. This can result in respiratory muscle fatigue in spontaneously breathing patients and difficulty in weaning ventilated patients.
- Surfactant production: starvation results in decreased surfactant production, which decreases lung compliance and increased work-of-breathing.
- Respiratory drive: starvation results in a decreased respiratory response to hypoxia.
- Pulmonary defense mechanisms: starvation results in an impaired immune response. The cause of death from starvation is often pneumonia.
- Colloid osmotic pressure: starvation results in a decreased circulating albumin, which decreases colloid osmotic pressure, increases lung water, and contributes to pulmonary edema.
- Airway epithelium: malnutrition may contribute to laryngeal ulceration with prolonged intubation.

where W is body mass (kg), H is height (cm), and A is age (years). The total daily caloric needs calculated from the Harris-Benedict equation are increased by an activity factor and an injury stress factor to determine the caloric needs of a patient. The activity factor is 20% if the patient is confined to bed and 30% if the patient is ambulatory. Typical stress factors are 10% to 30% for major trauma, 25% to 60% for sepsis, and 50% to 110% for burns.

The Ireton-Jones formula adjusts for obesity and mechanical ventilation. For the obese patient:

$$REE = [(606 \times G) + (9 \times W) - (12 \times A)] + (400 \times V) + 1444$$

where G is gender (male = 1, female = 0), W is actual body weight (kg), A is age (years), and V is ventilator (present = 1, absent = 0). The Ireton-Jones formula for ventilated patients is:

$$REE = 1925 - (10 \times A) + (5 \times W) + (281 \times G) + (292 \times T) + (851 \times B)$$

where T is for trauma (present = 1, absent = 2) and B is for burn (present = 1; absent = 0). Energy needs may also be estimated with calories per kilogram of body weight (usually 25-35 kcal/kg) if other data are unavailable.

Biochemical data are also useful in the assessment of nutritional status (Table 32-2). Albumin levels correlate with the degree of malnutrition, and decreased levels are associated with increased risk of morbidity and mortality. Because its half-life is about 20 days, albumin levels reflect chronic rather than acute protein depletion. Albumin is not considered a specific indicator of visceral protein status in critically ill patients. Transferrin is a more sensitive indicator of acute changes in nutritional status than albumin because its half-life is about 8 to 10 days. Thyroxine-binding prealbumin (transthyretin) is a sensitive indicator of visceral protein status, especially in acute stages of protein-energy malnutrition. An advantage of prealbumin as an indicator of nutritional status is its short half-life (2-3 days). Retinol binding protein is highly sensitive to changes in nutritional status, with a 12-hour half-life. However, it has limited use as an assessment parameter in renal failure because it is filtered by the glomerulus and metabolized by the kidney. The total lymphocyte count is useful as a nutritional screening parameter with noncritically ill patients, and it correlates with albumin in reference to postsurgical mortality and morbidity.

Table 32-2 Normal Values for Biochemical Data Used in Nutritional Assessment

Measurement	Normal	Deficient
Albumin	3.5-5 g/dL	< 2.5 g/dL
Transferrin	200-400 mg/dL	< 100 mg/dL
Prealbumin	10-20 mg/dL	≤ 10 mg/dL
Retinol binding protein	3-6 µg/dL	≤ 3 µg/dL
Total lymphocyte count	2000-3500 cells/mm³	≤ 1200 cells/mm³
Nitrogen balance	Positive	Negative

Nitrogen balance determines the amount of nitrogen (protein) required to maintain nitrogen equilibrium and reflects anabolism/catabolism and distribution of protein. It is determined as:

$$\text{N balance} = \text{nitrogen intake} - \text{nitrogen output}$$
$$= \text{protein intake}/6.25 - (\text{UUN} + 4)$$

where UUN is the urine urea nitrogen. The determination of nitrogen balance requires an accurate 24-hour urine collection, an accurate assessment of protein intake, and a creatinine clearance greater than 50 mL/min. Nitrogen balance is normally positive and becomes negative with inadequate caloric and/or protein intake and metabolic stress.

Indirect Calorimetry

Indirect calorimetry is the calculation of energy expenditure by the measurement of $\dot{V}o_2$ and/or $\dot{V}co_2$, which are converted to energy expenditure (Kcal/day) by the Weir method:

$$\text{Energy expenditure} = \dot{V}o_2 \times 3.941 + \dot{V}co_2 \times 1.11 \times 1440$$

Indirect calorimetry also allows calculation of the R. Indirect calorimeters operate by using an open- or a closed-circuit method.

Open-Circuit Method

The open-circuit method measures the concentrations and volumes of inspired and expired gases to determine $\dot{V}o_2$ and $\dot{V}co_2$. The principal components of an open-circuit calorimeter (metabolic cart) are the analyzers (O_2 and CO_2), a volume-measuring device, and a mixing chamber. The analyzers must be capable of measuring small changes in gas concentrations, and the volume monitor must be capable of accurately measuring volumes from 0.05 to 1 L. Exhaled gas from the patient is directed into a mixing chamber. At the outlet of the mixing chamber, a vacuum pump aspirates a small sample of gas for measurement of O_2 and CO_2. After analysis, this sample is returned to the mixing chamber. The entire volume of gas then exits through a volume monitor. Periodically, the analyzer also measures the inspired oxygen concentration. A microprocessor performs the necessary calculations. Meticulous attention to detail is required to obtain valid results using an open-circuit indirect calorimeter (Table 32-3).

Table 32-3 **Important Points That Must be Observed With the Open-Circuit Technique**

- The F_{IO_2} must be stable (±0.005%). An air-oxygen blender is often used to prevent fluctuations caused by the instability of gas mixing systems in mechanical ventilators.
- The F_{IO_2} must be ≤ 0.60. Open-circuit calorimeters measure $\dot{V}o_2$ inaccurately at high F_{IO_2}.
- The entire system must be leak free. This creates a problem with uncuffed airways, bronchopleural fistula, and if a sidestream capnograph is in line. Errors may also be introduced if the patient is undergoing renal dialysis.
- Inspired and expired gases must be completely separated. This can be a problem with a continuous bias flow in the system.

Closed-Circuit Method

The key components of the closed circuit calorimeter are a volumetric spirometer, a mixing chamber, a CO_2 analyzer, and a CO_2 absorber. The spirometer is filled with a known volume of oxygen and connected to the patient. As the patient rebreathes from the spirometer, O_2 is removed and CO_2 is added. The CO_2 is removed from the system by a CO_2 absorber before the gas is returned to the spirometer. The decrease in the volume of the system equals $\dot{V}O_2$. Gas from the patient flows into the mixing chamber, and a sample is aspirated for $\bar{FE}CO_2$ analysis. From the mixing chamber, gas flows through a CO_2 absorber and then to the spirometer. The volume of the spirometer is electronically monitored to measure tidal volume. The difference between end-expiratory volumes is calculated by a microprocessor to determine $\dot{V}O_2$. If the patient is mechanically ventilated, a bag-in-the-box system is used as a part of the inspiratory limb of the calorimeter. The bellows is pressurized by the ventilator to ventilate the patient. Measurement time is limited by FIO_2 and the volume of the spirometer. When the volume of the spirometer decreases to a critical level, the measurement is interrupted to refill the spirometer.

Leaks from the closed-circuit system will result in erroneously high $\dot{V}O_2$ measurements (uncuffed airway, bronchopleural fistula, sidestream capnograph). Another problem with this technique is that system compressible volume is increased and trigger sensitivity is decreased. The advantage of the closed-circuit method over the open-circuit method is its ability to make measurements at a high FIO_2 (up to 1).

Other Approaches

In patients with a pulmonary artery catheter, $\dot{V}O_2$ can be calculated from arterial oxygen content (CaO_2), mixed venous oxygen content ($C\bar{v}O_2$), and cardiac output ($\dot{Q}c$):

$$\dot{V}O_2 = \dot{Q}c \times (CaO_2 - C\bar{v}O_2)$$

Metabolic rate can then be calculated from the $\dot{V}O_2$:

$$REE = \dot{V}O_2 \times 4.83 \times 1440$$

Metabolic rate can also be calculated from $\dot{V}CO_2$, which can be used in conjunction with volumetric capnography:

$$REE = \dot{V}CO_2 \times 5.52 \times 1440$$

Normal $\dot{V}O_2$ is 250 mL/min and normal $\dot{V}CO_2$ is 200 mL/min (2.6 mL/kg/min).

General Considerations with Indirect Calorimetry

Because indirect calorimetry is labor intensive and expensive, it should be reserved for selected patients (Table 32-4). When measuring resting energy expenditure (REE)

Table 32-4 **Indications for Indirect Calorimetry**

- Patients with several nutritional stress factors (trauma, sepsis, burns, etc)
- Patients who are difficult to wean from mechanical ventilation
- Pediatric patients in whom caloric requirements are uncertain
- Obese patients in whom caloric requirements are uncertain
- Malnourished patients in whom caloric requirements are uncertain
- Patients who fail to respond appropriately to nutritional support

using indirect calorimetry, one must consider both the duration of each measurement and the number of measurements required for a reliable 24-hour estimate. Ideally, continuous 24-hour indirect calorimetry produces the best estimate of REE. For most critically ill patients, it is impossible to obtain measurements for longer than 15 to 30 minutes once every several days. It is important, however, to recognize that shorter and less frequent measurements will less reliably estimate REE. When indirect calorimetry is performed, the patient should be resting, undisturbed, motionless, supine, and aware of the surroundings (unless comatose). The patient should either be on continuous nutritional support or fasting for several hours before the measurement. Before indirect calorimetry is performed, there should have been no changes in ventilation for at least 90 minutes, no changes that affect $\dot{V}o_2$ for at least 60 minutes, and stable hemodynamics for at least 2 hours. Because REE is measured with the patient at rest, calories must be added due to patient activity. There may be considerable fluctuation in REE throughout the day and from day to day.

Nutritional Support in Mechanically Ventilated Patients

Enteral nutrition should always be considered when a patient has a functioning gastrointestinal (GI) tract. Nutrients absorbed via the portal system with delivery to the liver may allow for better absorption and result in enhanced immune competence. The presence of nutrients in the gut prevents intestinal atrophy and maintains the absorptive capacity of the GI mucosa. Enteral nutrition also helps preserve normal gut flora and gastric pH, which may guard against bacterial overgrowth in the small intestine and development of pneumonia. If enteral nutrition is administered appropriately, it is safer and less expensive than parenteral nutrition.

The preferred method of nutritional support is the oral route. However, it is practically impossible for most mechanically ventilated patients. In the mechanically ventilated patient, nasogastric or orogastric tubes are often used initially. These are used for short-term feeding and may be contraindicated in patients who have severe reflux, delayed gastric emptying, and are at risk of aspiration. A feeding tube placed into the small intestine should be considered for uninterrupted duodenal or jejunal feeding. It is generally assumed that feeding distal to the stomach decreases the risk of aspiration. Because of the risk of aspiration with enteral feeding, patients should be placed into the semirecumbent position (head elevated 30 degrees). In patients receiving mechanical ventilation and early enteral nutrition, the absence of gastric volume monitoring has been shown not to be inferior to routine residual gastric volume monitoring in terms of development of ventilator-associated pneumonia. Even minimal amounts of enteral feedings, called trophic nutrition, may have beneficial effects such as preserving intestinal epithelium. A study by the ARDS Network reported no significant difference in clinical outcomes among patients with acute lung injury initially provided trophic versus full enteral feeding for the first 6 days of mechanical ventilation.

The more distal to the stomach the feeding is delivered, the less likely aspiration related to the feeding. Thus, the optimal postpyloric tube placement is past the ligament of Treitz, or in the fourth portion of the duodenum. A Dobhoff tube is a small-bore, flexible, nasogastric feeding tube that is inserted by use of a stylet and typically has a weighted end that helps guide it through the digestive system.

If long-term feeding is needed, tubes can be placed through the skin into the stomach or small intestine by surgical, endoscopic, radiologic, or laparoscopic techniques. The percutaneous endoscopic gastrostomy (PEG) tube is placed endoscopically. These tubes are generally more comfortable than the nasogastric or enteric tubes.

Parenteral nutrition, which bypasses the GI tract, may be necessary when the GI tract is not functioning or if stimulation of the GI or pancreatic systems would worsen the condition of the patient. Placement of a central or peripheral venous catheter is required for parenteral nutrition. Central venous access is usually preferred because solutions of greater than 600 to 900 mOsm/L may be infused, the volume of fluid is unrestricted, and support may continue for a long time. Parenteral nutrition leaves the GI tract unstimulated, which can lead to gut atrophy, mucosal compromise, weakening of the gut barrier, and increased risk of pneumonia. The results of a randomized controlled trial suggest the clinical usefulness of complementing the energy delivery of insufficient enteral nutrition with a parenteral booster between days 4 and 8 after intensive care unit (ICU) admission. This approach reduced the risk of development of nosocomial infections, the number of antibiotic days, and the duration of mechanical ventilation. However, this is in contrast to another randomized controlled trial, which reported no benefit for early parenteral nutrition.

The objectives of nutritional support in mechanically ventilated patients are to preserve lean body mass, maintain immune function, and avert metabolic complications. Early nutritional support using the enteral route is a proactive strategy that may reduce disease severity, diminish complications, decrease length of stay in the ICU, and improve survival. A variety of nutritional supplements are commercially available. However, omega-3 and antioxidant supplementation in mechanically ventilated patients has not been found to provide benefit in terms of important patient outcomes. Glycemic control is important, but current evidence does not support tight glucose control in terms of improved outcomes and is associated with a higher risk of hypoglycemia. Guidelines for nutritional support of the Society of Critical Care Medicine that applies to mechanically ventilated patients are listed in Table 32-5.

Table 32-5 Guidelines for Nutritional Support in the Mechanically Ventilated Patient

- Enteral feeding should be started within the first 24-48 h after admission.
- Enteral feeding is the preferred route of feeding over parenteral nutrition for critically ill patient.
- In critically ill patients, neither the presence nor the absence of bowel sounds and evidence of passage of flatus and stool is required for the initiation of enteral feeding.
- Either gastric or small bowel feeding is acceptable.
- Critically ill patients should be fed via an enteral access tube placed in the small bowel if at high risk for aspiration or after showing intolerance to gastric feeding.
- If unable to meet energy requirements after 7-10 days by the enteral route alone, consider initiating supplemental parenteral nutrition.
- In the critically ill obese patient, permissive underfeeding or hypocaloric feeding with enteral nutrition is recommended.
- The following measures have been shown to reduce risk of aspiration: the head of the bed should be elevated 30-45 degrees; continuous infusion of enteral feeding; use of agents to promote motility; postpyloric tube placement.
- Blue food coloring and glucose oxidase strips as surrogate markers for aspiration should not be used in the critical care setting.
- Specialty high-lipid low-carbohydrate formulations designed to manipulate the respiratory quotient and reduce $\dot{V}\text{co}_2$ are not recommended for routine use.

Points to Remember

- There is a relationship between metabolism (energy expenditure), $\dot{V}\text{o}_2$, and $\dot{V}\text{co}_2$.
- R is dependent on substrate metabolized.
- Too few calories can result in respiratory muscle fatigue due to muscle catabolism, and too many calories can result in respiratory muscle fatigue due to a high ventilatory requirement.
- Methods used for nutritional assessment include anthropometric data, Harris-Benedict equation, biochemical data, and indirect calorimetry.
- Indirect calorimetry is the calculation of energy expenditure based on measurements of $\dot{V}\text{o}_2$ and $\dot{V}\text{co}_2$.
- Indirect calorimetry can be performed using open- or closed-circuit devices.
- Caloric requirements can be determined with measurement of $\dot{V}\text{o}_2$ alone, $\dot{V}\text{co}_2$ alone, or both $\dot{V}\text{o}_2$ and $\dot{V}\text{co}_2$.
- The enteral route of nutritional support is preferable to the parenteral route.

Additional Reading

Casaer MP, Mesotten D, Hermans G, et al. Early versus late parenteral nutrition in critically ill adults. *N Engl J Med.* 2011;365:506-517.

Dummler R, Zittermann A, Schafer M, et al. Postoperative assessment of daily energy expenditure. Comparison of two methods. *Anaesthesist.* 2013;62:20-26.

Flancbaum L, Choban PS, Sambucco S, et al. Comparison of indirect calorimetry, the Fick method, and prediction equations in estimating the energy requirements of critically ill patients. *Am J Clin Nutr.* 1999;69:461-466.

Heidegger CP, Berger MM, Graf S, et al. Optimization of energy provision with supplemental parenteral nutrition in critically ill patients: a randomized controlled clinical trial. *Lancet.* 2013;381:385-393.

Heyland DK, Cahill N, Day AG. Optimal amount of calories for critically ill patients: depends on how you slice the cake! *Crit Care Med.* 2011;39:2619-2626.

Huang YC, Yen CE, Cheng CH, et al. Nutritional status of mechanically ventilated critically ill patients: comparison of different types of nutritional support. *Clin Nutr.* 2000;19:101-107.

Joosten KF. Why indirect calorimetry in critically ill patients: what do we want to measure? *Intensive Care Med.* 2001;27:1107-1109.

Martindale RG, McClave SA, Vanek VW, et al. Guidelines for the provision and assessment of nutrition support therapy in the adult critically ill patient: Society of Critical Care Medicine and American Society for Parenteral and Enteral Nutrition: Executive Summary. *Crit Care Med.* 2009;37:1757-1761.

McArthur CD. Prediction equations to determine caloric requirements in critically ill patients. *Respir Care.* 2009;54,453-454.

McClave SA, Martindale RG, Vanek VW, et al. Guidelines for the provision and assessment of nutrition support therapy in the adult critically ill patient. *J Parenter Enteral Nutr.* 2009;33:277-316.

Petros S, Engelmann L. Validity of an abbreviated indirect calorimetry protocol for measurement of resting energy expenditure in mechanically ventilated and spontaneously breathing critically ill patients. *Intensive Care Med.* 2001;27:1164-1168.

Pirat A, Tucker AM, Taylor KA, et al. Comparison of measured versus predicted energy requirements in critically ill cancer patients. *Respir Care.* 2009;54:487-494.

Reignier J, Mercier E, Le Gouge A, et al. Effect of not monitoring residual gastric volume on risk of ventilator-associated pneumonia in adults receiving mechanical ventilation and early enteral feeding: a randomized controlled trial. *JAMA.* 2013;309:249-256.

Rice TW, Wheeler AP, Thompson BT, et al. Enteral omega-3 fatty acid, gamma-linolenic acid, and antioxidant supplementation in acute lung injury. *JAMA.* 2011;306:1574-1581.

Schulman RC, Mechanick JI. Metabolic and nutrition support in the chronic critical illness syndrome. *Respir Care.* 2012;57:958-978.

The National Heart, Lung, and Blood Institute Acute Respiratory Distress Syndrome (ARDS) Clinical Trials Network. Initial Trophic vs Full Enteral Feeding in Patients With Acute Lung Injury. The EDEN Randomized Trial. *JAMA.* 2012;307:795-803.

Walker RN, Heuberger RA. Predictive equations for energy needs for the critically ill. *Respir Care.* 2009;54:509-521.

Part 4
Topics Related to Mechanical Ventilation

Chapter 33
Airway Management

Objectives

1. List indications for an artificial airway.
2. List complications of artificial airways.
3. Assess patients for extubation and decannulation.
4. Compare endotracheal intubation and tracheostomy.
5. Describe the use of a speaking valve.

Introduction

Although noninvasive ventilation is used increasingly, many mechanically ventilated patients are managed with an endotracheal tube or tracheostomy. Thus, an understanding of airway management is important for those providing mechanical ventilation.

Indications for an Artificial Airway

There are four traditional indications for an artificial airway:

1. Provide ventilatory support.
2. Aid in the removal of secretions.
3. Bypass upper airway obstruction.
4. Prevent aspiration.

Each of these is a relative indication. For example, ventilatory support and airway clearance can be provided noninvasively. Massive aspiration can be minimized by use of an artificial airway, although microaspiration commonly occurs in the presence of a cuffed artificial airway.

Orotracheal Versus Nasotracheal Intubation

Potential advantages of nasotracheal intubation include greater tolerance in the patient who is awake, easier oral hygiene, ease of intubation in the patient with cervical spine injury, and decreased likelihood of self-extubation. However, the disadvantages of nasal intubation outweigh these advantages. Because nasotracheal intubation requires a narrower and longer tube, it increases airway resistance, makes suctioning and bronchoscopy more difficult, and increases the likelihood of sinusitis and otitis media. Accordingly, oral intubation is usually recommended, and the oral route is used in most intubated patients.

Complications of Airways

A life-threatening complication of airway management is misplacement of the tube (Table 33-1). Although many patients who experience an unplanned extubation do not require reintubation, there is significant morbidity and mortality associated with the

---

Table 33-1 **Complications of Artificial Airways**

- Misplacement of the tube
  - Unplanned extubation
  - Esophageal intubation
  - Mainstem intubation
- Airway trauma
  - Laryngeal
  - Tracheal
- Cuff leaks
- Aspiration and pneumonia
- Loss of upper airway functions
- Increased resistance of breathing
- Decreased ability to clear secretions

---

need for reintubation. Efforts to avoid unplanned extubation include securing the tube (around-the-head techniques are preferred), physical and chemical restraint when necessary, and vigilance of airway position when the patient or ventilator tubing is moved. The endotracheal tube can be misplaced into the esophagus or mainstem bronchus (usually the right). Although this usually occurs at the time of intubation, it can occur after intubation. The tip of the endotracheal tube can move several centimeters as the result of flexion and extension of the neck—flexion moves the endotracheal tube tip caudad and extension moves it cephalad.

As a landmark, the centimeter marking on the tube at the lip or nares should be recorded when proper tube position is determined and this landmark should be checked frequently. For the newly intubated patient, the oral endotracheal tube should generally be inserted 21 cm at the teeth for females and 23 cm for males. Tube position should be assessed frequently by auscultation and on a regular basis by chest X-ray. A thorough evaluation of endotracheal tube position should be performed immediately following intubation (Table 33-2).

The presence of the endotracheal tube is traumatic to the airway. The larynx and tracheal wall are particularly prone to injury, which may not be recognized until after extubation. Laryngeal injuries include edema, vocal cord paralysis, glottic stenosis, and granulation formation. Tracheal injuries include tracheal stenosis, tracheomalacia, and fistula formation to the esophagus or innominate artery. Tracheal injuries are usually related to compression of the tracheal mucosa by the endotracheal tube cuff. Tracheal wall injury can be ameliorated by avoidance of cuff overdistension, which is facilitated by cuff pressures of less than 30 cm H_2O. On the other hand, the risk of silent aspiration is increased with cuff pressures less than 20 cm H_2O. Thus, cuff pressures should be monitored at regular intervals and should be maintained in the range of 20 to 30 cm H_2O.

Cuff leaks occasionally occur. This can be due to cuff rupture, accidental severing of the pilot tube, or malfunction of the pilot balloon valve mechanism. Inability to maintain cuff inflation usually results in failure to adequately ventilate the patient and necessitates reintubation. Changing the endotracheal tube in critically ill patients is facilitated by use of a semirigid tube exchanger. Commercial tube exchangers are hollow and allow oxygen insufflation.

Table 33-2 **Techniques to Evaluate Endotracheal Tube Position**

- Auscultation: auscultate chest and epigastrium to differentiate tracheal versus esophageal intubation; auscultate right and left chest to differentiate tracheal versus bronchial intubation.
- Inspection: bilateral chest expansion should occur with tube in the trachea; condensation of moisture on the inside of endotracheal tube should occur with tracheal intubation.
- CO_2 detection: absent or low (< 5 mm Hg) exhaled CO_2 indicates esophageal intubation; this can be performed using a low-cost CO_2 detector and does not require the use of an expensive capnograph.
- Bronchoscopy: this allows direct visualization of tube placement and can be used to properly place the tube during difficult intubations.
- Light wand (lighted stylet): when passed to the tip of the endotracheal tube, these devices produce transillumination of the suprasternal notch when the tube is in proper position.
- Esophageal detector device: this is a squeeze bulb device that rapidly reinflates when attached to the endotracheal tube that is in the trachea.
- Chest X-ray: the tip of the tube should be above the carina and at mid-trachea; at the level of the aortic arch.

Intubation bypasses the normal filtering function of the upper airway, allowing contaminated aerosols to enter the lower respiratory tract. Intubation also bypasses the ability of the upper airway to warm and humidify the inspired gas. Bypass of the glottis with an artificial airway may result in a decrease in functional residual capacity. Although a positive end-expiratory pressure (PEEP) of 3 to 5 cm H_2O may be useful to maintain functional residual capacity in intubated patients, there is no basis for the term "physiologic PEEP." Bypass of the upper airway may be problematic in the patient with chronic obstructive pulmonary disease (COPD) due to inability to control exhalation by use of pursed lips.

The flow resistance through an endotracheal tube is greater than that through the native airway. Some clinicians use a low level of pressure support or tube compensation during a spontaneous breathing trial to overcome the resistance through the endotracheal tube. However, with a usual adult-size endotracheal tube and a minute ventilation compatible with spontaneous breathing, the resistance of the endotracheal tube may not be clinically important. Because of airway edema, the resistance through the endotracheal tube may be similar to the resistance through the upper airway following extubation. Nonetheless, prolonged spontaneous breathing through a small endotracheal tube is not desirable and should be supported with pressure support or tube compensation.

Extubation

Evaluation for Extubation

In many patients, extubation occurs when ventilatory support is no longer necessary. However, some patients need an artificial airway even though ventilatory support is no longer required. These include patients with upper airway obstruction, those unable

Table 33-3 **Complications of Extubation**

- Hoarseness
- Laryngeal edema
- Laryngospasm
- Stridor
- Vocal cord paralysis
- Glottic stenosis
- Granulation formation

to adequately clear secretions, and those unable to protect the lower respiratory tract from aspiration. Patients with a weak cough are five times more likely to fail extubation, patients with a large quantity of secretions are three times more likely to fail extubation, and patients who are unable to complete four simple tasks (open eyes, follow with eyes, grasp hand, stick out tongue) are four times as likely to fail extubation. Patients with any two of these risks are nearly seven time more likely to fail extubation.

One concern before extubation is whether the upper airway is free of swelling and inflammation. This is often assessed as the amount of leak around the endotracheal tube during positive pressure ventilation with the cuff deflated (leak test). Although patients who develop upper airway obstruction after extubation may have a failed leak test, absence of a leak with the cuff deflated may also occur in many patients who are successfully extubated.

Complications of Extubation

Complications of extubation are listed in Table 33-3. Failed extubation occurs in 10% to 25% of patients. Noninvasive ventilation reduces the rate of reintubation in patients at risk for extubation failure. Hoarseness is common after extubation and is usually short term and benign. For postextubation stridor due to upper airway swelling, cool mist therapy, aerosolized racemic epinephrine, parenteral steroids, and heliox therapy can be used. These treatments are only useful, however, for acute reversible swelling that responds relatively quickly to therapy. For irreversible postextubation obstruction (eg, vocal cord paralysis), the patient must be reintubated and tracheostomy may be required.

Tracheostomy

Timing of Tracheostomy

There are both advantages and disadvantages of tracheostomy compared with translaryngeal intubation (Table 33-4). No clear evidence or consensus exists for when a tracheostomy should replace an endotracheal tube. Using percutaneous techniques, the modern tracheostomy procedure is a relatively simple bedside procedure. Although many patients tolerate endotracheal intubation for weeks without complications, prolonged intubation increases the risk of glottic injury. On the other hand, tracheostomy increases the risk of tracheal stenosis. Tracheostomy is usually reserved for patients requiring long-term ventilatory support and for those needing long-term airway protection (eg, patients with neurologic disease) or those with multiple failed attempts to extubate. Some failure-to-wean patients may be successfully liberated from mechanical ventilation after

Table 33-4 **Comparison of Advantages of Translaryngeal Intubation and Tracheostomy During Prolonged Ventilatory Support**

Translaryngeal intubation	Tracheostomy
Easy and rapid initial insertion	Ease of reinsertion if dislodged
Avoids surgical procedure	Reduced laryngeal injury
Lower cost of initial placement	Better secretion removal with suctioning
	Lower incidence of tube obstruction
	Less oral injury
	Improved patient comfort
	Better oral hygiene
	Improved ability to speak
	Preservation of glottic competence
	Better swallow allowing oral feeding
	Lower resistance to air flow
	Less tube dead space
	Lower work of spontaneous breathing
	More rapid weaning from mechanical ventilation

Modified with permission from Jaeger JM, Littlewood KA, Durbin CG. The role of tracheostomy in weaning from mechanical ventilation. *Respir Care.* 2002; Apr;47(4):469-480.

tracheostomy. This may relate to less resistance through the tracheostomy tube, less dead space, increased ability to remove secretions, and improved patient comfort.

Types of Tracheostomy Tubes

Tracheostomy tubes are available in a variety of sizes and styles from several manufacturers. The dimensions of tracheostomy tubes are given by their inner diameter, outer diameter, length, and curvature. Proper fit of the tube is an important consideration, as a poorly fitting tube can lead to distal obstruction in the trachea and the formation of granulation tissue. Tracheostomy tubes can be angled or curved to improve the fit of the tube in the trachea. Extra proximal length tubes facilitate placement in patients with large necks, and extra distal length tubes facilitate placement in patients with tracheal anomalies. Some tubes have a spiral wire reinforced flexible design, and some have an adjustable flange design to allow bedside adjustments to meet extra length tracheostomy tube needs. An inner cannula is used on some tracheostomy tube designs. The inner cannula can be removed for cleaning. Cuffs on tracheostomy tubes include high-volume low-pressure cuffs, tight-to-shaft cuffs, and foam cuffs. The fenestrated tracheostomy tube has an opening in the posterior portion of the tube, above the cuff, which allows the patient to breathe through the upper airway when the inner cannula is removed. Some tracheostomy tubes have a port above the cuff that allows subglottic aspiration of secretions.

Speaking With a Tracheostomy Tube

For mechanically ventilated patients with a tracheostomy, the cuff is deflated and the leak that results through the upper airway can be used to facilitate speech. Good-quality voice can result in many patients by using higher levels of PEEP (which increases leak during exhalation), a longer inspiratory time, and a higher tidal volume set on the ventilator to compensate for the volume lost due to leak. For many patients voice quality is adequate without the need for a speaking valve, improving safety if the upper airway becomes obstructed when a speaking valve is used.

A speaking valve allows the patient to inhale through the tracheostomy tube but exhale through the upper airway. A speaking valve is more commonly used when the patient no longer requires positive pressure ventilation. When a speaking valve is placed, it is important that the patient can adequately exhale through the upper airway. This can be assessed by measurement of tracheal pressure when the valve is placed. If the expiratory tracheal pressure is greater than 10 cm H_2O, the placement of a smaller tube or the presence of upper airway pathology should be considered.

For patients who do not tolerate cuff deflation, a speaking tracheostomy tube can be used. With this tube, gas flow is introduced above the cuff to provide flow past the vocal cords and, thus, allow speech. Cuff deflation, with or without a speaking valve, usually produces better voice than a speaking tracheostomy tube.

Decannulation

In patients no longer requiring mechanical ventilation, level of consciousness, cough effectiveness, secretions, and oxygenation are considered important determinants of decannulation readiness. A stepwise approach is usually followed. The patient is first observed for tolerance of cuff deflation, followed by tolerance of a speaking valve and tolerance of capping. If the patient tolerates a capped tracheostomy tube for 24 to 72 hours, strong consideration should be given to decannulation. Decannulation failure is commonly defined as the need to reinsert an artificial airway within 48 to 96 hours following planned tracheostomy removal.

Miscellaneous Airway Appliances

Alternative airway management equipment includes esophageal obturator airways, pharyngotracheal lumen airways, and esophageal-tracheal Combitubes. These devices, however, should not be used beyond the period of initial resuscitation. Another supraglottic airway is the laryngeal mask airway. It is inserted without a laryngoscope and has an inflatable rim that provides a low-pressure seal over the glottic opening. It is used for short-term ventilation when an intubated airway cannot be secured, and should be changed to an endotracheal tube as soon as possible. Video laryngoscopy can be used to accomplish endotracheal intubation. Video laryngoscopes are grouped into three different designs: stylets, guide channels, and video modifications of the traditional (usually Macintosh) laryngoscope blades.

Points to Remember

- The indications for an artificial airway are to provide ventilatory support, aid in the removal of secretions, bypass upper airway obstruction, and to prevent aspiration.
- Oral intubation is preferable to nasal intubation because a shorter tube is used, the oral endotracheal tube has a larger internal diameter, and kinking is less likely with the orotracheal tube.

- Complications of artificial airways include misplacement of the tube, trauma to the airway, cuff leaks, pneumonia, bypass of normal upper airway and glottic functions, decreased ability to clear secretions, and aspiration.
- Techniques to evaluate tracheal intubation include auscultation, inspection, CO_2 detection, bronchoscopy, and chest X-ray.
- Complications of extubation include hoarseness, stridor, laryngeal edema, laryngospasm, vocal cord paralysis, glottic stenosis, and granuloma formation.
- Many patients tolerate endotracheal intubation for several weeks with minimal complications.
- It is important that a tracheostomy tube is selected that fits well in the trachea.
- For mechanically ventilated patients with a tracheostomy tube, speech is facilitated by deflating the cuff and adjusting the ventilator to balance leak and ventilation.
- A speaking valve forces exhalation through the upper airway and thus allows the patient to speak.
- In patients no longer requiring mechanical ventilation, level of consciousness, cough effectiveness, secretions, and oxygenation are considered important determinants of decannulation readiness.
- Devices such as the laryngeal mask are never preferable to an endotracheal tube unless intubation is impossible.

Additional Reading

Bittner EA, Schmidt UH. The ventilator liberation process: update on technique, timing, and termination of tracheostomy. *Respir Care.* 2012;57:1626-1634.

Durbin CG. Early complications of tracheostomy. *Respir Care.* 2005;50:511-515.

Durbin CG. Indications for and timing of tracheostomy. *Respir Care.* 2005;50:483-487.

Durbin CG. Techniques for performing tracheostomy. *Respir Care.* 2005;50:488-496.

Durbin CG. Tracheostomy: why, when, and how? *Respir Care.* 2010;55:1056-1068.

Durbin CG, Perkins MP, Moores LK. Should tracheostomy be performed as early as 72 hours in patients requiring prolonged mechanical ventilation? *Respir Care.* 2010;5:76-87.

Epstein SK. Decision to extubate. *Intensive Care Med.* 2002; 28:535-546.

Epstein SK. Extubation. *Respir Care.* 2002; 47:483-495.

Epstein SK, Nevins ML, Chung J. Effect of unplanned extubation on outcome of mechanical ventilation. *Am J Respir Crit Care Med.* 2000; 161:1912-1916.

Fisher DF, Kondili D, Williams J, et al. Tracheostomy tube change before day 7 is associated with earlier use of speaking valve and earlier oral intake. *Respir Care.* 2013;58:257-263.

Hess DR. Facilitating speech in the patient with a tracheostomy. *Respir Care.* 2005;50:519-525.

Hess DR. Tracheostomy tubes and related appliances. *Respir Care.* 2005;50, 497-510.

Hoit JD, Banzett RB, Lohmeier HL, et al. Clinical ventilator adjustments that improve speech. *Chest.* 2003;124:1512-1521.

Hurford WE. The video revolution: a new view of laryngoscopy. *Respir Care.* 2010;55:1036-1045.

Jaeger JM, Littlewood KA, Durbin CG. The role of tracheostomy in weaning from mechanical ventilation. *Respir Care.* 2002; 47:469-482.

O'Connor HH, White AC. Tracheostomy decannulation. *Respir Care.* 2010;55:1076-1081.

Schmidt U, Hess D, Kwo J, et al. Tracheostomy tube malposition in patients admitted to a respiratory acute care unit following prolonged ventilation. *Chest.* 2008;134:288-294.

Stelfox HT, Crimi C, Berra, L, et al. Determinants of tracheostomy decannulation: an international survey. *Crit Care.* 2008;12:R26.

Stelfox HT, Hess DR, Schmidt UH. A North American survey of respiratory therapist and physician tracheostomy decannulation practices. *Respir Care.* 2009;54:1658-1664.

Terragni PP, Antonelli M, Fumagalli R, et al. Early vs late tracheotomy for prevention of pneumonia in mechanically ventilated adult ICU patients: a randomized controlled trial. *JAMA.* 2010;303(15):1483-1489.

White AC, Kher S, O'Connor HH. When to change a tracheostomy tube. *Respir Care.* 2010;55:1069-1075.

Young D, Harrison DA, Cuthbertson BH, Rowan K; TracMan Collaborators. Effect of early vs late tracheostomy placement on survival in patients receiving mechanical ventilation: the TracMan randomized trial. JAMA. 2013;309:2121-2129.

Chapter 34
Airway Clearance

> ### Objectives
>
> 1. Describe techniques for airway clearance in mechanically ventilated patients.
> 2. List complications of endotracheal suction.
> 3. List techniques to reduce suction-related complications in mechanically ventilated patients.
> 4. Describe the effects of lateral and prone positioning on oxygenation.

Introduction

Airway clearance is important in the care of mechanically ventilated patients. These therapies include suctioning, saline instillation, bronchoscopy, postural drainage therapy, and positioning. Failure to adequately attend to the bronchial hygiene needs of the patient can complicate the course of mechanical ventilation.

Airway Clearance

Airway clearance is impaired in intubated patients due to decreased mucociliary activity and inability to cough effectively. Mucociliary activity is impaired due to the presence of the artificial airway, airway trauma due to suctioning, inadequate humidification, high F_{IO_2}, drugs (eg, narcotics), and underlying pulmonary disease. Cough effectiveness is impaired due to the presence of the artificial airway and depressed neurologic status. Methods commonly used to improve secretion clearance in intubated patients include suctioning, postural drainage therapy with or without percussion and/or vibration, positioning, and bronchoscopy.

Hyperinflation Therapy

Hyperinflation of the lungs with a manual ventilator is a technique that has been used to facilitate secretion clearance in intubated patients. However, high level evidence is lacking that this technique improves secretion clearance. Moreover, it may increase the likelihood of lung injury and hemodynamic complications due to the high airway pressures that might be applied during hyperinflation therapy.

Suctioning

Although not a benign procedure, suctioning is an important aspect of airway care. Complications of endotracheal suctioning are listed in Table 34-1. Suction-related complications can often be avoided by use of appropriate technique (Table 34-2). Techniques to facilitate selective endobronchial suctioning (particularly of the left) include use of curved tip catheters, turning the patient's head to the side (eg, turning the head to the right to facilitate suctioning of the left bronchus), and lateral positioning. Of these, the use of a curved tip catheter is most successful.

Table 34-1 **Complications of Suctioning**

- Hypoxemia
- Atelectasis
- Airway trauma
- Contamination
- Cardiac arrhythmias
- Selective secretion clearance from the right bronchus
- Increased intracranial pressure
- Coughing and bronchospasm

The closed-suction system consists of a catheter within a protective sheath that fits between the ventilator circuit and the airway. The catheter thus becomes part of the ventilator circuit. The sheath protects the catheter from external contamination, and the patient is suctioned without removal from the ventilator. Closed suction prevents alveolar de-recruitment during suctioning and prevents contamination of clinicians during the suction procedure. Because the closed-suction catheter is used repeatedly and because it does not need to be changed at regular intervals, its use is also cost-effective.

Saline Instillation

In the past, saline was often instilled during suctioning to facilitate secretion removal. However, more saline is instilled than is removed during subsequent suctioning. This may increase the volume of secretions and may worsen airway obstruction. Care must be taken to avoid contamination of the airway during saline instillation. Saline instillation can also produce airway irritation, coughing, and bronchospasm. It may be useful for selected patients with tenacious secretions but should not be a routine procedure.

Mucus Shaver

The mucus shaver is a concentric inflatable catheter that is used for removal of mucus and secretions from the interior surface of the endotracheal tube. The mucus shaver is advanced to the distal endotracheal tube tip, inflated, and subsequently withdrawn. This device may be useful when accumulation of secretions in the airway is suspected (Figure 34-1).

Table 34-2 **Techniques to Avoid Suctioning-Related Complications**

- Hyperoxygenation with $F_{IO_2} = 1$
- Use closed-suction catheter
- Use proper catheter size
- Use least amount of vacuum necessary to evacuate secretions
- Use a gentle technique
- Limit the time of each suction attempt
- Suction only during withdrawal of the catheter

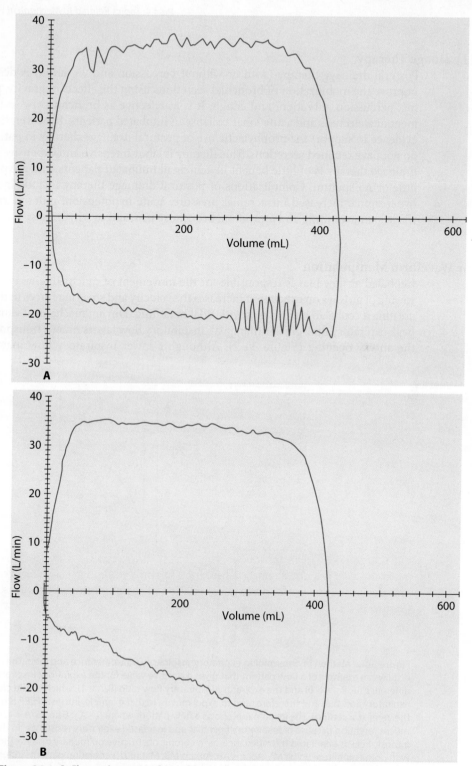

Figure 34-1 A. Flow-volume waveforms from a patient with significant obstruction of the endotracheal tube with secretions. **B.** Flow-volume waveforms immediately after use of the mucus shaver.

Postural Drainage Therapy

Postural drainage therapy (with or without percussion and vibration) is designed to improve the mobilization of bronchial secretions using the effects of gravity, positioning, percussion, vibration, and cough. It is as effective as bronchoscopy in the treatment of atelectasis and acute lobar collapse in intubated patients. However, there is no evidence to support the prophylactic use of postural drainage therapy in patients who do not have retained secretions. This therapy is labor intensive and expensive. Postural drainage therapy is of little benefit in acutely ill intubated patients who are producing little or no sputum. Complications of postural drainage therapy include hypoxemia, hypercapnia, increased intracranial pressure, acute hypotension, pulmonary hemorrhage, pain, vomiting and aspiration, bronchospasm, and dysrhythmias.

Ventilator Waveform Manipulation

Cephalad airflow bias is responsible for the movement of mucus in airways. The narrowing of airways on exhalation increases the velocity and shearing forces in the airway, creating a cephalad airflow bias with tidal breathing. During mechanical ventilation, a peak expiratory flow greater than peak inspiratory flow favors mucus transport toward the airway opening (Figure 34-2). Although a lower inspiratory flow may facilitate

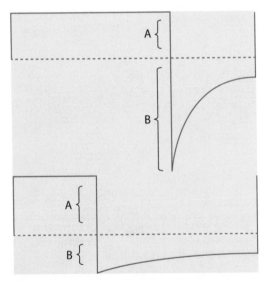

Figure 34-2 Method of determining expiratory-inspiratory flow difference and ratio. The upper panel displays an example of a flow pattern that gives a positive value for the expiratory-inspiratory flow difference (ie, B – A > 0) and the expiratory-inspiratory flow ratio (B/A > 1), which would create an expiratory flow bias and therefore tend to expel mucus. In that example, intrinsic PEEP is generated by the ventilator settings. The lower panel shows a flow pattern where B – A < 0 and B/A < 1, which favors mucus retention because of inspiratory flow bias and increased expiratory resistance. In that example, intrinsic PEEP is generated by impedance, as in chronic obstructive pulmonary disease. (Reproduced with permission from Volpe MS, Adams AB, Amato MB, Marini JJ. Ventilation patterns influence airway secretion movement. *Respir Care.* 2008; Oct;53(10):1287-1294.)

airway clearance, it has the potential to cause flow asynchrony or auto-positive end-expiratory pressure (auto-PEEP).

Cough Assist

The mechanical insufflation-exsufflator (MIE), also called the Cough Assist, is a device that inflates the lungs with positive pressure followed by a negative pressure to simulate a cough. Treatment consists of several cycles of MIE and is repeated as necessary until secretions are cleared. For each cycle, the inspiratory pressure is 25 to 35 cm H_2O for 1 to 2 seconds, followed by an expiratory pressure of -30 to -40 cm H_2O for 2 to 4 seconds. The MIE can be used with an oronasal mask or attached to an artificial airway. Combining manual abdominal thrusts with this technique can help increase expiratory flow expulsion of secretions. This procedure has been shown to be effective in patients with neuromuscular disease. In patients with bulbar disease who are not intubated, use of the MIE can be limited by upper airway closure during the active negative pressure expiratory phase.

Bronchoscopy

The most common indication for bronchoscopy in intubated patients is the diagnosis of ventilator-associated pneumonia using a protected specimen brush or bronchoalveolar lavage (BAL). Fiberoptic bronchoscopy may also be used to clear secretions in intubated patients (Table 34-3). However, it is invasive and should be reserved for cases in which atelectasis persists despite conservative methods (ie, cough assist and suctioning).

Nonbronchoscopic Bronchoalveolar Lavage

Mini-BAL is a nonbronchoscopic procedure for small-volume BAL to guide antibiotic therapy prescribed for patients suspected of ventilator-associated pneumonia. The catheter has a smaller diameter than a bronchoscope, so the risk of complications is minimized. Some mini-BAL catheters are directional, meaning that they can be

Table 34-3 Indications and Complications of Fiberoptic Bronchoscopy in Intubated Patients

Indications	Complications
• Obtain lower respiratory tract secretions for diagnosis of pneumonia	• Hypoxemia
• Clearing of secretions that are not adequately cleared by more conservative methods	• Hypercarbia
• Persistent atelectasis that fails to respond to conservative treatment	• Air-trapping with bronchoscope in airway (particularly with small endotracheal tube)
• Assess upper airway patency	• Bronchospasm
• Assess hemoptysis	• Contamination of lower respiratory tract
• Determine the location and extent of injury from toxic inhalation or aspiration	• Pneumothorax
• Perform difficult intubation	• Hemoptysis
• Remove aspirated foreign body	• Arrhythmias

theoretically directed into one lung or the other. However, the procedure is blind, so the user has no means of confirming the actual catheter location. Other mini-BAL catheters have a plugged tip to avoid upper airway contamination. A polyethylene-glycol tip protects the inner sampling catheter from contamination. Unlike bronchoscopy, the mini-BAL procedure is used only for diagnostic purposes; it cannot be used for therapeutic airway clearance.

Positioning

Physiologic Effects

With normal lung function, ventilation is greater in the dependent lung zones due to the pleural pressure gradient (pleural pressure is more negative at the bottom of the lungs) that places dependent alveoli on a more compliant part of the pressure-volume curve. This may not be the case with pathologic conditions such acute respiratory distress syndrome (ARDS), in which the injury and edema are often greatest in the dorsal lung regions. When these patients are turned from a supine to a prone position, there is often an improvement in oxygenation. This is related to the gravitational effects on blood flow and the pleural pressure gradient, resulting in an improvement in $\dot{V}/\dot{Q}$. This effect does not always occur, with about 25% of patients failing to respond. For some patients, the improvement in Pao_2 allows reduction in Fio_2 and PEEP. Prone positioning is technically difficult and care must be observed to avoid dislodgement of the airway and vascular lines. Beds to facilitate prone position are commercially available. Chest wall compliance may decrease in the prone position, resulting in an increase in airway pressure with volume ventilation or a decrease in tidal volume with pressure ventilation. Facial edema and anterior pressure sores also may occur when the patient is placed prone. The length of time that patients should remain in the prone position is unclear. Evidence suggests that prone positioning not only improves Pao_2, but it may improve survival in patients with severe ARDS. Prone position should be considered in patients with ARDS when the Pao_2/Fio_2 is less than 150 after an appropriate PEEP titration.

Lateral positioning can be useful in patients with unilateral lung disease. Positioning with the good lung down results in a higher Pao_2. Because gravity causes greater blood flow to dependent lung zones, positioning the good lung down presumably improves $\dot{V}/\dot{Q}$ by placing the more ventilated lung in the area of greatest blood flow. Positioning may be more effective than PEEP to improve Pao_2 in patients with unilateral lung disease. PEEP may adversely affect arterial oxygenation with unilateral lung disease because it shunts pulmonary blood flow away from the healthy lung to the diseased lung.

Kinetic Bed Therapy

Kinetic therapy is the use of a bed that automatically and continuously turns the patient from side to side. These beds have been shown to decrease the incidence of pneumonia but have not been shown to affect outcome and cost. Although these beds are popular in some hospitals, their impact on the management of mechanically ventilated patients remains unclear and may increase the cost of care.

Points to Remember

- Suctioning-related complications can usually be avoided by use of appropriate technique.
- Closed suction is preferable to open suction in mechanically ventilated patients.
- Saline instillation may be useful for selected patients but should not be a routine procedure.
- Postural drainage therapy is of little benefit in acutely ill patients who are producing little or no sputum.
- Manual hyperinflation therapy is of little benefit as a secretion clearance technique.
- Manipulation of the ventilator waveform such that expiratory flow exceeds inspiratory flow might facilitate cephalad movement of airway secretions.
- Indications for bronchoscopy in intubated patients are secretion clearance and the diagnosis of ventilator-associated pneumonia.
- Mini-BAL is a nonbronchoscopic procedure to guide antibiotic therapy prescribed for patients suspected of ventilator-associated pneumonia.
- The MIE is a device that inflates the lungs with positive pressure followed by a negative pressure to simulate a cough.
- When patients with ARDS are turned from a supine to a prone position, there is often an improvement in oxygenation.
- Prone position might improve survival in patients with severe ARDS.
- Lateral positioning with the good lung down is useful in patients with unilateral lung disease.
- Kinetic bed therapy has been shown to decrease the incidence of pneumonia but has not been shown to affect outcome and cost.

Additional Reading

AARC Clinical Practice Guidelines. Endotracheal suctioning of mechanically ventilated patients with artificial airways. *Respir Care.* 2010;55:758-764.

Berra L, Coppadoro A, Bittner EA, et al. A clinical assessment of the mucus shaver: a device to keep the endotracheal tube free from secretions. *Crit Care Med.* 2012;40:119-124.

Branson RD. Secretion management in the mechanically ventilated patient. *Respir Care.* 2007;52:1328-1347.

Cereda M, Villa F, Colonbo E, et al. Closed system suctioning maintains lung volume during volume-controlled mechanical ventilation. *Intensive Care Med.* 2001;27:648-654.

Gattinoni L, Carlesso E, Taccone P, et al. Prone positioning improves survival in severe ARDS: a pathophysiologic review and individual patient meta-analysis. *Minerva Anestesiol.* 2010;76:448-454.

Guérin C. Prone position. *Curr Opin Crit Care.* 2014;20:92-97.

Guérin C, Reignier J, Richard JC, et al. Prone positioning in severe acute respiratory distress syndrome. *N Engl J Med.* 2013;368:2159-2168.

Hess DR. Airway clearance: physiology, pharmacology, techniques, and practice. *Respir Care.* 2007;52:1392-1396.

Hess DR. Patient positioning and ventilator-associated pneumonia. *Respir Care.* 2005;50:892-898.

Hess DR. The evidence for secretion clearance techniques. *Respir Care.* 2001;46:1276-1292.

Li Bassi G, Saucedo L, Marti JD, et al. Effects of duty cycle and positive end-expiratory pressure on mucus clearance during mechanical ventilation. *Crit Care Med.* 2012;40:895-902.

Lorente L, Lecuona M, Jiménez A, et al. Tracheal suction by closed system without daily change versus open system. *Intensive Care Med.* 2006;32:538-544.

Maggiore SM, Iacobone E, Zito G, Antonelli M, Proietti R. Closed versus open suctioning techniques. *Minerva Anestesiol.* 2002;68:360-364.

Ntoumenopoulos G, Shannon H, Main E. Do commonly used ventilator settings for mechanically ventilated adults have the potential to embed secretions or promote clearance? *Respir Care.* 2011;56:1887-1892.

Paulus F, Binnekade JM, Vroom MB, Schultz MJ. Benefits and risks of manual hyperinflation in intubated and mechanically ventilated intensive care unit patients: a systematic review. *Crit Care.* 2012;16:R145.

Siempos II, Vardakas KZ, Falagas ME. Closed tracheal suction systems for prevention of ventilator-associated pneumonia. *Br J Anaesth.* 2008;100:299-306.

Strickland SL, Rubin BK, Drescher GS, et al. AARC clinical practice guideline: effectiveness of nonpharmacologic airway clearance therapies in hospitalized patients. *Respir Care.* 2013;58:2187-2193.

Volpe MS, Adams AB, Amato MB, Marini JJ. Ventilation patterns influence airway secretion movement. *Respir Care.* 2008;53:1287-1294.

Chapter 35
Inhaled Drug Delivery

Objectives

1. List drugs commonly administered by inhalation to mechanically ventilated patients.
2. Describe the use of inhaled nitric oxide (iNO), heliox, and volatile anesthetics during mechanical ventilation.
3. Compare the use of nebulizers and metered dose inhalers (MDIs) in mechanically ventilated patients.
4. Select an appropriate aerosol delivery device for use during mechanical ventilation.

Introduction

Oxygen and air are mixed to provide the prescribed F_{IO_2}. Rarely, nitric oxide, helium, or volatile anesthetics are added to the inspired gas. Aerosol medication can also be added to the inspired gas. This chapter covers aspects of inhaled gas and aerosol administration.

Inhaled Gases

Nitric Oxide

Inhaled nitric oxide (iNO) is a selective pulmonary vasodilator. As such, improved blood flow in ventilated lung units may occur, often resulting in improved ventilation-perfusion mismatch, better oxygenation, and lower pulmonary arterial pressure. In adults with acute respiratory distress syndrome (ARDS), iNO is associated with a transient improvement in oxygenation. However, no survival benefit or reduction in ventilator-free days has been reported with use of iNO for ARDS. With iNO, there is an increased risk of developing renal dysfunction. Although iNO may result in systemic methemoglobinemia or in generation of inhaled nitrogen dioxide, these effects are rare unless high doses are used. Oxygenation benefit typically occurs with an iNO dose of 20 ppm or less. Rebound hypoxemia can occur when iNO is discontinued. Despite the lack of evidence that iNO improves important outcomes, it is used as rescue therapy for refractory hypoxemia. The cost of iNO in the United States is very high and is not offset by third-party reimbursement or in cost savings from fewer days on the ventilator.

Heliox

Heliox is a mixture of helium (60%-80%) with oxygen (20%-40%). The use of heliox in severe asthma can improve gas exchange and decrease the work-of-breathing. Heliox has also been used with invasive and noninvasive ventilation (NIV) in patients with chronic obstructive pulmonary disease (COPD) exacerbation. The low density of helium reduces the pressure required for flow through a partially obstructed airway. Ideally, a gas mixture containing 80% helium is preferred, but improved clinical status may occur with as low as 40% helium. Heliox can be administered through some mechanical ventilators, but it adversely affects the function of others. High-level evidence is lacking to support improved outcome in patients with obstructive lung disease (eg, asthma and COPD). There is contradictory evidence related to the benefit of heliox to improve aerosol delivery; heliox may improve aerosol delivery, but it is unclear whether this improves patient outcomes. Heliox might be considered in patients who develop postextubation stridor, but there is concern that the heliox will mask the symptoms with progression to life-threatening airway obstruction.

Volatile Anesthetics

Inhaled anesthetic agents have been used to achieve improved gas exchange in patients with severe acute asthma. Inhaled anesthetics have bronchodilatory properties, which is the basis for their use in the setting. The anesthetic properties of these agents also provide sedation to facilitate synchrony. Halothane, enflurane, sevoflurane, or isoflurane have been used in adult patients with asthma refractory to traditional therapies. Isoflurane is most commonly used, primarily due to its safety profile relative to other agents. The use of inhaled anesthetics for the treatment of acute asthma is uncommon due to the need for experienced providers and appropriate equipment for the delivery and scavenging of volatile agents. Integration of ventilator technology and capabilities in modern anesthesia machines may allow for safer delivery of these agents in the intensive care unit (ICU). However, evidence is lacking that the use of these agents improves important outcomes such as mortality, ventilator days, or complications of mechanical ventilation.

Inhaled Aerosol Delivery

Therapeutic aerosols are often used in mechanically ventilated patients, most commonly to administer beta-agonist bronchodilators. However, beta-agonists should be avoided in ARDS, in which they have been shown to increase mortality. Other aerosols that might be administered during mechanical ventilation included anticholinergics, steroids, antibiotics, and prostacyclins. Therapeutic aerosols can be delivered using a nebulizer or MDI. A variety of factors affect aerosol delivery during mechanical ventilation (Table 35-1).

Nebulizer

With the traditional jet nebulizer, about 5% of the dose placed into the device is deposited in the lower respiratory tract. There are a number of disadvantages associated with jet nebulizer use during mechanical ventilation. Contamination of the lower respiratory tract can occur if the nebulizer is the source of bacterial aerosols. The continuous flow from the nebulizer may increase tidal volume during volume ventilation or pressure during pressure ventilation. Continuous flow from the nebulizer makes triggering more difficult and increases resistance of expiratory filters and pneumotachometers. Some of these disadvantages can be offset by using the nebulizer control of the ventilator, which powers the nebulizer only during inspiration and may compensate for the additional flow added by the nebulizer.

Table 35-1 **Important Technical Factors That Affect Aerosol Delivery During Mechanical Ventilation.**

Nebulizer

Type of nebulizer: much variability exists among jet nebulizers of different manufacturers; mesh nebulizer is generally superior to jet nebulizer.

Position in circuit: jet nebulizer should be at least 15 cm from the endotracheal tube; mesh nebulizer should be between ventilator and humidifier.

Breath actuation: dose delivery is increased when nebulizer is actuated only during inspiratory phase.

Flow and fill volume: for jet nebulizer, flow should be 6-8 L/min and fill volume 4-5 mL.

Duration of nebulization: greater dose is delivered with continuous nebulization.

Inspiratory time: greater dose is delivered with longer inspiratory time.

Metered dose inhaler (MDI)

Chamber device: dose delivery is greater with an inline chamber device.

Actuation: the MDI should be actuated at the onset of inspiration.

Nebulizer or MDI

Humidity: greater aerosol is delivered if inspired gas is not humidified, but this increases the risk of endotracheal tube occlusion.

Tube size: less aerosol dose is delivered with a smaller endotracheal tube or smaller tracheostomy tube.

Gas density: greater aerosol might be delivered with lower-density gas (eg, heliox).

Leak port: for noninvasive ventilation, greater dose is delivered with device between leak port and interface.

Dose: more drug is delivered with higher dose.

Patient factors: severity of obstruction, asynchrony.

The vibrating mesh nebulizer uses a mesh or plate with multiple apertures to produce an aerosol. They require electric power for operation of the control unit. These devices have a high drug output, and their residual volume is negligible. The mesh nebulizer overcomes some of the issues associated with the jet nebulizer because it adds no gas flow into the circuit and the device can remain in the circuit between treatments. The mesh nebulizer is placed between the ventilator and the humidifier (Figure 35-1). Aerosol delivery is more efficient with the mesh nebulizer compared to the jet nebulizer.

Continuous Aerosol Delivery

Continuous aerosols can be delivered into the ventilator circuit using a mesh nebulizer and syringe pump. Continuous aerosol bronchodilators are used for severe acute asthma. Continuous aerosol vasodilators (eg, prostacyclin) are used to improve oxygenation with refractory hypoxemia and to decrease pulmonary artery pressure with pulmonary hypertension.

Metered Dose Inhaler

Many of the complications of jet nebulizer during mechanical ventilation are avoided by use of a MDI. Pulmonary deposition from a MDI is similar to the jet nebulizer (5%).

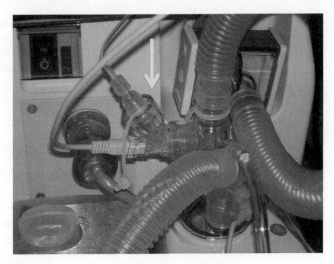

Figure 35-1 Mesh nebulizer position at inlet of heated humidifier.

Either MDI or nebulizer can be used effectively in mechanically ventilated patients. The MDI can be introduced into the ventilator circuit using an elbow adapter, inline adapter, or chamber adapter. However, for the same number of actuations, the greatest pulmonary deposition occurs with the chamber adapter. To maximize delivery, the MDI should be actuated at the beginning of inhalation. As with the nebulizer, the endotracheal tube is a formidable barrier to aerosol penetration. An issue with the newest generation of MDIs is their cost, which is high compared to that of a nebulizer.

Dosing

The usual dose from a nebulizer is about 10 times the dose with a MDI. Because the usual dose from the MDI is only a fraction of that with a nebulizer and the deposition from each is similar, more drug may be deposited in the lungs with the nebulizer—particularly with a mesh nebulizer. Thus, the mesh nebulizer may be more effective and convenient than MDI if high doses are required (eg, status asthmaticus). The dose of inhaled medications (nebulizer or MDI) may need to be increased in intubated patients due to the decreased pulmonary deposition secondary to the endotracheal tube.

Evaluation of Response

Response to an inhaled bronchodilator includes decreased peak airway pressure, plateau pressure, auto-PEEP, and resistive pressure (peak minus plateau pressure). More sophisticated measurements such as airway resistance and flow-volume loops may be useful in selected patients to evaluate bronchodilator response.

Aerosol Delivery During Noninvasive Ventilation

Aerosol therapy during noninvasive ventilation (NIV) can be delivered by MDI with a chamber spacer or nebulizer. A number of factors affect aerosol delivery during NIV.

These include the type of ventilator, mode of ventilation, circuit conditions, type of interface, type of aerosol generator, drug-related factors, breathing parameter, and patient-related factors. Despite the effects of continuous flow, high inspiratory flow, leaks, humidity, and asynchrony, significant therapeutic effects have been reported with inhaled bronchodilator administration during NIV. Careful attention to the technique is required to optimize therapeutic effects of inhaled therapies during NIV.

Points to Remember

- Inhaled pulmonary vasodilators improve oxygenation in some patients with ARDS, but their effect on mortality is unclear.
- Heliox may improve gas exchange and aerosol delivery in patients with obstructive lung disease, but it is unclear that it reduces ventilator days.
- Heliox can affect the performance of ventilators and other respiratory care equipment.
- Evidence is lacking that the use of volatile anesthetics in patients with asthma improves important outcomes.
- About 5% of the dose from jet nebulizer or MDI is deposited in the lungs of intubated patients.
- Aerosol delivery with mesh nebulizer is greater than that with a jet nebulizer.
- Either MDI or nebulizer can be used effectively in mechanically ventilated patients.
- Chamber adapters deliver a greater dose from a MDI than in-line or elbow devices.
- Response to inhaled bronchodilator therapy is assessed as a decrease in peak airway pressure, plateau pressure, and auto-positive end-expiratory pressure (auto-PEEP).
- Continuous aerosol therapy can be used to deliver bronchodilators or pulmonary vasodilators.
- Either nebulizer or MDI can be used to deliver aerosols during NIV.

Additional Reading

Adhikari NK, Burns KE, Friedrich JO, et al. Effect of nitric oxide on oxygenation and mortality in acute lung injury: systematic review and meta-analysis. *BMJ.* 2007;334:779.

Afshari A, Brok J, Møller AM, Wetterslev J. Aerosolized prostacyclin for acute lung injury (ALI) and acute respiratory distress syndrome (ARDS). *Cochrane Database Syst Rev.* 2010:CD007733.

Afshari A, Brok J, Møller AM, Wetterslev J. Inhaled nitric oxide for acute respiratory distress syndrome and acute lung injury in adults and children: a systematic review with meta-analysis and trial sequential analysis. *Anesth Analg.* 2011;112:1411-1421.

Ari A, Fink JB, Dhand R. Inhalation therapy in patients receiving mechanical ventilation: an update. *J Aerosol Med Pulm Drug Deliv.* 2012;25:319-332.

Char DS, Ibsen LM, Ramamoorthy C, Bratton SL. Volatile anesthetic rescue therapy in children with acute asthma: innovative but costly or just costly? *Pediatr Crit Care Med.* 2013;14:343-350.

Dhand R. Aerosol delivery during mechanical ventilation: from basic techniques to new devices. *J Aerosol Med Pulm Drug Deliv.* 2008;21:45-60.

Dhand R. Aerosol therapy in patients receiving noninvasive positive pressure ventilation. *J Aerosol Med Pulm Drug Deliv.* 2012;25:63-78.

Dhand R, Guntur VP. How best to deliver aerosol medications to mechanically ventilated patients. *Clin Chest Med.* 2008;29:277-296.

Dolovich MB, Ahrens RC, Hess DR, et al. Device selection and outcomes of aerosol therapy: evidence-based guidelines. *Chest.* 2005;127:335-371.

Gao Smith F, Perkins GD, Gates S, et al. Effect of intravenous β-2 agonist treatment on clinical outcomes in acute respiratory distress syndrome (BALTI-2): a multicentre, randomised controlled trial. *Lancet.* 2012;379:229-235.

Hess DR. Aerosol delivery during mechanical ventilation. *Minerva Anestesiol.* 2002;68:321-325.

Hess DR. Heliox and noninvasive positive-pressure ventilation: a role for heliox in exacerbations of chronic obstructive pulmonary disease? *Respir Care.* 2006;51:640-650.

Hess DR. Nebulizers: principles and performance. *Respir Care.* 2000;45:609-622.

Hess DR. The mask for noninvasive ventilation: principles of design and effects on aerosol delivery. *J Aerosol Med.* 2007;20(Suppl 1):S85-S99.

Hess DR, Fink JB, Venkataraman ST, et al. The history and physics of heliox. *Respir Care.* 2006;51:608-612.

Matthay MA, Brower RG, Carson S, et al. Randomized, placebo-controlled clinical trial of an aerosolized β_2-agonist for treatment of acute lung injury. *Am J Respir Crit Care Med.* 2011;184:561-568.

Vaschetto R, Bellotti E, Turucz E, et al. Inhalational anesthetics in acute severe asthma. *Curr Drug Targets.* 2009;10:826-832.

Venkataraman ST. Heliox during mechanical ventilation. *Respir Care.* 2006;51:632-639.

Chapter 36
Emergency Ventilation and Ventilation in a Disaster

> ### Objectives
>
> 1. Compare techniques for exhaled gas ventilation.
> 2. Compare self-inflating and flow-inflating manual ventilators.
> 3. Discuss issues related to mechanical ventilation and disaster preparedness.
> 4. Describe ventilators that can be used for mass casualty respiratory failure (MCRF).

Introduction

Techniques available for emergency ventilation include exhaled gas ventilation techniques, manual ventilation devices, and oxygen-powered demand valves. Some of these methods (eg, exhaled-gas techniques) may be used by nonprofessional laypersons. Others (eg, manual ventilators) are used during emergency ventilation (eg, cardiopulmonary resuscitation). In recent years, concern has been raised regarding ventilation in the setting of a disaster.

Exhaled Gas Ventilation Techniques

Mouth-to-Mouth Ventilation

Advantages of mouth-to-mouth ventilation are ease-of-use, availability, universal application, no equipment requirement, and a large reservoir volume (the delivered volume is limited only by the rescuer's vital capacity). However, there are important problems related to mouth-to-mouth ventilation. Gastric insufflation occurs with the high pharyngeal pressures associated with high airway resistance (eg, obstructed airway), low lung compliance, short inspiratory times (which produce high inspiratory flows), and rapid respiratory rates (which does not allow adequate time for lung deflation between breaths and the development of auto-PEEP). With mouth-to-mouth ventilation, the delivered oxygen concentration is about 16% and the delivered carbon dioxide concentration is about 5%. A major concern related to the use of mouth-to-mouth ventilation is the potential for disease transmission. It is therefore prudent to use a protective barrier device during emergency ventilation. Mouth-to-mouth ventilation is discouraged, and alternative ventilation devices (eg, bag-valve-mask) should be used whenever possible.

Face Shield Barrier Devices

Face shield devices use a flexible plastic sheet that contains a valve and/or filter to separate the rescuer from the patient. These devices make the task of exhaled gas ventilation more pleasant for the rescuer. Their ability to prevent disease transmission is unclear. Many of the limitations of mouth-to-mouth ventilation (eg, difficulty using the device effectively, gastric insufflation, low inspired oxygen) also apply to these devices.

Mouth-to-Mask Ventilation

These devices provide a barrier between the rescuer and the patient to prevent infectious disease transmission during emergency ventilation. The mask should provide an adequate seal using an air-filled resilient cuff on the mask and should have a port for administration of supplemental oxygen. It should be constructed of a transparent material to allow visual detection of regurgitation. A one-way valve or filter should be attached to the mask to protect the rescuer from contamination with the patient's exhaled gas or vomitus. An extension tube may also be used as an additional barrier between the rescuer and the patient, and the exhaled gas of the patient should be vented away from the rescuer. The valve or filter should not jam in the presence of vomitus or humidity, and it should have minimal airflow resistance. The dead space of the mask should be as small as possible.

It is important that correct technique is used to hold the mask. The rescuer should be positioned at the head of the patient. The mask is placed over the patient's nose and mouth and held with the rescuer's thumbs. The first fingers of each hand are placed under the patient's mandible, and the mandible is lifted as the head is tilted back. The mask is sealed with the rescuer's thumbs. An alternative method is to hold the mask with the thumb and the first finger of each hand, using the other fingers to lift the mandible and hyperextend the head. With either method, both of the rescuer's hands are used to hold the mask and open the patient's airway. For patients with cervical spine injury, the mandible should be lifted without tilting the head.

Manual Ventilation Techniques

Self-Inflating Manual Ventilators

Manual ventilators are commonly used during resuscitation and during patient transport. Because they are self-inflating, they do not require a supplemental flow of oxygen to inflate the bag. These devices can be used with a mask or attached directly to an endotracheal or tracheostomy tube. Four critical performance criteria for manual bag-valve ventilation devices are ventilation capability (rate and tidal volume), oxygen delivery, valve performance, and durability.

The bag-valve manual ventilator consists of a self-inflating bag, an oxygen reservoir, and a non-rebreathing valve (Figure 36-1). The bag is squeezed by the operator to ventilate the patient. The bag volume varies among manufacturers and ranges from about 1 to 2 L. One-way valves are used to produce unidirectional flow from the bag, thus drawing gas into the bag when it inflates, directing gas out of the bag to the patient when it is compressed, and preventing rebreathing of exhaled gas.

The bag-valve ventilator allows the operator to feel changes in impedance such as might occur with changes in airways resistance or lung compliance. The non-rebreathing

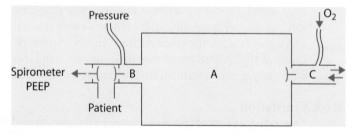

Figure 36-1 Schematic illustration of a bag-valve ventilator. **A.** Self-inflating bag. **B.** Non-rebreathing valve. **C.** Oxygen reservoir.

valve should have a low resistance, it should not jam with high oxygen flows, its dead space should be as low as possible, and there should be no forward or backward leak through the valve. It should be possible to attach a pressure manometer to monitor airway pressure and the exhalation port should allow attachment of a spirometer and/or PEEP valve. If the patient breathes spontaneously, the exhalation valve should close so that the patient breathes oxygen from the bag. However, allowing spontaneous breathing through the bag-valve ventilator is discouraged due to the high work imposed by the valve resistance. The patient connection should have a standard adapter (15 mm inside diameter and 22 mm outside diameter) to attach to a mask or artificial airway.

Bag-valve-mask ventilation requires proper technique (Figure 36-2). It is important to recognize that the entire volume of the bag is not delivered to the patient when the bag is compressed. A number of factors affect volume delivery from a manual bag-valve ventilator (Table 36-1). It can be difficult for a single person to deliver an appropriate tidal volume with a bag-valve mask. This is due to the inability to maintain an adequate mask seal and an open airway using one hand, while squeezing an adequate volume from the bag with the other hand.

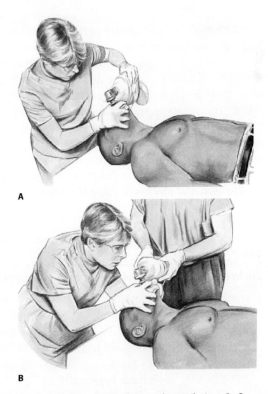

A

B

Figure 36-2 Technique used to perform bag-valve mask ventilation. **A.** One-person technique. **B.** Two-person technique. (Reproduced with permission form American Heart Association: Guidelines 2000 for Cardiopulmonary Resuscitation and Emergency Cardiovascular Care. Part 3: adult basic life support. The American Heart Association in collaboration with the International Liaison Committee on Resuscitation, Circulation 2000; Aug 22;102[8 Suppl]:I22-I59.)

Table 36-1 **Factors Affecting the Tidal Volume Delivered by Bag-Valve Manual Ventilators**

Factor	Comments
Mask vs endotracheal tube	Volumes delivered during bag-valve-mask ventilation are often inadequate; gastric insufflation possible with bag-valve mask
One hand vs two hands	Higher volumes delivered with two hands than with one hand squeezing the bag
Hand size	Higher volumes can be delivered by persons with larger hands
Lung impedance	Delivered volumes decrease with an increase in airway resistance and a decrease in lung compliance
Resuscitator brand	Differences exist for delivered volumes among commercially available devices
Fatigue	Delivered volumes may decrease during prolonged bag-valve ventilation
Gloves	Wearing medical gloves does *not* affect delivered tidal volume delivery

Although not commonly performed, monitoring of exhaled tidal volumes during bag-valve ventilation may be desirable. Monitoring of airway pressure during manual ventilation is also important if the patient is at risk of air leak (eg, post-thoracotomy). A variety of factors affect the delivered oxygen concentrations from bag-valve ventilators (Table 36-2). A delivered oxygen concentration of nearly 100% should be available during resuscitation, suctioning, patient transport, and special procedures.

Gastric insufflation can be a significant problem during bag-valve-mask ventilation. Gastric insufflation increases with an increase in ventilation pressure, as may occur with low lung compliance. The risk of gastric insufflation is decreased by use of a slower inspiratory flow. The Sellick maneuver (firm pressure against the cricoid cartilage) can be used, but its effectiveness is unclear.

Table 36-2 **Factors Affecting Oxygen Concentration Delivered From Manual Bag-Valve Ventilators**

Factor	Comments
Oxygen flow	A low oxygen flow decreases delivered oxygen concentration; flows of 15 L/min should be used with adult bag-valve ventilators
Oxygen reservoir	A smaller reservoir volume decreases the delivered oxygen concentration; ideally, the reservoir volume should exceed the volume of the device
Oxygen supply valve	An oxygen supply valve will allow the delivery of 100% oxygen but may impede bag reinflation
Bag recoil time	A slower bag recoil time will increase the delivered oxygen concentration
Resuscitator brand	Differences in delivered oxygen concentration exist between commercially available devices

A manual ventilator should be at the bedside of all mechanically ventilated patients so that it can be used in the event of a ventilator failure. Bedside manual ventilators can be a source of bacterial contamination. Care should be taken to avoid contamination of these devices, and they should be replaced if they become grossly contaminated.

Flow-Inflating Manual Ventilators

Flow-inflating bags are not commonly used in adult critical care. They are continuous-flow, semi-open, breathing systems that lack a non-rebreathing valve. The circuit consists of a thin-walled anesthesia bag, an endotracheal tube or mask connector, an oxygen flow, and a bleed-off at the tail of the bag. Inflation of the bag is controlled by the oxygen flow and the bleed-off. The oxygen flow and bleed-off also control the pressure in the bag. Thus, the bag can be used to provide PEEP as well as ventilation, and it can be fitted with a manometer and a pressure pop-off. Because the patient exhales into the bag, the oxygen flow must be high enough to prevent CO_2 accumulation. The bleed-off from the bag can produce significant expiratory resistance. Disadvantages of this system are that a source of compressed gas is required, and this system is more difficult to use than a self-inflating bag-valve resuscitator.

Oxygen-Powered Demand Valves

Although not commonly used in the hospital, oxygen-powered demand valves are used by emergency care personnel in the field. These devices are powered by a pressurized gas source and cannot be used in the absence of this gas source. These devices deliver 100% oxygen when the device is triggered by the operator (resuscitator function) or when triggered by the patient (demand-valve function). They can be used with a face-mask or with an artificial airway. They do not provide the operator with a sense of lung impedance. Use of these devices is discouraged due to their likelihood of producing overventilation and gastric insufflation.

Mechanical Ventilation in a Disaster

Natural disasters, the threat of terrorism, and concerns regarding severe febrile respiratory illness brought attention to the requirements for mass casualty mechanical ventilation. Mechanical ventilation in a mass casualty scenario requires a substantial increase in the capacity for mechanical ventilation to prevent unnecessary mortality. Ventilators may be needed for mass casualty care for movement of patients from the scene of an accident, for movement of patients between facilities, and for in-patient care of critically ill and injured patients.

Ventilators for Mass Casualty Respiratory Failure

Desirable characteristics of a ventilator for mass casualty respiratory failure (MCRF) are listed in Table 36-3. Automatic resuscitators, pneumatically or electrically powered portable ventilators, critical care ventilators, and ventilators designed for noninvasive ventilation (NIV) can be used in the setting of MCRF.

Table 36-3 Performance Characteristics of Ventilators for Mass Casualty Respiratory Failure

Characteristic	Rationale	Capabilities	
		Mandatory	Desirable
FDA-approved for adults and pediatric patients	Natural disasters, pandemics, and chemical/bioterrorism will also affect children	Ventilate 10-kg patient	Ventilate 5-kg patient
Ability to operate without 50-psig compressed gas	The redundancy for electrical power in hospitals far exceeds oxygen stores and redundancy.	Operate without 50-psig input	Operate from a 50-psig gas source or alternating-current power, whichever is available
	In the absence of high-pressure oxygen, low-flow oxygen from a flow meter can be used to increase F_{IO_2}.	F_{IO_2} from 0.21 to 1.0	
Battery life ≥ 4 h	Allow for transport from facility to facility. Provide continuous support during intermittent power failure	4 h of operation at nominal settings	> 4 h operation at nominal settings
Constant volume delivery	Meet guidelines for V_T delivery, as dictated by the ARDS Network protocol Reduce potential for ventilator-induced lung injury Provide age-appropriate setting	Volume control ventilation (250–750 mL)	Pressure control and volume control ventilation
Mode: CMV	Meet ARDS Network guidelines Ensure minimum ventilation in a situation of multiple patients and a shortage of caregivers	CMV	CMV, IMV, and pressure support
PEEP	Meet ARDS Network guidelines Prevent ventilator-induced lung injury Reverse hypoxemia	Adjustable: 5–15 cm H_2O	Adjustable: 5–20 cm H_2O
Separate controls for respiratory rate and V_T	Meet ARDS Network guidelines Ensure minute ventilation in apneic patients	Respiratory rate 6–35 breaths/min	Respiratory rate 6–75 breaths/min (for pediatric patients)
Monitor airway pressure and V_T	Meet ARDS Network guidelines Provide assessment of patient's lung compliance Patient safety: prevent overdistention	Monitor peak inspiratory pressure and delivered V_T	Monitor plateau pressure and patient V_T
Appropriate alarm	Patient safety Improve ability to monitor large numbers of patients with reduced staff	Alarms for: Circuit disconnect High airway pressure Low airway pressure (leak) Loss of electrical power Loss of high-pressure source gas	Alarms for: High V_T in pressure modes Low minute ventilation Remote alarms

Reproduced with permission from Branson RD, Johannigman JA, Daugherty EL, Rubinson L. Surge capacity mechanical ventilation. *Respir Care.* 2008; Jan;53(1):78-88.

ARDS = acute respiratory distress syndrome
CMV = continuous mandatory ventilation
FDA = Food and Drug Administration
F_{IO_2} = fraction of inspired oxygen
IMV = intermittent mandatory ventilation
PEEP = positive end-expiratory pressure

An automatic resuscitator is designed to replace manual ventilators. These devices are pneumatically powered and pressure-cycled. They have few to no alarms, cannot provide a constant tidal volume (V_T), do not allow setting of rate and tidal volume separately, and commonly provide 100% oxygen or a lower concentration with the use of an air-entrainment mechanism. Sophisticated pneumatically powered portable ventilators have the ability to provide continuous mandatory ventilation with PEEP, and allow separate control of V_T and respiratory rate. Electrically powered portable ventilators are most often used in the home and for in-hospital transport. Critical care ventilators are capable of managing all types of respiratory failure but are not recommended for MCRF due to their large size, high cost, and complexity.

The use of NIV in MCRF is controversial. Many patients with MCRF may have acute respiratory distress syndrome (ARDS), and the role of NIV in ARDS is limited; NIV is not recommended for severe ARDS. There is also concern that NIV is an aerosol-producing procedure that possibly increases the risk of caregiver exposure. Some ventilators designed primarily for NIV are also approved for invasive mechanical ventilation.

A concern is the availability of sufficient numbers of ventilators in the setting of a disaster. Possible sources of additional ventilators in a MCRF scenario are shown in Table 36-4. Every community should have a plan in place so that a sufficient number of ventilators are available should a local disaster occur.

Table 36-4 Possible Sources of Additional Ventilators in a Mass Casualty Respiratory Failure Scenario

Source	Strategy	Possible Problems
Affected hospital	Cancel elective surgeries Repurpose anesthesia workstations as mechanical ventilators and intensive care unit monitoring (during nontrauma disasters)	Number of anesthesia machines is limited. If the duration of mechanical ventilation is prolonged, anesthesia machines will be needed when surgeries and other procedures are re-initiated.
Unaffected hospital	Redistribute available equipment from unaffected hospitals to those in need	There are few extra available ventilators at most hospitals, even during usual conditions. Delayed situation awareness may reduce willingness of unaffected hospitals to share equipment.
Mechanical ventilator rental services	Obtain additional ventilators from a rental company	The same company may have contracts with a number of affected hospitals, so the total number of additional ventilators may be limited. Logistical delays may be encountered when sending ventilators from distant geographic areas.
Strategic National Stockpile	Deploy mechanical ventilators to states or cities in need	Delay in distribution because most states still have limited capacity to distribute equipment from the Strategic National Stockpile Unclear how distribution will be prioritized when multiple hospitals request ventilators at the same time

Reproduced with permission from Branson RD, Johannigman JA, Daugherty EL, Rubinson L. Surge capacity mechanical ventilation. *Respir Care*. 2008; Jan;53(1):78-88.

> ### Points to Remember
>
> - Limitations of mouth-to-mouth ventilation are its potential for disease transmission, improper performance, delivery of a low oxygen concentration, and its common association with gastric insufflation.
> - Mouth-to-mask devices provide a barrier between the rescuer and the patient.
> - Self-inflating bag-valve ventilators are capable of delivering high oxygen concentrations.
> - Because of the valve resistance, patients should not be allowed to spontaneously breathe from a bag-valve ventilator.
> - Flow-inflating manual ventilators are more difficult to use than self-inflating devices.
> - Automatic resuscitators, pneumatically or electrically powered portable ventilators, critical care ventilators, and ventilators designed for NIV can be used in the setting of MCRF.
> - Every community should have a plan in place so that a sufficient number of ventilators are available should a local disaster occur.

Additional Reading

Adelborg K, Dalgas C, Grove EL, et al. Mouth-to-mouth ventilation is superior to mouth-to-pocket mask and bag-valve-mask ventilation during lifeguard CPR: a randomized study. *Resuscitation.* 2011;82:618-622.

AriñoIrujo JJ, Velasco JM, Moral P, et al. Delivered oxygen fraction during simulated cardiopulmonary resuscitation depending on the kind of resuscitation bag and oxygen flow. *Eur J Emerg Med.* 2012;19:359-362.

Barnes TA, Catino ME, Burns EC, et al. Comparison of an oxygen-powered flow-limited resuscitator to manual ventilation with an adult 1,000-mL self-inflating bag. *Respir Care.* 2005;50:1445-1450.

Bergrath S, Rossaint R, Biermann H, et al. Comparison of manually triggered ventilation and bag-valve-mask ventilation during cardiopulmonary resuscitation in a manikin model. *Resuscitation.* 2012;83:488-493.

Blakeman TC, Rodriquez D, Dorlac WC, et al. Performance of portable ventilators for mass-casualty care. *Prehosp Disaster Med.* 2011;26:330-334.

Branson RD, Johannigman JA, Daugherty EL, Rubinson L. Surge capacity mechanical ventilation. *Respir Care.* 2008;53:78-88.

Branson RD, Rubinson L. Mechanical ventilation in mass casualty scenarios. *Respir Care.* 2008;53:38-39.

Carter BG, Fairbank B, Tibballs J, et al. Oxygen delivery using self-inflating resuscitation bags. *Pediatr Crit Care Med.* 2005;6:125-128.

Godoy AC, Vieira RJ, De Capitani EM. Alterations in peak inspiratory pressure and tidal volume delivered by manually operated self-inflating resuscitation bags as a function of the oxygen supply rate. *J Bras Pneumol.* 2008;34:817-821.

Neumar RW, Otto CW, Link MS, et al. Part 8: Adult Advanced Cardiovascular Life Support: 2010 American Heart Association Guidelines for Cardiopulmonary Resuscitation and Emergency Cardiovascular Care. *Circulation.* 2010;122:S729-S767.

Rabus FC, Luebbers HT, Graetz KW, Mutzbauer TS. Comparison of different flow-reducing bag-valve ventilation devices regarding respiratory mechanics and gastric inflation in an unprotected airway model. *Resuscitation.* 2008;78:224-229.

Rubinson L, Hick JL, Curtis JR, et al. Definitive care for the critically ill during a disaster: medical resources for surge capacity: from a Task Force for Mass Critical Care summit meeting, January 26-27, 2007, Chicago, IL. *Chest.* 2008;133:32S-50S.

Schumacher J, Weidelt L, Gray SA, Brinker A. Evaluation of bag-valve-mask ventilation by paramedics in simulated chemical, biological, radiological, or nuclear environments. *Prehosp Disaster Med.* 2009;24:398-401.

Von Goedecke A, Wagner-Berger HG, Stadlbauer KH, et al. Effects of decreasing peak flow rate on stomach inflation during bag-valve-mask ventilation. *Resuscitation.* 2004;63:131-136.

Chapter 37
Mobilization and Portable Ventilation

Objectives

1. Discuss the rationale for mobilization and ambulation of mechanically ventilated patients.
2. Describe the approach to ambulation of the mechanically ventilated patient.
3. Describe the characteristics of a portable ventilator.

Introduction

In recent years, there has been increasing interest in mobilization and ambulation of mechanically ventilated patients. This therapy requires the use of a portable ventilator. Portable ventilators are also used for intra- and inter-hospital transport. This chapter covers aspects of mobilization and ambulation of mechanically ventilated patients, as well as the use of portable ventilators for transport.

Mobilization

Survivors of critical illness who have been mechanically ventilated can have muscle wasting and fatigue. Survivors of acute respiratory distress syndrome (ARDS) may have persistent physical disability for years after ICU (intensive care unit) discharge. The consequences of these acquired deficits may lead to disability, social isolation, institutionalization, and a significant economic burden for society. A variety of factors are responsible for these physical deficits, including severity of illness, acute inflammation, corticosteroid administration, and use of neuromuscular blockers. Perhaps the most important risk factor is prolonged bed rest.

Daily awakening and spontaneous breathing trials lead to fewer ventilator days, and there is accumulating evidence supporting early physical activity for mechanically ventilated patients. The ABCDE bundle is an evidence-based organizational approach for the management of critically ill mechanically ventilated patients: awakening and breathing coordination of daily sedation and spontaneous breathing trials, choice of sedative or analgesic agents, delirium monitoring, and early mobility and exercise.

Approaches to Mobilization and Ambulation of the Mechanically Ventilated Patient

Prior to ambulation, there are specific factors that need to be considered. It is important to consider the amount of sedation the patient is receiving. In addition to having a more alert and responsive patient, less sedation also frequently allows the patient to be extubated sooner. The patient also needs to be hemodynamically stable. While it may be tempting to move quickly to full ambulation, patients should be allowed to progress more slowly, first sitting up and dangling their legs from the bed, then standing and then taking a few steps at the bedside and moving into a chair before progressing to more ambitious goals.

When considering mobilizing and ambulating patients who are mechanically ventilated, it is important to remember that with respiratory compromise, the patient's ventilatory status and reserve can limit their exercise capacity. This means that, in some cases, respiratory support may need to be increased in order to improve the patient's ability to mobilize and ambulate. Also, because exercise demands an increase in oxygen requirement of the respiratory muscles, it can steal oxygen from other skeletal muscles, causing additional limitation of mobility and ambulation. This effect can be addressed by increasing the amount of support during mobility and ambulation, to allow increased ventilation without increased oxygen demand by the respiratory muscles.

Despite concerns that have been raised about the safety of mobilizing and ambulating patients with critical illness, few serious adverse events have been reported. For early mobilization and ambulation to be a success, there also must be a collaborative consensus that ambulation can proceed safely, and that consensus should include collaboration among all the members of the patient's team, including physicians, nurses, and physical and respiratory therapists. The level of ventilator support should not be a limiting factor. Patients who are on high F_{IO_2} and a high level of positive end-expiratory pressure (PEEP) can be ambulated safely. The limiting factor is the amount of sedation the patient is receiving, not the settings on the ventilator.

The success of early mobilization and ambulation programs requires significant multidisciplinary teamwork and coordination from all staff members, from attending physicians, residents and fellows, to nurses, physical therapists, respiratory therapists, and critical care technicians. Typically, the nurse manages the catheters and monitor, the physical therapist manages the patient's activity, the respiratory therapist manages the ventilator, and a critical care technician assists as needed.

For successful ambulation, the ventilator must have a sufficient amount of battery power. Most of the portable ventilators that are commercially available have hours of internal battery power, and those batteries must be kept fully charged. Lacking a sufficient battery, a long extension cord may be used when necessary, but caution to avoid tripping over the cord or accidentally unplugging it must be exercised. It is important to use modes of ventilation that promote synchrony. When a patient begins ambulation, the team should consider whether changes need to be made on the ventilator settings so that the patient will be synchronous with the ventilator during that activity.

In addition to a walker, it is important to have the ventilator and oxygen cylinders on a movable wheelbase, and to have a ventilator circuit with sufficient length to allow for movement. There are a number of commercially available portable ventilators designed for patient transport that can be used for ambulation of patients. A pulse oximeter is also important to monitor the patient's oxygen saturation and titrate the ventilator settings accordingly, and to monitor the patient's heart rate.

For patients who are too unstable to be awakened for active mobilization, passive range-of-motion and positioning exercises are important to minimize the development of joint contractures. Neuromuscular electrical stimulation and passive cycling are modalities that may be increasingly available in the future.

Portable Ventilators

Critically ill patients commonly require diagnostic tests and therapeutic procedures that cannot be performed at the bedside. When the critically ill patient requires transport, every effort should be made to take the ICU with the patient. For the mechanically ventilated patient, that means personnel who are familiar with the patient, monitoring equipment, airway equipment, and a means of providing ventilation (Table 37-1). Ventilation during transport can be provided by using either a manual ventilator or a portable ventilator. Use of a portable ventilator is superior to manual ventilation because it provides a more consistent level of ventilation and frees a clinician to perform other tasks.

Characteristics of a Portable Ventilator

There are available very sophisticated microprocessor-controlled portable ventilators. Ideally, the ventilator should be capable of providing modes that are commonly used in the ICU. There should be separate controls for respiratory rate and tidal volume. The ventilator should be able to provide either volume- or pressure-controlled ventilation. It should be possible to control the F_{IO_2}. PEEP must be available, and the trigger sensitivity must be PEEP-compensated. High pressure and disconnect alarms should be provided.

Table 37-1 Transport Equipment and Supplies

Type	Examples
Monitoring equipment	Electrocardiograph leads and cables, pulse oximetry probes and cables, thermometer, stethoscope, blood pressure cuff
Suction equipment	Suction catheters, Yankauer, suction tubing
Intravenous/intraosseous equipment	Angiocatheters, arm boards, intraosseous needles, tourniquets, tape, tegaderm, gauze
Chest tube/needle drainage equipment	Chest tubes, pleurovacs, syringes, stopcocks
Nasogastric/urinary equipment	Feeding tubes, nasogastric tubes, Foley catheters, syringes
Sterile field supplies	Betadine, chlorhexidine, alcohol wipes, sterile gloves, sterile drapes
Communication equipment	Cell phones, 2-way radios
Intubation equipment	Endotracheal tubes, nasal and oral airways, CO_2 detectors, stylets, laryngeal mask airways, tape, Magill forceps, commercial tube holders, tracheostomy tubes
Laryngoscopy equipment	Laryngoscope blades and handles, batteries, bulbs
Oxygen-related equipment	Nasal cannulas, oxygen tubing, flow meters, head hood, self-inflating bags, resuscitation masks, simple masks, Venturi masks, non-rebreather masks
Aerosol equipment	Aerosol mask, tracheostomy mask, aerosol tubing, sterile water, nebulizers
Miscellaneous	Defibrillator pads, tape, needles, cervical collars, butterfly catheters, syringes, blankets

Data from Horowitz R, Rosenfeld RA. Pediatric critical care interfacility transport. *Clin Pediatr Emerg Med.* 2007;8(3):190-202.

A major consideration is portability. The ventilator should be lightweight. The ventilator's dimensions should make it easy to transport with the patient (eg, place on the bed). Transport ventilators may be either pneumatically or electronically powered. A major disadvantage of pneumatically controlled transport ventilators is that they consume gas for operation, thus depleting the gas source very quickly. Microprocessor-controlled portable ventilators typically provide more precise control settings, are affected less by fluctuations in source-gas pressure, and do not consume as much gas for their operation. Battery-operated ventilators should have a battery life of at least 4 hours and the battery should recharge quickly.

A unique challenge occurs when mechanically ventilated patients require transport for magnetic resonance imaging. Operation of the magnetic resonance imager creates a strong magnetic field. Thus, devices (including ventilators) that have ferromagnetic components cannot be used. Patients can be ventilated using either a manual ventilator, or a ventilator specifically designed for use during magnetic resonance imaging. Also, aluminum oxygen cylinders and aluminum regulators are necessary for oxygen delivery.

Points to Remember

- Mobility and ambulation results in improved outcomes of mechanically ventilated patients.
- Prior to ambulation, the patient should be alert and hemodynamically stable.
- The level of ventilator support may need to be increased during mobilization and ambulation.
- Mobilization and ambulation of mechanically ventilated patients requires a multidisciplinary approach.
- Use of a portable ventilator is superior to manual ventilation because it provides a more consistent level of ventilation and frees a clinician to perform other tasks.
- Portable ventilators should provide the same level of ventilation that is provided in the ICU.

Additional Reading

Bailey PP, Miller RR 3rd, Clemmer TP. Culture of early mobility in mechanically ventilated patients. *Crit Care Med.* 2009;37:S429-S435.

Blakeman TC, Branson RD. Evaluation of 4 new generation portable ventilators. *Respir Care.* 2013;58:264-272.

Blakeman TC, Branson RD. Inter- and intra-hospital transport of the critically ill. *Respir Care.* 2013;58:1008-1023.

Blakeman TC, Rodriquez D, Dorlac WC, et al. Performance of portable ventilators for mass-casualty care. *Prehosp Disaster Med.* 2011;26:330-334.

Chipman DW, Caramez MP, Miyoshi E, et al. Performance comparison of 15 transport ventilators. *Respir Care.* 2007;52:740-751.

Kress JP. Clinical trials of early mobilization of critically ill patients. *Crit Care Med.* 2009;37:S442-S447.

Kress JP. Sedation and mobility: changing the paradigm. *Crit Care Clin.* 2013;29:67-75.

Mendez-Tellez PA, Needham DM. Early physical rehabilitation in the ICU and ventilator liberation. *Respir Care.* 2012;57:1663-1669.

Morandi A, Brummel NE, Ely EW. Sedation, delirium and mechanical ventilation: the 'ABCDE' approach. *Curr Opin Crit Care.* 2011;17:43-49.

Schweickert WD, Kress JP. Implementing early mobilization interventions in mechanically ventilated patients in the ICU. *Chest.* 2011;140:1612-1617.

Schweickert WD, Pohlman MC, Pohlman AS, et al. Early physical and occupational therapy in mechanically ventilated, critically ill patients: a randomized controlled trial. *Lancet.* 2009;373:1874-1882.

Chapter 38
Extracorporeal Life Support

Introduction

The concept of extracorporeal life support (ECLS, commonly called extracorporeal membrane oxygenation [ECMO]) has been available since the introduction of cardiac bypass during cardiac surgery. The first use of ECMO outside of the operating room occurred in the late 1960s. These first applications were to patients with severe refractory hypoxemia and the acute respiratory distress system (ARDS). Based on the initial successful application of ECMO to patients with ARDS in the 1970s, a randomized controlled trial comparing the use of ECMO to standard conventional management in patients with ARDS was conducted. This study failed to show benefit for the use of ECMO, with mortality in each group of about 90%. As a result, the use of ECMO in adult ARDS was not considered an option by most centers. In the 1980s a number of groups began using neonatal ECMO in an attempt to reduce the mortality in near-term infants from meconium aspiration, diaphragmatic hernia, sepsis, pneumonia, and other causes of severe respiratory failure. By the 1990s, based on the success of ECMO in neonates, more centers began using ECMO in pediatric and adult patients with severe respiratory failure. By 2000, the use of ECMO expanded to cardiac patients in all age groups. The increased use of ECMO in ARDS has been supported in recent years by the successful use of ECMO in the H1N1 epidemic of 2009. Today, ECMO is also used as a bridge to lung and heart transplantation and as a means of ensuring lung protective ventilation in patients in whom CO_2 elimination is markedly compromised.

Types of Extracorporeal Life Support

There are two approaches to ECLS: VV and VA. With VV ECMO, blood is removed from a major vein, passed through a pump and oxygenator, and back to the patient via a major vein. In VA ECMO, blood is removed from a major vein but, after passing through a pump and oxygenator, is returned via a major artery.

Venovenous ECMO

This approach to ECMO is primarily designed to support the respiratory system. Blood is removed from a large vein, usually a femoral vein with the catheter frequently

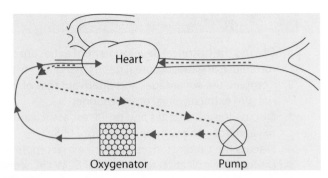

Figure 38-1 Venovenous ECMO. Blood is removed from a vein and returned via a vein. (From Turner DA, Cheifetz IM. Extracorporeal membrane oxygenation for adult respiratory failure. *Respir Care*. 2013; 58:1038-1052.)

extending into the inferior vena cava, and returned to another large vein, the contralateral femoral or the superior vena cava via the jugular vein (Figure 38-1). Since the arterial circulation is not affected, normal pulsatile blood flow is maintained. This approach requires a normal functioning heart. Thus, blood flows through the pulmonary circulation. Gas exchange is a combination of the effect of gas exchange via the ECMO system and the respiratory system. The amount of gas exchange occurring in each area is dependent on the amount of blood flow diverted through the ECMO circuit. The greater the ECMO blood flow, the less contribution to gas exchange by the respiratory system.

VV ECMO has the advantage of not invading the arterial circulation, so the risk of air embolism is minimized. Pulmonary perfusion is also maintained, and pulsatile blood flow is maintained to the kidneys. The major disadvantages to this approach are that cardiac function must be relatively normal. Patients with severely compromised cardiac function are not candidates for VV ECMO. Catheter position is critical. Recirculation can occur, nullifying the effects of ECMO. Careful monitoring of the oxygenation and ventilation is important. The ability of VV ECMO to oxygenate the patient is less than that of VA ECMO for the same blood volume diverted to the ECMO system. The patient must be anticoagulated, and bleeding is a major potential complication.

Venoarterial (VA) ECMO

With venoarterial (VA) ECMO, blood is removed from a large vein (femoral or jugular) similar to VV ECMO, but blood is returned to circulation via a large artery, frequently the carotid artery in neonates and children or the femoral artery in adults (Figure 38-2). VA ECMO is designed to support the failing heart. With this approach, essentially 100% of the cardiac output can be diverted through the ECMO system. As a result, pulsatile blood flow is lost. All gas exchange occurs via the ECMO system.

The advantages of this approach are independence from cardiac function, ability to divert the entire blood volume, maximized oxygenation capability, and a marked decrease in the need for ventilatory support. The major disadvantages are the need to invade the arterial circulation and the risk of air embolism. Pulsatile blood flow is

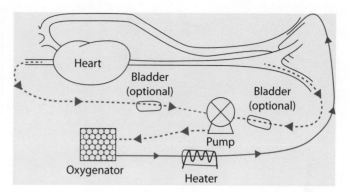

Figure 38-2 Venoarterial ECMO. Blood is removed via a vein and returned via an artery. (From Turner DA, Cheifetz IM. Extracorporeal membrane oxygenation for adult respiratory failure. *Respir Care.* 2013; 58: 1038-1052.)

lost, and thus, pulse oximeters do not work. Normal pulmonary and renal pulsatile flow is lost. The patient must be anticoagulated, and thus, bleeding is a major potential complication.

Pumps, Oxygenators, and Catheters

There are three parts of an ECMO system regardless of the approach used to provide ECMO: the pump, the oxygenator, and the cannulas used to establish vascular access. Original ECMO systems used roller pumps to move blood through the circuit. These pumps are still in use for neonates. However, most adult and pediatric ECMO systems use a centrifugal pump. The major problem with roller pumps is that blood is moved by compressing the circuit between the roller and its casing as the pump rotates. This places stress on the circuit and can potentially cause circuit leaks. In addition, the compression destroys red blood cells and platelets, requiring transfusions. Neither of these concerns exists with centrifugal pumps.

Original oxygenators were very large—some a meter in diameter. Newer models are much smaller, approximately 25 cm long and 5 in in diameter. All oxygenators operate by the countercurrent principle; that is, blood flows in one direction on one side of a semipermeable membrane and gas moves in the opposite direction on the other side of the membrane. Oxygen and carbon dioxide move across the membrane in opposite directions. Oxygen diffuses from the gas to the blood, and carbon dioxide diffuses from the blood to the gas. The gas flowing through the oxygenator is referred to as the sweep flow. Dependent on the specific oxygenator, sweep flows of up to 15 L/min can be set. Because of the physiology of oxygen transport by the blood, compared to carbon dioxide, oxygenators are more efficient in removing carbon dioxide than adding oxygen. In some cases with VV ECMO in which the oxygenation needs are great, carbon dioxide is added to the sweep flow to avoid severe hypercapnia and alkalosis. Efficient carbon dioxide removal is a reason that VV ECMO has been recently promoted for the management of patients with chronic obstructive pulmonary disease (COPD) in severe hypercapnic respiratory failure.

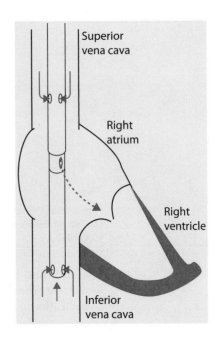

Figure 38-3 Graphic depiction of the double-lumen bicaval cannula. Blood is removed form the superior vena cava and inferior vena cava, and returned adjacent to the tricuspid valve, directing returned blood into the right ventricle. (From Turner DA, Cheifetz IM. Extracorporeal membrane oxygenation for adult respiratory failure. Respir Care. 2013; 58:1038-1052.)

A number of monitors can be added to the ECMO system to ensure safety. Pre- and post-membrane pressure and blood gases can be measured continuously, and a blood warmer is added to the system to maintain the returning blood at body temperature. The ECMO system can be used to rapidly adjust a patient's body temperature. With VA ECMO diverting nearly 100% of the blood volume, body temperature can be changed in a short time.

A number of different types of cannulas have been designed for ECMO. Most are single-lumen cannulas. Recently a double-lumen bicaval cannula has become popular for VV ECMO where the goal is to mobilize the patient after stabilization of ECMO. This cannula is placed into the external jugular vein and passed into the vena cava. It drains blood from both the superior and inferior vena cava, and directs the return of blood directly across the tricuspid valve (Figure 38-3). The major concern with this type of cannula is recirculation of blood if the catheter is not correctly placed. The advantage to this type of cannula is mobility. Patients can be mobilized with less concern regarding altered blood flow resulting from kinking of the catheter, as would occur with a femoral catheter.

Extracorporeal CO$_2$ Removal

VV or VA ECMO is very effective in removing CO$_2$. The CO$_2$ level in blood returning from an ECMO system can be decreased to almost zero. As a result, it does not require a large diversion of the cardiac output by a VV ECMO system to markedly reduce the Paco$_2$. The movement of 1 to 2 L/min of cardiac output through a VV ECMO system can decrease the $Paco_2$ by 20 mm Hg or more. Experimental pump-less VV ECMO systems might be used to manage the hypercarbia common in patients in an exacerbation of COPD, severe acute asthma, severe ARDS where lung protective ventilation is at its limit, and in patients awaiting lung transplantation who require rehabilitation. The systems that are being developed require adequate cardiovascular reserves and have very low resistance to blood flow ($\leq$ 15-mm Hg pressure drop across the oxygenator at 3 L/min flow).

Indications for ECMO

ECMO is used with neonates, children, and adults. ECMO was originally designed for management of severe respiratory failure. However, there is an increasing trend for the use of ECMO in patients with cardiac failure and chronic respiratory failure (Table 38-1).

Neonates

ECMO was first used primarily in neonates. The overall number of neonates having received ECMO is much larger than that of pediatric and adult patients combined, but the use of ECMO in neonates is decreasing. This is attributed to better overall management of neonates with cardiopulmonary failure. The introduction of surfactant and lung protective ventilatory strategies, as well as improvement in the medical management of neonates, has reduced the yearly number of patients requiring ECMO since its peak in the mid 1990s. The primary indications for ECMO in neonates are congenital diaphragmatic hernia, meconium aspiration, persistent pulmonary hypertension of the newborn, respiratory distress syndrome, sepsis, and severe cardiac anomalies/cardiac surgery.

Table 38-1 Indications for ECMO

Neonates
Congenital diaphragmatic hernia
Meconium aspiration
Persistent pulmonary hypertension of the newborn
Respiratory distress syndrome
Postcardiac surgery
Pediatrics
Postcardiac surgery
Pneumonia
ARDS
Non-ARDS respiratory failure
Adults
Severe heart failure
Postcardiac surgery
Bridge to transplantation
Management of severe hypercapnia
Management of severe refractory hypoxemia

Pediatrics

The number of pediatric patients treated with ECMO has increased each year since the mid-1980s. Early use of ECMO in pediatric patients has been primarily for severe respiratory failure whether it was from ARDS, pneumonia, or other causes. However, today the primary reason that pediatric patients are placed on ECMO is postcardiac surgery, in most cases for the correction of severe cardiac anomalies.

Adults

Few ECMO cases in adults were reported before 1990. However, by the mid 1990s, the number of adult ECMO cases started to rise and there has been major growth in the number of adult ECMO cases since 2009. This is due to the positive results reported by many centers on the use of ECMO for the management of severely ill patients as a result of the H1N1 epidemic of 2009, and the increase in the use of ECMO to manage patients with heart failure. In addition, centers are using ECMO as a bridge to transplantation, and for the management of exacerbations of COPD and asthma.

The Future

The number of pediatric patients, and adults, managed with ECMO is expected to continue to rise as the number of centers offering ECMO increases. This increase in the use of ECMO will be in three specific patient populations. The first and largest increase will be in patients with heart failure. Many centers with a large heart failure/cardiac surgical program will likely develop ECMO programs. The second area of increase will be in patients with acute hypercapnia who cannot be adequately managed with lung protective ventilation, or in patients with chronic lung disease failing conventional management or requiring rehabilitation as transplant candidates. The third area will be the management of severe refractory hypoxemia of any cause. Clinical challenges such as the H1N1 epidemic will continue to promote the use of ECMO in this group of patients. The expectation is that the number of centers offering ECMO will continue to increase.

Points to Remember

- The two approaches to ECMO are VV and VA.
- VV ECMO is primarily for respiratory support.
- VA ECMO is primarily for cardiovascular support.
- Gas exchange with ECMO is caused by the countercurrent principle.
- VV ECMO is more effective in removing CO_2 than oxygenating the blood.
- Centrifugal pumps are primarily used today for pediatric and adult ECMO; neonatal ECMO is still preformed with roller pumps.
- The major concern with VV ECMO is recirculation, and this concern is increased with the use of double-lumen catheters.

- The primary concern with VA ECMO is air emboli with a system leak.
- Bleeding is a major concern with VV and VA ECMO because of the need for anti-coagulation.
- Experimental pump-less ECMO systems are being used for CO_2 removal.
- The use of ECMO in neonates can be expected to decrease except for cardiac anomalies and cardiac surgery.
- Pediatric and especially adult ECMO cases and centers will increase.
- The primary use of ECMO in pediatrics and adults is for cardiovascular support, management of hypercapnia, and management of severe refractory hypoxemia.

Additional Reading

Abrams DC, Brenner K, Burkart KM, et al. Pilot study of extracorporeal carbon dioxide removal to facilitate extubation and ambulation in exacerbations of chronic obstructive pulmonary disease. *Ann Am Thorac Soc.* 2013;10:307-314.

Brown KL, Ichord R, Marino BS, Thiagarajan RR. Outcomes following extracorporeal membrane oxygenation in children with cardiac disease. *Pediatr Crit Care Med.* 2013;14(5 Suppl 1):S73-S83.

Burki NK, Mani RK, Herth FJ, et al. A novel extracorporeal CO_2 removal system: results of a pilot study of hypercapnic respiratory failure in patients with COPD. *Chest.* 2013;143:678-686.

Dalton HJ. Extracorporeal life support: moving at the speed of light. *Respir Care.* 2011;56:1445-1453.

Davies A, Jones D, Bailey M, et al. Extracorporeal membrane oxygenation for 2009 influenza A(H1N1) acute respiratory distress syndrome. *JAMA.* 2009;302:1888-1895.

Elbourne D, Field D, Mugford M. Extracorporeal membrane oxygenation for severe respiratory failure in newborn infants [review]. *Cochrane Database Syst Rev.* 2002;(1):CD001340. Update in *Cochrane Database Syst Rev.* 2008;(3):CD001340.

Hayes D Jr, Tobias JD, Kukreja J, et al. Extracorporeal life support for acute respiratory distress syndromes. *Ann Thorac Med.* 2013;8:133-141.

Luyt CE, Comes A, Becquemin MH, et al. Long-term outcomes of pandemic 2009 influenza A(H1N1)-associated severe ARDS. *Chest.* 2012;142:583-592.

MacLaren G, Dodge-Khatami A, Dalton HJ, et al. Joint statement on mechanical circulatory support in children: a consensus review from the Pediatric Cardiac Intensive Care Society and Extracorporeal Life Support Organization. *Pediar Crit Care Med.* 2013;14 (5 Suppl 1):S1-S2.

Noah MA, Peek GJ, Finney SJ, et al. Referral to an extracorporeal membrane oxygenation center and mortality among patients with severe 2009 influenza A(H1N1). *JAMA.* 2011;306:1659-1668.

Patroniti N, Zangrillo A, Pappalardo F, et al. The Italian ECMO network experience during the 2009 influenza A(H1N1) pandemic: preparation for severe respiratory emergency outbreaks. *Intensive Care Med.* 2011;37:1447-1457.

Peek GJ, Mugford M, Tiruvoipati R, et al. Efficacy and economic assessment of conventional ventilatory support versus extracorporeal membrane oxygenation for severe adult respiratory failure (CESAR): a multicentre randomised controlled trial. *Lancet.* 2009;374:1351-1363.

Pham T, Combes A, Roze H, et al. Extracorporeal membrane oxygenation for pandemic influenza A(H1N1)-induced acute respiratory distress syndrome: a cohort study and propensity-matched analysis. *Am J Respir Crit Care Med.* 2013;187:276-285.

Terragni P, Faggiano C, Ranieri VM. Extracorporeal membrane oxygenation in adult patients with acute respiratory distress syndrome. *Curr Opin Crit Care.* 2014;20:86-91.

Turner DA, Cheifetz IM. Extracorporeal membrane oxygenation for adult respiratory failure. *Respir Care.* 2013;58:1038-1052.

Index

Note: Page numbers followed by *f* and *t* indicate figures and tables, respectively.